NOVEL FRONTIERS OF ADVANCED NEUROIMAGING

Edited by **Kostas N. Fountas**

Novel Frontiers of Advanced Neuroimaging
http://dx.doi.org/10.5772/2558
Edited by Kostas N. Fountas

Contributors

G. García-Martí, A. Alberich-Bayarri, L. Martí-Bonmatí, Evanthia Kousi, Ioannis Tsougos, Kapsalaki Eftychia, Maria de la Iglesia-Vaya, Jose Molina-Mateo, Mª Jose Escarti-Fabra, Ahmad S. Kanaan, Hiroyuki Kato, Masahiro Izumiyama, Hoan Tran, Howard Yonas, Peter Walla, Jaak Panksepp, Aimee Mavratzakis, Shannon Bosshard, Elias P. Casula, Vincenza Tarantino, Demis Basso, Patrizia S. Bisiacchi, Claudio Irace, A. Bican, İ. Bora, O. Algın, B. Hakyemez, V. Özkol, E. Alper, Robert P. Granacher, Jr.

Published by InTech

Janeza Trdine 9, 51000 Rijeka, Croatia

Publishing Process Manager Iva Simcic
Technical Editor InTech Prepress, Novi Sad
Cover InTech Design team

Additional hard copies can be obtained from orders@intechopen.com

Novel Frontiers of Advanced Neuroimaging, Edited by Kostas N. Fountas
p. cm.
ISBN 978-953-51-0923-5

For EU product safety concerns:
IN TECH d.o.o., Prolaz Marije Krucifikse Kozulić 3, 51000 Rijeka, Croatia,
info@intechopen.com or visit our website at intechopen.com.

Meet the editor

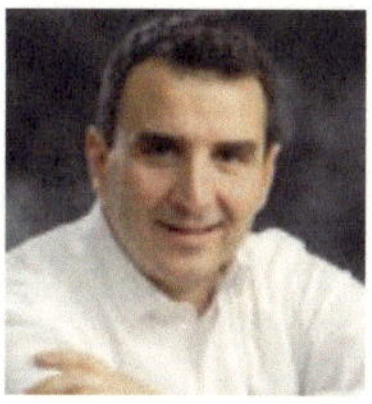

Kostas N. Fountas has earned his Medical Degree from the National and Capodistrian University of Athens, Greece. He completed his neurosurgical training at the Medical Center of Central Georgia and the Medical College of Georgia in Augusta, GA, USA.
He has joined the Faculty of Medicine, School of Health Sciences of the University of Thessaly, in Larisa, Greece since 2007. He has been the Head of the Department of Neurosurgery of the University Hospital of Larisa, since 2009.
His scientific interests are focused on functional imaging, electrophysiology, and neuro-oncology. He has contributed 120 publications in peer-reviewed journals, as well as 20 chapters in textbooks. Dr. Fountas has given more than 250 oral and poster presentations in national and international scientific meetings.

Contents

Preface

The book you are holding in your hands is a quite unusual neuroimaging textbook. The participating authors attempted to provide the reader with a preview of the emerging applications of novel but also established neuroimaging techniques. The book is divided into three sections. The first section includes advanced MR-based techniques such as task-generated and resting functional imaging, brain morphometry, diffusion tensor imaging and fractional anisotropy tractography, and proton spectroscopy, in evaluating brain anatomical structure and connectivity, but also various intracranial pathological entities. The second part presents a novel implementation of advanced neuroimaging techniques in evaluating the brain's affective processing. The third section describes the applications of traditional and novel imaging techniques in clarifying various legal issues, while it outlines the role of neuroimaging in forensic medicine.

Dr. Kostas N. Fountas
Assistant professor of Neurosurgery,
University of Thessaly, School of Medicine, Larissa,
Greece

Section 1

Advanced MR-Based Imaging Techniques

Chapter 1

Brain Structure MR Imaging Methods: Morphometry and Tractography

G. García-Martí, A. Alberich-Bayarri and L. Martí-Bonmatí

Additional information is available at the end of the chapter

http://dx.doi.org/10.5772/53079

1. Introduction

Brain morphology is in constant change from the very beginning of the neurodevelopment in human beings. The characterization of the brain morphology and its biological implications on a specific subject is a complex task which requires efficient computational approaches. Radiology has traditionally assessed the main brain changes in different alterations from a macroscopic point of view, thus, not considering subtle changes as a results of neuronal plasticity. In conjunction with functional information, the structural neuroimaging methods have established as the key in the diagnosis of several central nervous system disorders, including tumours, neurodegenerative disorders and psychiatric diseases.

2. Brain morphometry

2.1. Introduction

Morphometry techniques use statistical methods to detect and to quantify subtle structural abnormalities that appear when comparing different populations. Nowadays, there are several methodologies which have been designed to achieve these goals. The fast evolution in terms of spatial resolution and signal-to-noise ratio in Magnetic Resonance (MR) scanners as well as the improvements on new imaging techniques and data processing algorithms, help to developing studies that increase the knowledge over many fields of neuroimaging. This section describes the scope of these new methodologies and the main processes related with their implementation.

2.2. Morphometric methods

The first method developed in order to measure anatomical differences was based on the manual delineation of brain structures and their analysis by defining regions of interest

(ROI). Although its main advantage is the anatomical accuracy of the measures, there are some assumptions that should be taken into account, including high variability, poor reproducibility, the need for previous hypotheses about the anatomical areas and regions to study and computational requirements needed to study a large number of subjects.

In order to supply these restrictions, semiautomatic methods have been developed. These methodologies perform a fully computerized treatment of different brain areas, providing a reproducible way to define exploratory analysis without *a priori* knowledge about the spatial distribution of the potentially affected areas.

2.2.1. Deformation-based morphometry

Models based on deformation fields use the spatial transformations needed to register an image to a template. In this registration process, a three-dimensional nonlinear deformation map is generated, which contains the adjusted parameters obtained by the fitting process between both, the image and the template. The deformation-based morphometry (DBM) (Gaser et al., 2001) is therefore a useful methodology to find differences at the macroscopic level.

To obtain the deformation field, the algorithm is initialized and a first mesh is generated. At each iteration, this mesh is fitted to achieve the required target varying from low to high detail by a coarse to fine minimization strategy. This registration is followed by an estimation of the nonlinear deformations which are composed by a linear combination of 3D discrete cosine (DC) transform basis functions. Displacement vectors are then smoothed with and 8 x 8 x 8 mm Full Width at Half Maximum (FWHM) filter.

The statistical analysis of these parameters helps to determine whether there are specific differences between subjects. The deformation field provides information about both volume and position differences, and can be studied by analyzing the displacement vectors for each point or by quantifying the local signal variation. Multivariate statistical models are needed in order to make inferences about the differences between groups.

2.2.2. Tensor-based morphometry

Tensor-based morphometry (TBM) (Kipps et al., 2005) is a morphometric method which uses tensor magnitudes to identify regional changes in anatomical areas The estimation of these differences is based on the small variations that are generated when normalizing each voxel of an image (i_a, i_b, i_c) to a template reference (j_a, j_b, j_c).

By using the deformation fields, the determinants of the Jacobian matrix (J) can be estimated. This matrix is equivalent to a second-order tensor that provides univariate (point to point) information about how the brain shape varies from the original image to the template. This feature improves the use of the DBM method, because it avoids the use of the entire deformation field (multivariate approach) in order to determine if there are specific (local) differences between images.

For each voxel, the Jacobian matrix contains information about translation, rotation and shear transformations:

$$J = \begin{bmatrix} \partial i_a / \partial j_a & \partial i_a / \partial j_b & \partial i_a / \partial j_c \\ \partial i_b / \partial j_a & \partial i_b / \partial j_b & \partial i_b / \partial j_c \\ \partial i_c / \partial j_a & \partial i_c / \partial j_b & \partial i_c / \partial j_c \end{bmatrix}$$

In order to perform the statistical analysis to detect differences between subjects, the J matrix can be decomposed into a rotation matrix (R) and symmetric positive-definite matrices (U or V), to satisfy the following axioms:

$$J = RU = VR$$

$$U = \sqrt{\left(J^T J\right)}$$

$$V = \sqrt{\left(JJ^T\right)}$$

$$R = JU^{-1} = V^{-1}J$$

In the normalization process which applies rigid transformations, it holds that U = V = I, where I is the identity matrix. If U and V matrices are different from the matrix I, there is a change in the shape which can be encoded by the tensor E. For a given deformation, there are infinite ways to express the associated tensors in terms of an n-parameter:

$$\begin{cases} n \neq 0 \quad \Rightarrow \quad E^n = n^{-1}(U^n - 1) \\ \\ n = 0 \quad \Rightarrow \quad E^n = \ln(U) \end{cases}$$

When n = 0, the obtained tensor is the Hencky tensor, which is useful to express local brain volume increases or decreases relative to the template. From these calculations, a comparison between images of many subjects can be done by extracting different variables (area, length and volume) and analyzing those using statistical models.

2.2.3. *Diffeomorphic morphometry*

This methodology is based on registering an image with a template using a flow field that encodes the geometric transformation required to normalize an image to another. A large deformation framework is used in order to conserve topology, obtaining a diffeomorphic and invertible deformation (Ashburner, 2007).

If there are two images A and B (with the same dimensions) and a function f which takes points from A and put those on B, then f can be considered as a translator; i. e. for each point of A provides the corresponding B-point. In order to maintain the diffeomorphic propriety, this function must be bijective; i. e. the relationship between A and B points must be 1 to 1 (a specific point of A only can be associated to a specific point of B and vice versa).

$$\begin{cases} f : A \rightarrow B \\ f^{-1} : B \rightarrow A \end{cases}$$

where the transformation is diffeomorphic if there is a smooth bijective function f that transforms A into B and vice versa. The last step is to estimate a statistical model to detect significant changes between groups.

2.2.4. *Voxel-based morphometry*

The voxel-based morphometry (VBM) technique (Ashburner and Friston, 2000) is based on the normalization of several individual brains with to a specific template. These normalized images are voxel-by-voxel analyzed to detect variations of local tissue. Unlike other morphometric techniques, VBM is based on applying a mass univariate statistical analysis for each voxel. Typically, the brain is previously segmented into gray matter (GM), white matter (WM) and cerebrospinal fluid (CSF) maps. These calculations need a prior preprocessing to normalize the data in a common stereotactic space. The purpose of these processes is the minimization of the anatomical variability between different subjects, discounting macroscopic factors and allowing a statistical analysis to obtain subtle differences that can be attributed only to the anatomical variability between groups.

2.2.4.1. *Signal heterogeneity*

This step aims to minimize the bias field contained in the MR images. The lack of signal homogeneity, which may result from factors such as static magnetic field inhomogeneities, sensitivity of transmit and receiving coils and dielectric effect, directly affects the voxel intensities. In order to quantitatively evaluate the data, differences in the brightness between voxels of a particular region or area can be a source of bias for the algorithms convergence criteria (figure 1).

Figure 1. Low-frequency bias field estimated from brain MR images

For these reasons, it is necessary to correct this inhomogeneity and there are several approaches, including modeling of field heterogeneity by DC basis functions (Ashburner and Friston, 2000), the use of Legendre polynomial basis functions (Brechbühler et al., 1996) or the Gaussian deconvolution on the histogram of the image (Sled et al., 1998). There are also methods which model the field by a linear combination of low frequency functions based on cubic B-splines adjusted by a cost function based on the intensity and the gradient of the image (Manjón et al., 2007).

2.2.4.2. *Non-linear normalization*

The nonlinear normalization (or warping) normalizes an image to a template by applying transformations that do not preserve the proportions of the original image. The main aim is to perform a deformation of an original image with a template to facilitate a high precise comparison within brain regions between different subjects.

The algorithm tries to reduce the difference between original and template images, using a standard least-squares minimization (Mean Square Error, MSE):

$$MSE = \sum_{i} \left(f(x_i, y_i, z_i) - w \cdot g(x_i', y_i' z_i') \right)^2$$

where $f(x_i, y_i, z_i)$ represents the value of the voxel i in the coordinate (x,y,z) of the original image f, $g(x_i', y_i', z_i')$ is the value of the voxel i in the coordinate (x',y',z') of the template g and w represents a weighting factor.

2.2.4.3. *Segmentation*

The segmentation process aims to classify the MR brain images into GM, WM, CSF and other cortical and subcortical areas. Although there are many algorithms for brain segmentation, there is an efficient strategy commonly used by neuroimaging applications that in practice gives good results but theoretically is slightly away from the pure concept of segmentation. This method does not obtain the real tissue-intensity extracted from the image but a probability map for each class. Each voxel in these maps has a normalized brightness value in the range [0 ... 1], that reflects the probability of belonging to a particular tissue.

In order to identify and classify the different tissues, the algorithm analyzes the range of the brightness values of each voxel in the original image. If n is the number of bits of the image, then the intensity values can be assigned in the range [0 ... 2^n-1]. For example, a coded image with 8 bits, has a brightness value between 0 and 255, with 0 black (no light) and 255 white (figure 2). With this approach, it is possible to represent images using cumulative graphs (histograms) in which each point represents the number of voxels with a given brightness level.

Figure 2. Gray scale with 256 potential values (0 black, 255 white)

The intensities can be modeled by its mean and variance, adjusting the image histogram by a Gaussian-mixture function,. The algorithm performs a separate treatment for each tissue, assigning a different group (class) to each voxel (figure 3). Initially, these voxels are assigned to an initial value defined by *a priori* knowledge. Then, the algorithm obtains the total number of voxels in each group and their mean and variance. With these data, new iterations are recalculated:

$$p_{i,k} = \frac{1}{\sqrt{(2\pi\, c_k)}} \exp\left(\frac{-(f(x_i) - v_k)^2}{2c_k} \right)$$

where $p_{i,k}$ represents the probability that the voxel i is assigned to the k-tissue, c_k is the variance of the tissue k, $f(x_i)$ represents the brightness of the i-voxel in the image f and v_k is the mean of the k-tissue. With the new probabilities, the algorithm continues until either the convergence criterion is achieved or the fixed number of iterations is exceeded.

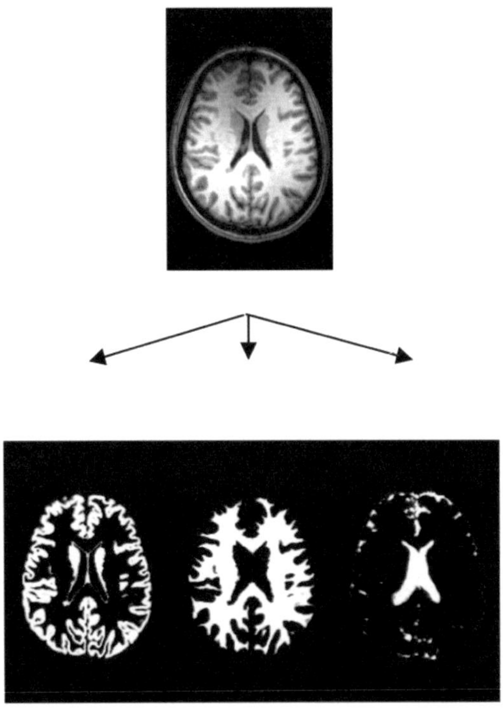

Figure 3. Segmentation process. Top: original image. Bottom (from left to right): gray matter, white matter and cerebrospinal fluid probability maps.

2.2.4.4. Smoothing

The main purpose of the smoothing process is to increase the signal-to-noise ratio by reducing the high-frequency random noise. Additionally, smoothing involves other advantages such as increasing the normality of the data and the minimization of inter-subject anatomical differences. The smoothing kernel fixes the brightness of each voxel taking into account the Gaussian average of their adjacent voxels (neighbors). The filtered image is then blurred, mainly in edge and contour areas because the high-frequency signals are removed while the low-frequency bands are preserved (figure 4). The main parameter which defines the shape of the filter is the standard deviation (σ) expressed as the total amplitude at FWHM:

$$FWHM = \sigma\sqrt{(8 \cdot \log(2))}$$

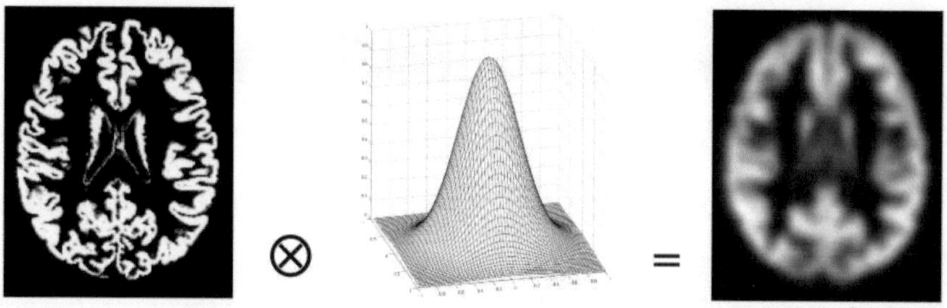

Figure 4. Smoothing of an image. From left to right: original image, 2D Gaussian kernel and smoothed image.

2.2.5. Statistics and results

Usually, the statistical analysis that follows the application of morphometric techniques is based on the General Linear Model (GLM) (Friston et al., 1995). This model allows statistical inferences selecting specific effects of interest in the study groups and is based on an equation that defines the measured signals by a linear combination of explanatory variables plus an error whose distribution is (assumed) Gaussian:

$$Y = X\beta + \varepsilon$$

where Y represents the measured data, X models the design matrix, β represents the estimated parameters and ε is the error.

This structure allows the definition of a measured variable Y as a linear combination of explanatory variables plus an error. It is assumed that this error is independent and follows a Gaussian distribution with zero mean. The design matrix X is a model structure which includes covariates of interest that could potentially influence the results (age, sex, clinical scales, overall tissue volume,...).

By using a voxel-by-voxel approach, multiple statistical comparisons are tested. So, it is necessary to apply additional corrections to minimize the presence of false positives (type I errors). This problem can be solved by applying specific corrections to ensure the reliability of the results. In this sense, the Bonferroni correction based on setting the significance criteria to α / number of observations or the False Discovery Rate (FDR) (Genovese et al.,

2002) that controls the fraction of false positives, can be used. The obtained maps are then colored and overlaid over a high resolution T1 image showing the morphometric differences between groups (figure 5).

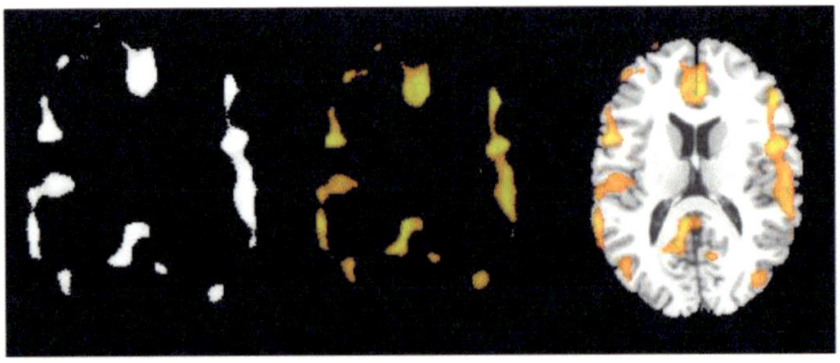

Figure 5. From left to right: original statistic map, colored statistic map and overlay over a T1 axial MR image.

2.3. Structured report

The final step of the morphometric procedure is to include all the information in a structured, concise and brief report (Marti-Bonnmati L., 2011). This report lists all the variables and numerical data calculated in the different processes:

- Parametric data
- The report should include the parameters used in the morphometric method (type of technique, normalization, segmentation, smoothing, templates…) and statistical information (type of test, thresholds, p-values,…).
- Volumetric measures
- Overall volumes of GM, WM and CSF and absolute (ml) and relative (%) values must be included. Furthermore, volumetric measurements for subcortical areas (for example, basal ganglia) are desirable. These values are compared with normal values (obtained from healthy subjects) after discounting potentially relevant sources of bias (age, sex, laterality,…)
- Figures, coordinates and labels for each area of interest
- The final report should also incorporate the significant areas showing differences between groups and their associated values and coordinates. If any, these areas should be overlaid onto a T1 template and detailed in a table which shows statistic values, location of the affected regions (including Brodmann areas) and cluster volumes.

3. White matter tractography

3.1. Introduction

The diffusion tensor magnetic resonance imaging (DT-MRI, DTI) technique is widely used nowadays to explore the anatomy of white matter tracts in the human brain *in vivo*. The DTI is a non-invasive technique that permits the visualization of white matter fiber bundles by the reconstruction of their trajectories in a voxel-by-voxel basis through the measurement of water diffusion along different directions. Water molecules movement in white matter is restricted by the axon and the longitudinal arrangement of myelin covering the axon. In these situations, where a main direction predominates over the others, the water molecules movement has a high anisotropy.

The DTI technique permits the acquisition of MR diffusion images with different orientations of the magnetic field gradients, thus, obtaining a set of images with information of the water movement directionalities for each anatomical cut. The number of gradient orientations is a key parameter in the acquisition of DTI data and, although it is mathematically enough to have 6 directions in order to calculate a tensor, a higher number of directions provide a higher directional resolution.

The computational processing of the DTI data permits the calculation of the orientation and fractional anisotropy (FA) voxelwise. In fact, FA parametric maps can be generated to depict the main orientation of the white matter structure. Computational algorithms specially designed for fiber tracking can be applied to the orientation and anisotropy data in order to reconstruct the trajectory of white matter tracts.

The DTI has a unique view of the tissue architecture of neurons and changes associated with various pathophysiological alterations. There is an increase in the use of this technique for the analysis of white matter alterations produced by tumours and the corresponding surgery planning. Also, the study of congenital abnormalities of the corpus callosum and cerebellum, epilepsy, schizophrenia and early and late Alzheimer's disease is being widely assessed by this technique (Catani M., 2006).

The DTI can be combined with other MRI techniques, such as conventional T1 and T2 images, MR perfusion studies or the results of the concentration of metabolites composing fiber bundles obtained from MR spectroscopy.

3.2. Principles of diffusion tensor MRI

The phenomenon of molecular thermal motion results in random movement of molecules in the three directions of space. These displacements are considered, in general, as translational motions of molecules characterized by Brownian nature. This movement or molecular diffusion in the human body takes place mostly between water molecules.

In some tissues of the human body, water molecules can present a free movement without barriers, also known as free diffusion, or a movement which is limited by the structure of the neighbouring tissues, known as restricted diffusion. The figure 6, shows both concepts.

In general, diffusion measurements express the effective displacement in space of the water molecules in a certain time interval (Le Bihan D., 1988). Although temperature modulates the molecular motion of water molecules (approximately 2.4% per degree Celsius) (Tofts

PS., 2000), that thermal influence is not significant in the study of diffusion, as there are other biophysical properties that have a significant effect on the mobility of tissue water.

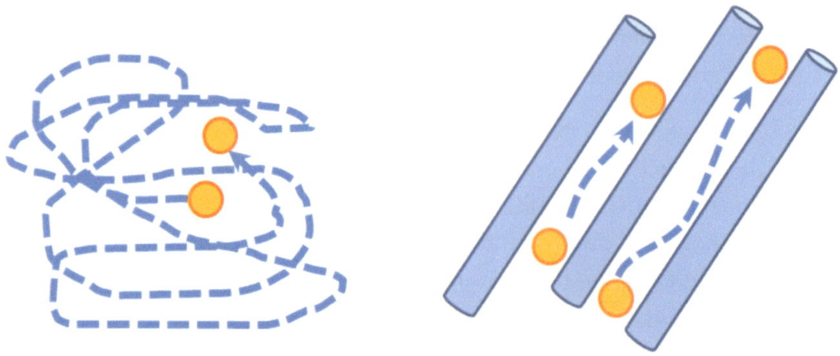

Figure 6. Schematics of diffusion of water molecules in a free environment (left) and in a restricted environment (right).

If pure water is used as a reference standard, the average displacement of the water molecules in a range of about 50ms does not exceed 20μm. Because this dimension is comparable to the cell dimensions, there is a high probability that the water molecules also interact with intracellular components, hydrophobic membranes and macromolecules that impede the movement of water. Therefore, the "apparent" diffusion is several times lower than in the case of pure water. In biological systems, diffusion comprises a complex mixture of single thermal diffusion with exchange between the intracellular and extracellular compartments through cell membranes and tortuosity of the interstitial space, which is conditioned by cell size, organization and density clustering.

To understand diffusion and its quantification, it is assumed that in the initial time we have a group of molecules concentrated at one point. If we wait a time t, without exerting any action on the molecules, they will have expanded in the three dimensions following the Einstein's equation of diffusion:

$$r^2 = 6 \cdot D \cdot t$$

where t is the time interval and r is the average radius of the distribution. As can be deduced, the diffusion coefficient D is expressed as units of distance squared per unit time. For use in radiology or clinical applications, it is usually expressed in mm^2/s.

In order to study the physical diffusion properties explained above, MRI is the only imaging modality that allows visualization and calculation of molecular diffusion *in vivo* directly from molecular translational movement of water.

MR signal is sensitive to microscopic movements water molecules. During the de-phase of the spins after the radio frequency (RF) pulse, phase incoherencies appear in the spins relaxation due to thermal agitation of the water molecules, which accelerates the loss of spins synchronism and reduces the relaxation time. Moreover, the repeated movement of water molecules cause the nuclear spins displacement to other regions in which magnetic field differs from the original value, thus causing a frequency modulation of relaxation.

In order to quantify the displacement movement of the spins independently, a gradient in one direction can be applied immediately after the pulse. In this situation, the water molecules which have been moved in the direction of the gradient will be under a magnetic field be farther more of the original and therefore the signal drop faster.

The free diffusion approximation of light in the previous sections cannot be assumed in biological tissues, because sometimes, the movement of water molecules is restricted or defined to a certain direction. In the latter case, in which a molecule is most likely to move in one direction than another, one speaks of an anisotropic diffusion. The most obvious example (as will be seen below) takes place in the cerebral white matter, where the water molecules tend to move along axonal tracts of the different fascicles brain.

This anisotropy of diffusion can be characterized mathematically, considering a diffusion tensor in the following matrix form:

$$\begin{pmatrix} D_{xx} & D_{xy} & D_{xz} \\ D_{yx} & D_{yy} & D_{yz} \\ D_{zx} & D_{zy} & D_{zz} \end{pmatrix}$$

Since the matrix is symmetric, ie Dxy = Dyx; Dyz = Dzy and dxz = Dzx, simply calculate 6 of the 9 parameters. Therefore, we can deduce that to extract directional properties of diffusion, it will require at least 6 different gradient directions.

An example of 6 acquisitions can be appreciated in figure 7.

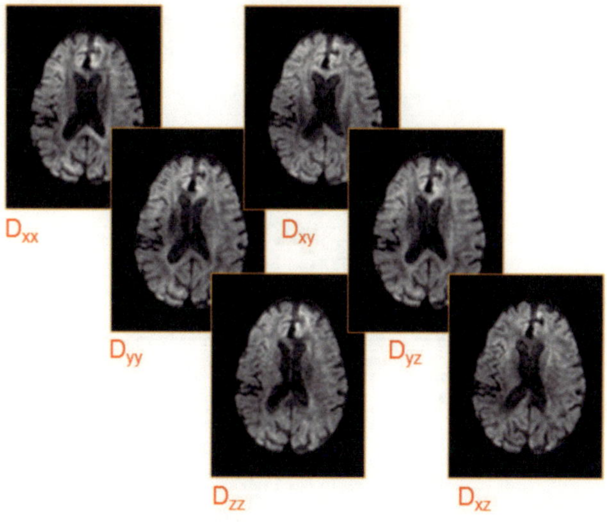

Figure 7. Diffusion images acquired in different magnetic field gradient orientations for the calculation of the diffusion tensor.

The eigenvector of the diffusion matrix provide the information about main orientation of the water molecules movement in each voxel. An example of orientation maps at different detail scales can be appreciated in figure 8:

From the diffusion matrix, the fractional anisotropy (FA) parameter can be calculated from the expression:

$$F_f = \sqrt{\frac{(\lambda_1 - \bar{\lambda})^2 + (\lambda_2 - \bar{\lambda})^2 + (\lambda_3 - \bar{\lambda})^2}{\lambda_1^2 + \lambda_2^2 + \lambda_3^2}}$$

Being λ_1, λ_2 and λ_3 the eigenvalues of the diffusion matrix, and the average value of the eigenvalues. An example of the combination of both orientation and FA information in a voxel-by-voxel basis may be appreciated in figure 9.

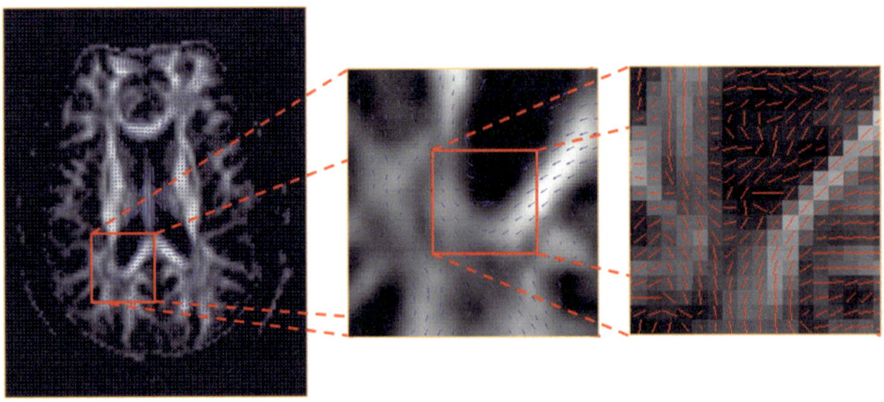

Figure 8. Orientation maps calculated from the diffusion matrix. From left to right: full brain map showing the vector field with the main orientations for each region. Detail of the vector field in a selected region. Voxel-by-voxel representation of the main diffusion orientation.

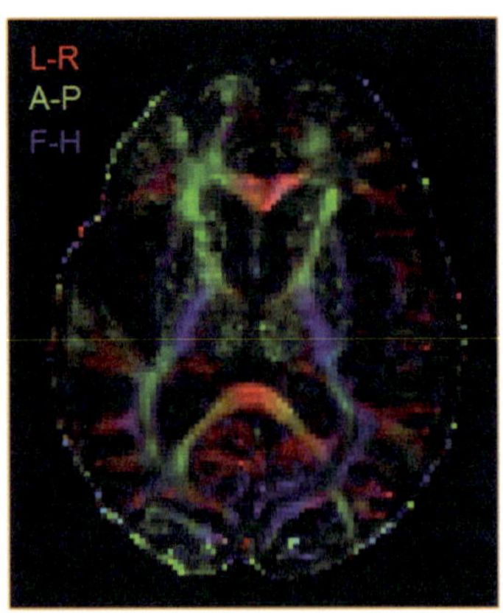

Figure 9. Combined fractional anisotropy (FA) and orientation map. The level of intensity expresses the FA value, while the color indicates the main orientation (LR: left-right, AP: anterior-posterior, FH: foot-head).

3.3. Fiber segmentation

Different segmentation strategies exist for white matter tractography reconstructions of the fibers. The main segmentation techniques can be divided in seed based segmentation, regions of interest segmentation and white matter atlas segmentation.

3.3.1. Seed segmentation

This technique considers an initial point in a 3D space with a given orientation and FA. Thus, the algorithm will initiate a path by the neighbouring voxels showing similar orientations. This trajectory will be calculated until a too sharp angle exists between the orientation of the current voxel and the following. The fiber trajectory calculated will be reconstructed unless if it accomplishes also the condition of the minimum length, which is another parameter imposed in the segmentation to avoid the reconstruction of small fibers from random noise.

3.3.2. Regions of interest segmentation

This is the technique with a higher use in clinical routine nowadays. White matter fibers are reconstructed from regions of interest (ROIs) which are placed according to the user anatomical knowledge. This technique allows for the calculation of the fibers that pass through the ROIs that have been introduced. Exclusive ROIs can also be placed in order to avoid the reconstruction of fibers bundles which are adjacent to the one of interest.

An example of this technique can be appreciated in figure 10, where the uncinate fasciculus is reconstructed. Two ROIs are placed in order to exclusively reconstruct fibers crossing both regions.

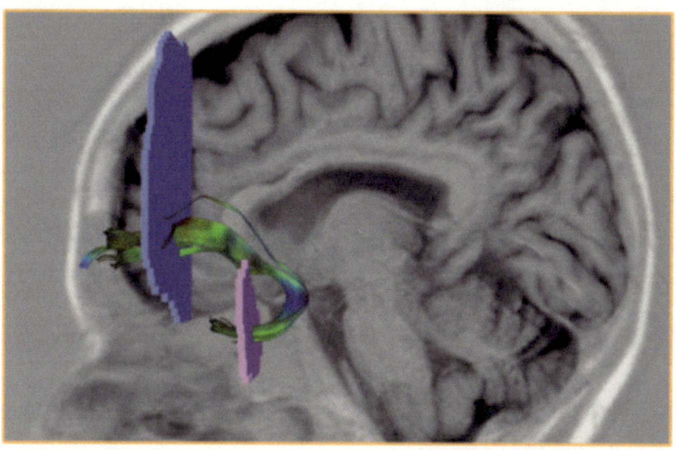

Figure 10. Segmentation of the uncinate fasciculus by the placement of two ROIs, in the frontal and temporal lobes.

3.3.3. Atlas based segmentation

The tracts segmentation using white matter atlas has a higher complexity. In general terms, the main basis of the method consists in the calculation of the orientation and FA maps for large series of subjects. All these data is anatomically co-registered and a final expert anatomical labelling is performed (O'Donnell LJ., 2007).

3.4. Extracted parameters

The main white matter tracts can be segmented routinely by ROI segmentation for clinical applications. The authors suggest the segmentation of the following white matter fasciculum according to experience with pre-surgical evaluation and study of neurodegenerative disorders:

- Corpus callosum
- Cingulate fasciculus
- Uncinate fasciculus
- Corticospinal fasciculus
- Inferior longitudinal fasciculus
- Superior longitudinal fasciculus

In figure 11, examples of fiber reconstructions in different pathologic conditions can be appreciated.

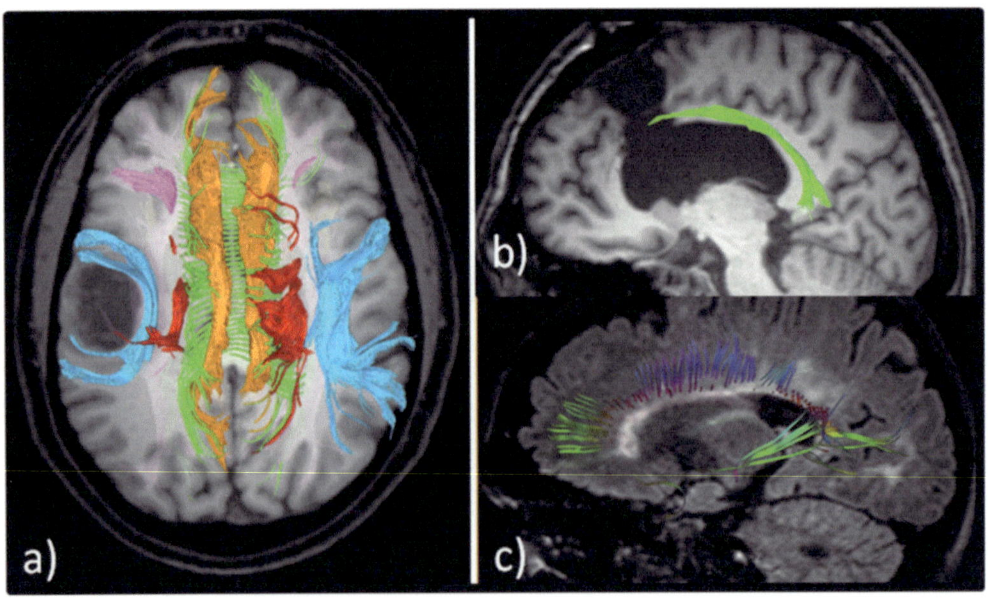

Figure 11. White matter fasciculus reconstruction in different clinical cases. In a), main white matter fibers segmentation for the pre-surgical evaluation of a glioblastoma multiforme. The right superior longitudinal fasciculus, in blue, can be appreciated to be attached to the tumour periphery. In b), the reconstruction of a sectioned cingulum is observed in a patient after an emergency intervention due to an acute hydrocephaly. In c), corpus callosum fibers shortening due to advanced multiple sclerosis lesions.

In each reconstructed fiber bundle we can extract a set of parameters related to the microstructure:

- Fractional anisotropy (FA): its value ranges from 0 (pure isotropic) to 1 (highly anisotropic) and shows the degree of existence of a preferential diffusion direction within the voxel.
- Mean diffusivity (D): it is measured in mm^2/s and expresses the degree of restriction to water molecules movement in a voxel. High D values reflect low degree of restriction to movement, while low D values show a restricted diffusion of molecules due to a higher cell density and reduced interstitial space.
- Number of fibers (NF): it is the total number of fibers that have been reconstructed in a certain fasciculum.
- Average length (L): it is mostly expressed in centimetres and provides the average length of the fibers of the reconstructed fasciculum.

3.5. Structured report

An adequate tractography report should be brief and concise (Marti-Bonmati L., 2011), and include:

- Parametric data: the results of the parameters presented in the anterior section (FA, D, NF, L) for each reconstructed white matter fasciculum. These values should be compared to values obtained in a large series of age-matched healthy subjects.
- Figures: representative figures of the main white matter tracts superimposed on anatomical images.

4. Conclusions and future challenges

The brain morphometry and tractography techniques have established as the main image processing methodologies for the characterization of brain structure in all types of central nervous system disorders. Although many centres benefit from their application to different clinical cases, large population studies have been mainly limited due to lack of standardization in the acquisition, processing and reporting techniques. The future challenges for these techniques have to be focused in multi-centre initiatives that facilitate the protocols sharing, the standardization of analysis procedures and the way this information is presented in adequate structured reports.

Author details

G. García-Martí
Department of Radiology, Hospital Quirón Valencia, Valencia, Spain
CIBERSAM, Universitat de Valencia, Valencia, Spain

A. Alberich-Bayarri
Department of Radiology, Hospital Quirón Valencia, Valencia, Spain
Consortium for the Assessment of Cardiovascular Remodelling (cvREMOD), Valencia, Spain

L. Martí-Bonmatí
Department of Radiology, Hospital Quirón Valencia, Valencia, Spain
Consortium for the Assessment of Cardiovascular Remodelling (cvREMOD), Valencia, Spain
Radiology Unit. Department of Medicine. Universitat de València, Valencia, Spain

5. References

Ashburner J, Friston KJ. Voxel-Based Morphometry – The methods. Neuroimage. 2000; 11: 805-821.

Ashburner J. A fast diffeomorphic image registration algorithm. Neuroimage. 2007; 38: 95-113.

Brechbuhler C, Gerig G, Szekely G. Compensation of spatial inhomogeneity in MRI based on a parametric field estimate. Visualisation in Biomedical Computation (VBC96). 1996; 141–146.

Catani M. Diffusion tensor magnetic resonance imaging tractography in cognitive disorders. Curr Opin Neurol. 2006;19:599-606.

Friston LJ, Holmes AP, Worsley LJ, Poline JP, Frith CD, Frackowiak RSJ. Statistical parametric maps in functional imaging. A general linear approach. Human Brain Mapping. 1995; 2: 189-210.

Gaser C, Nenadic I, Buchsbaum BR, Hazlett EA., Buchsbaum MS. Deformation-Based Morphometry and Its Relation to Conventional Volumetry of Brain Lateral Ventricles in MRI. Neuroimage. 2001; 13: 1140-1145.

Genovese CR, Lazar NA, Nichols T. Thresholding of Statistical Maps in Functional Neuroimaging Using the False Discovery Rate. Neuroimage. 2002; 15: 870-878.

Kipps CM, Duggins AJ, Mahant N, Gomes L, Ashburner J, McCusker EA. Progression of structural neuropathology in preclinical Huntington's disease: a tensor based morphometry study. J. Neurol., Neurosurg. Psychiatry. 2005; 76: 650–655.

Le Bihan D, Breton E, Lallemand D, Aubin ML, Vignaud J, Laval-Jeantet M. Separation of diffusion and perfusion in intravoxel incoherent motion MR imaging. Radiology. 1988;168:497-505.

Manjón JV, Lull JJ, Carbonell-Caballero J, García-Martí G, Martí-Bonmatí L, Robles M. A nonparametric MRI inhomogeneity correction method. Med Image Anal. 2007; 11: 336-345.

Martí Bonmatí L, Alberich-Bayarri A, García-Martí G, Sanz Requena R, Pérez Castillo C, Carot Sierra JM, Manjón Herrera JV. Imaging biomarkers, quantitative imaging, and bioengineering. Radiologia 2011. Jul 4. [Epub ahead of print].

O'Donell LJ, Westin CF. Automatic Tractography Segmentation Using a High-Dimensional White Matter Atlas. IEEE Trans Med Imag. 2007;26:1562:1575.

Sled J, Zijdenbos A, Evans A. A nonparametric method for automatic correction of intensity nonuniformity in MRI data. IEEE Trans. Med. Imaging. 1998; 17: 87–97.

Tofts PS, Lloyd D, Clark CA, Barker GJ, Parker GJ, McConville P, Baldock C, Pope JM. Test liquids for quantitative MRI measurements of self-diffusion coefficients in vivo. Magn Reson Med. 2000;43:368-374.

Chapter 2

Proton Magnetic Resonance Spectroscopy of the Central Nervous System

Evanthia Kousi, Ioannis Tsougos and Kapsalaki Eftychia

Additional information is available at the end of the chapter

http://dx.doi.org/10.5772/53892

1. Introduction

Early and accurate diagnosis of patients with cerebral demyelinating or infection diseases, space occupying mass lesions and neurological deficits, is essential for optimum treatment decision concerning the administration of specific medication or chemotherapeutic agents, radiation therapy and/or surgical resection.

Currently, conventional MR imaging (MRI) is considered to be an established and useful tool in brain disease detection and it is widely chosen as the initial examination step in patients suspected of brain lesions as it is effective in simultaneously characterizing the soft tissue, cerebrospinal fluid (CSF) spaces, and blood vessels. It is a flexible imaging modality for which contrast can be extensively manipulated without patient burdening by ionizing radiation. Nevertheless, the accurate characterization of brain lesions with MR imaging remains problematic in several cases as the sensitivity and specificity with which this modality defines several brain lesions remains limited [1].

To overcome the aforementioned limitation, the development of new imaging techniques is required, in order to highlight functional or metabolic properties of brain tissue. Proton Magnetic resonance spectroscopy (^{1}H-MRS) is one such technique which provides a non-invasive method for characterizing the cellular biochemistry which underlies brain pathologies, as well as for monitoring the biochemical changes after treatment in vivo. It is considered as a bridge between metabolism and the anatomic and physiological studies available from MRI [2].

Until now, ^{1}H-MRS has been used as both a research and a clinical tool for detecting abnormalities -visible or not yet visible- on conventional MRI. Suggestively, Moller-Hartman et al. reported that when only the MR images used for radiological diagnosis of focal intracranial mass lesions, their type and grade were correctly identified in 55% of the cases, however, the addition of MR spectroscopic information significantly raised the proportion of correctly diagnosed cases to 71% [3].

^{1}H-MRS has been always challenging in terms of its technical requisites (field strength, gradients, coils and software), as well as the accurate metabolic interpretation with regards to pathologic processes. However, the clinical applications of ^{1}H-MRS are continuously increasing as the clinical hardware have become more robust and user-friendly along with improved data analysis, spectra post-processing techniques and metabolite interpretation confidence.

The purpose of this chapter is to provide a thorough review concerning the current status of ^{1}H-MRS in terms of its clinical usefulness as well as its technical prerequisites.

2. Basic principles

In order to introduce the basic concepts and terminology of ^{1}H -MRS, the basic principles of MRS are briefly described below.

Proton is a charged particle with spin, and exhibits the electromagnetic properties of a dipole magnet. When protons are placed in an external magnetic field B_0, they align themselves along the direction of the field (either parallel or anti-parallel) and demonstrate a circular oscillation. The frequency of this circular motion (called Larmor frequency) is dependent on the strength of the local magnetic field and the molecular structures at which protons belong. This can be expressed by the Larmor equation:

$$\omega_0 = \gamma \mathbf{B}_0$$

where ω_0 is the Larmor frequency, γ is the gyromagnetic ratio specific for the nuclei, and $\mathbf{B}_0$ is the strength of the external magnetic field.

When electromagnetic energy (in the form of a RF pulse) is supplied at this frequency, the molecules absorb this energy and change their alignment. When the RF pulse is switched off, the molecules realign themselves to the magnetic field by releasing their absorbed energy. This released energy is the basis of the MR signal [4].

^{1}H-MRS uses the same hardware as conventional MRI, however, their main difference is that the frequency of the MR signal is used to encode different types of information. MRI generates structural images, whereas ^{1}H-MRS provides chemical information about the tissue under study.

Although recent studies have shown promise for the use of ^{1}H-MRS to investigate malignant processes to prostate [5], breast [6], skeletal muscles [7], cervical and ovarian cancer [8], the overwhelming number of applications have been demonstrated in the brain, due to the absence of free lipid signals in normal cerebrum, relative ease of shimming, and lack of inherent motion artifacts.

The output of ^{1}H-MRS is a spectrum which is described by two axes as it is illustrated in figure 1. The vertical axis (y) represents the signal intensity or relative concentration for the various cerebral metabolites and the horizontal axis (x) serves to describe the frequency chemical shift in parts per million (ppm). The nature of the chemical shift effect is to produce a change in the resonant frequency for nuclei of the same type attached to different chemical species. It is due to variations in surrounding electron clouds of neighboring atoms, which shield nuclei from the main magnetic field (B_0). The resulting frequency difference can be used to identify the presence of important chemical compounds. Within the spectrum, metabolites are characterized by one or more peaks with a certain resonance frequency, line width (full width at half maximum of the peak's height, FWHM), line shape (e.g., lorentzian or Gaussian), phase, and peak area according to the number of protons that contribute to the observed signal. By monitoring those peak factors, ^{1}H-MRS can provide a qualitative and/or a quantitative analysis of a number of metabolites within the brain if a reference of known metabolite concentration is used at a particular field strength [9].

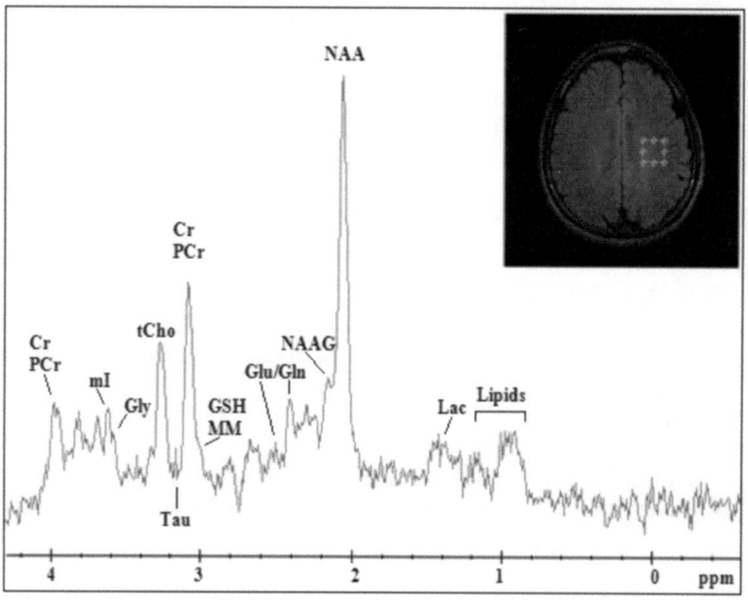

Figure 1. Proton MR spectrum from Parietal White Metter measured at 3T in the normal human brain of a 19-year-old volunteer.

3. Neurospectroscopy biochemical features and their clinical significance

Accurate classification of cerebral lesions by in-vivo ^{1}H-MRS requires determination of the relationship between metabolic profile and pathologic processes.

The assignment and clinical significance of the basic resonances in a spectrum as well as the less commonly detected compounds are discussed below:

N-Acetyl Aspartate (NAA) in ^{1}H-MR spectra of normal cerebral tissue, is the most prominent resonance which originates from the methyl group of NAA at 2.01ppm with a contribution from neurotransmitter N-aspartyl-glutamate (NAAG) (figure 1). NAA is exclusively localized in central and peripheral nervous system and it is synthesized in brain mitochondria. Its concentration subtly varies in different parts of the brain [10] and undergoes large developmental changes, increasing from 4.82mM at birth to 8.89mM in adulthood. Although NAA is considered as a neuronal marker and equate with neuronal density and viability, its exact function remains largely unknown.

The utility of NAA, as an axonal marker is supported by the loss of NAA in many white matter diseases, including leukodystrophies [11], multiple sclerosis (MS) [12] and hypoxic encephalopathy [13], chronic stages of stoke [14] and tumors [1, 2, 9]. However, there are cases when the abnormal levels of NAA do not reflect changes in neuronal density, but rather a perturbation of the synthetic and degradation pathways of NAA metabolism. For instance, in Canavan's disease high levels of intracellular NAA [15] are due to aspartoacylase (ASPA) deficiency, which is the enzyme that degrades NAA to acetate and aspartate.

Further examples that show the lack of direct relationship of NAA to neuronal integrity include various pathologies such as temporal lobe epilepsy (TLE) [16] or amyotrophic lateral sclerosis (ALS) [17], which exhibit spontaneous or treatment reversals of NAA to normal levels.

Choline-containing compounds comprise signals from free choline (Cho), phosphocholine (PC) and glycerophosphocholine (GPC), with a resonant peak located at 3.22 ppm. Since the resonance contains contributions from several methyl proton choline-containing compounds, it is often referred as "total Choline" (tCho). tCho is involved in pathways of phospholipid synthesis and degradation thus reflecting a metabolic index of membrane density and integrity as well as membrane turnover [1, 2, 9].

Consistent changes of tCho signal have been observed in a large number of cerebral diseases. Processes that lead to elevation of tCho include accelerated membrane synthesis of rapidly dividing cancer cells in brain tumors [1, 2, 9], cerebral infractions, infectious diseases [18], and inflammatory-demyelinating diseases [19].

Unlike to NAA, which is distributed almost homogeneously throughout the healthy brain, tCho exhibits a marked regional variability with higher concentrations observed in the pons and lower levels in the vermis and dentate [20]. Therefore, detailed knowledge about regional variations of tCho is necessary for an accurate interpretation of the metabolite's levels, especially in diseases such as epilepsy and psychiatric disorders where tCho is subtly different to normal levels.

Creatine (Cr) and Phosphocreatine (PCr) together they are often referred as total creatine (tCr) because they cannot be distinguished with standard clinical MR unit (up to 7T) and their sum is thus mentioned. Cr and PCr arise from the methyl and methylene protons of Cr and phosphorylated Cr. Within the ^{1}H-MR spectrum, tCr is located at 3.03 ppm and 3.93 ppm resonant frequencies.

In the brain tCr is present in both neuronal and glial cells and is involved in energy metabolism serving as an energy buffer via the creatine kinase reaction retaining constant

ATP levels and as an energy shuttle, diffusing from the energy producing (i.e. mitochondria) to energy utilizing sites (i.e. nerve terminals in brain) [21]. As tCr is not naturally produced in the brain, its concentration is assumed to be stable with no changes reported with age or a variety of diseases and is used for calculating metabolite ratios (NAA/Cr, tCho/Cr etc) [21]. Nevertheless, the use of tCr as an internal concentration reference should be used with caution as decreased tCr levels have been observed in the chronic phases of many pathologies including tumors [22], stroke [23] and gliosis [24].

myo-inositol (mI) is a cyclic sugar alcohol that gives rise to four groups of resonances with the larger and most important signal occurring at 3.56 ppm. It is observable on short time echo (TE) spectra as it exhibits short T2 relaxation times and is susceptible to dephasing effects due to J-coupling. The exact function of mI is uncertain, however it has been proposed as a glial marker and an increase of mI levels is believed to represent glial proliferation or an increase in glial cell size, both of which may occur in inflammation [2]. Additionally, this metabolite is involved in the activation of protein C kinase which leads to production of proteolytic enzymes found in malignant and aggressive cerebral tumors, serving as a possible index for glioma grading [25]. mI has also been labeled as a breakdown product of myelin. Thus, altered levels of mI have been also encountered in patients with degenerative and demyelinating diseases [12, 15].

Lactate and Lipids, in the normal brain should be maintained below or at the limit of detectability within the ^{1}H-MR spectrum, overlapping with macromolecule (MM) resonances at 1.33ppm (doublet) and 0.9-1.3 ppm respectively. Any detectable increase in lactate and lipids can therefore be considered abnormal. Lactate is present in both intracellular and extracellular spaces and provides an index of metabolic rate and clearance [22]. As an end-product of anaerobic glycolysis, increased lactate levels have been observed in a wide variety of conditions in which oxygen supply is restricted such as in both acute and chronic ischemia [14], metabolic disorders [2], and tumors [1, 2, 9, 22]. Lactate also accumulates in tissues that have poor washout like cysts [26] and normal pressure hydrocephalus [27]. However, in CSF, lactate may be detectable at low levels in normal subjects with prominent ventricles [4].

The spectral region between 0.9ppm and 1.3ppm as referred above; represents the methylene (1.3ppm) and the methyl (0.9ppm) groups of fatty acids. It is during membrane breakdown when fractured proteins and lipid layers become visible. Regardless of the exact molecular source, an elevation of lipid resonances indicates cerebral tissue destruction such as infarction [14], acute inflammation [28] and necrosis [18]. In addition, lipid signals have been observed in patients with several metabolic disorders such as Zellweger syndrome and Refsum's disease [29].

Glutamate (Glu) and Glutamine (Gln) together they form a complex of peaks (Glx complex) between 2.15 ppm and 2.45 ppm, as their similar chemical structures, renders their distinction difficult within a proton spectra at 1.5T. However, at 3T and above Glu and Gln start to become resolved [30] and at magnetic fields of 7T and higher, the Glu and Gln resonances are visually separated leading to big quantification accuracy [21]. Glu is the major excitatory neurotransmitter in mammalian brain and the direct precursor for the major inhibitory neurotransmitter, γ-aminobutyric acid (GABA). The amino acid Gln, is an important component of intermediary metabolism, is primarily located in astroglia and it is synthesized from Glu [21].

The Glx complex plays a role in detoxification and regulation of neurotransmitters. Increased levels of Glx complex are markers of epileptogenic processes [31] and low levels of Glx have been observed in Alzheimer Dementia and patients with chronic Schizophrenia [32]. Glx complex increment, has been also observed in the peritumoral brain edema correlated with neuronal loss and demyelination [33]. As reported by Malhorta et al., Glx might be used as an in vivo index of inflammation since they observed elevated Glx levels in acute MS plaques but not in chronic ones [34].

Alanine (Ala) is an amino acid present in the normal brain, resonating at 1.47 ppm. It is frequently considered as a specific metabolic charecteristic of meningiomas, however, its identification rate varies from 32% to 100% [3, 22]. It can be also presented in neurocytomas [35], gliomas and PNETs [36]. In vivo ^{1}H-MRS at 1.5T often cannot provide a distinction between Ala and Lac peaks as they resonate in neighboring frequencies. When both metabolites are present they produce a triplet peak located between 1.3 ppm and 1.5 ppm [37] observed at 3T and higher.

Glycine (Gly) is the simplest amino acid and possible antioxidant, distributing mainly in astrocytes and glycinergic neurons, where it is regulated due to its neuroactive properties as an inhibitory neurotrasmitter [28]. It resonates at 3.55 ppm and it overlaps with mI rendering the observation of Gly impossible in a non-processed spectrum. In cases of mI absence, the even low Gly levels can be quantified [38].

High levels of Gly have been observed in glioblastomas, medulloblastomas, ependymomas and neurocytomas [28]. It has also been reported that this metabolite may provide a noticeable metabolic index for the differentiation of glioblastomas from lower grade astrocytomas, primary gliomas from recurrence [38] and glial tumors from metastatic brain tumors [36].

Taurine (Tau) gives two triplets at 3.25 ppm and 3.42 ppm, which can be observed at higher magnetic fields [21] as they significantly overlap with Cho and mI. Tau is an inhibitory neurotransmitter that activates GABA-a receptors or strychnine-sensitive glycine receptors and it has also been proposed as an osmoregulator and a modulator of neurotransmitter action [21]. High levels of Tau have been observed in medulloblastoma, pituitary adenoma and metastatic renal cell carcinoma [39]. Shirayama et al have been also reported increased levels of Tau in the medial prefrontal cortex in schizophrenic patients [40].

Glutathione (GSH) is the major protective molecule of living cells assigned to 2.9 ppm. It serves as an antioxidant and detoxifier thus having an important role against oxidative stress [41]. Glutathione also plays a role in apoptosis and amino acid transport [42].

Altered levels of this metabolite have been reported in acute ischemic stroke patients as ischemia is associated with significant oxidative stress [41], in Parkinson's disease and other neurodegenerative diseases affecting the basal ganglia [21]. GSH has been also found to be significantly elevated in meningiomas when compared to other tumors [42], showing as well an inverse relationship with glioma malignancy.

Several other amino Acids such as Succinate at 2.4 ppm, Acetate at 1.92 ppm, Valine and Leucine at 0.9 ppm together with Alanine and Lactate, are the major spectral findings of bacterial and parasitic diseases. Acetate and Succinate are presumably originating from enhanced glycolysis of the bacterial organism [9]. The amino acids Valine and Leukine are known to be the end-products of proteolysis by enzymes released in pus [9]. Specifically, Leucine and Valine peaks have been detected in cystercercosis lesions, however they have not been reported in proton MR spectra of brain tumors [9].

4. Technical considerations

In order to precisely identify the metabolite peaks within a spectrum, several technical considerations should be taken into account concerning the applied magnetic field, the shimming procedures as well as the adequate voxel positioning and the available ^{1}H-MRS techniques , which all highly affect the quality of the yielded spectrum before any post-processing intervention.

4.1. Field strength

In ^{1}H-MRS clinical applications, it is not the signals of water and fat that are of interest, but rather the smaller signals of metabolites, thus a magnetic field of sufficient strength is required. Therefore, most clinical ^{1}H-MRS measurements are performed using MR systems with field strengths of 1.5T and higher. Although more powerful 4-, 6-, 7- , and even 8T MR body scanners are currently in use, the most common high field systems operate at 3T. The main advantage of increasing magnetic field strength is the subsequent increase of the signal-to-noise ratio (SNR). Theoretically, SNR increases proportionally to field strength, however, when put into clinical practice, the study of Barker et al [43], demonstrated a 28% increase in SNR at 3T compared to that of 1.5T at short TEs, appreciably less than the theoretical 100% improvement. Another advantage of magnetic field increment, is the proportional increase of the Chemical Shift, from 220 Hz at 1.5T to 440 Hz at 3T. This is reflected by more effective water suppression and improved baseline separation of J-coupled metabolites such as glutamate, glutamine and GABA, without the need of sophisticated spectral editing techniques [44]. The improvement in spectral resolution is further evident at 7T where weakly represented neurochemicals with important clinical impact, such as scyllo-Ins, aspartate, taurine and NAAG, can be clearly visible [44].

On the other hand, the aforementioned advantages may be hampered by intrinsic field-dependent technical difficulties that should be considered. When the frequency shift between two adjacent nuclei is large enough, a measurable alteration of MR signal, used to encode the x- and y-axis spatial coordinates, will occur producing a spatial misregistration. This means that the volume of MRS information may not be the same as that displayed on the localizer MR image [45]. J-modulation anomalies represent another difficulty encountered at high magnetic fields. The large separation of coupled resonances such as Lactate can result in incomplete inversion of the coupled spin over a large portion of the selected volume, resulting in anomalous intensity losses at long echo times. Strategies to quantify the lactate signal loss have been previously discussed by Lange et al. [46]. Magnetic susceptibility from paramagnetic substances and blood products, are sensibly increased with increasing magnetic field strength. Consequently, magnetic field inhomogeneity and susceptibility artifacts makes more difficult to obtain good-quality spectra, especially from largely heterogeneous lesions [45]. Improved local shimming methods can alleviate the problem.

4.2. Shimming

Shimming refers to the process of adjusting field gradients, either manually or automatically, in order to optimize the magnetic field homogeneity over the volume under study. Magnetic field inhomogeneities result primarily from susceptibility differences between different tissues and between tissue and air cavities, which are scaled non-linearly in ultra-high magnetic fields [47]. Thus, voxels that are placed in inhomogeneous regions of the brain, such as the temporal poles, are difficult to shim due to their close proximity to the sinuses.

Field homogeneity is specified by measuring the full width at half maximum (FWHM) of the water resonance, which determines the spectral resolution. Special emphasis, especially when field is increased, must be placed on shimming, as it increases both sensitivity and spectral resolution. This is why most devices come equipped with second or third order shimming by monitoring either the time domain or frequency domain of the ^{1}H-MRS signal [48]. Some times 4-order shimming might be necessary [49], especially in cases when field homogeneity should be reached in large volumes of interest during magnetic resonance spectroscopic imaging (MRSI).

Effective shimming requires methods for mapping field's strength variations over the area under study. Methods that have been developed for field mapping can be grouped in two categories: those which are based on 3D field mapping [49] and those which map the magnetic field along projections [50]. In both shimming methods, information about the magnetic field variation is calculated from phase differences acquired during the evolution of the magnetization in a non-homogeneous field.

4.3. Voxel positioning

For a meaningful in vivo ^{1}H-MRS, it is important to locate the voxel in the appropriate region for a reliable metabolic characterization of a lesion [48].

First and foremost, cautious spatial localization is used to remove unwanted signals from outside the ROI, like extracranial lipids and to avoid "partial volume effects", thereby providing a more genuine tissue characterization. Additional benefits from careful spatial voxel localization, originate from the fact that variations in the main magnetic field and magnetic field gradients, are greatly reduced, thereby providing narrower spectral lines and more uniform proton excitation.

Several lesions and stroke infarcts do not always place themselves in positions that are easy to shim such as temporal lobes, the base of the brain and the cortex near the scull. Small voxels is those regions are easier to shim, but the signal also depends on volume so a voxel with 1-cm sides is often considered the practical minimum size to achieve a reasonable SNR [51].

4.4. ^{1}H-MR spectroscopy data acquisition techniques

Spectra can be acquired either with a single voxel (SV) technique (single voxel spectroscopy, SVS) or multiple voxels technique, known as either magnetic resonance spectroscopic imaging (MRSI) or chemical shift imaging (CSI) in two or three dimensions. SVS is based on the stimulated echo acquisition mode (STEAM) [52] or the point resolved spectroscopy (PRESS) [53] pulse sequences while MRSI uses a variety of pulse sequences (Spin Echo, PRESS etc.) [54].

SVS acquires a spectrum from a small volume of tissue located at the intersection of three mutual orthogonal slice-selective pulses as depicted in figure 2. The pulse sequence is designed to collect only the echo signal from the point where all three slices intersect [53].

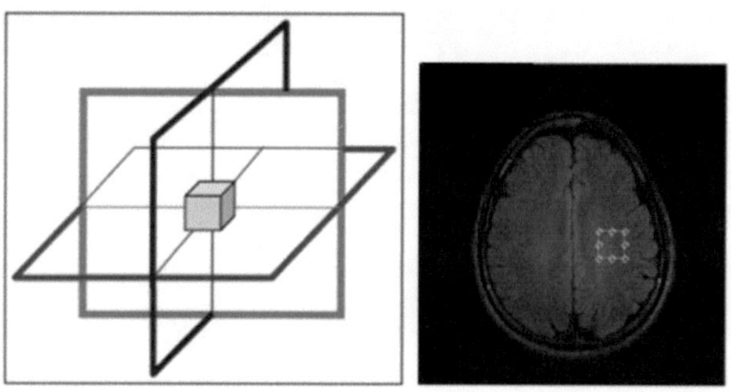

Figure 2. Schematic representation of the three orthogonal SV slice selective pulses (left) resulting in the signal collection only from the rectangular region of interest.

The advantages of this approach are that:

1. the volume is typically well-defined with minimal contamination (e.g. extracranial lipids),
2. the magnetic field homogeneity across the volume can be readily optimized, leading to
3. improved water suppression and spectral resolution.

The main disadvantage of SVS is that it does not address spatial heterogeneity of spectral patterns and in the context of brain tumors, these factors are particularly important for treatment planning such as radiation or surgical resection.

Lesion's heterogeneity is better assessed by MRSI. MRSI techniques have been extended to two dimensions (2D) by using phase-encoding gradients in two directions, or, subsequently, three-dimensional (3D) encoding [55]. Thus, the detection of localized ^{1}H-MR spectra from a multidimensional array of locations is allowed (Figure 3). While technically more challenging -due to (1) significant magnetic field inhomogeneity across the entire area of interest, (2) spectral degradation due to intervoxel contamination the so called "voxel bleed", (3) long data acquisition times and (4) post-processing of large multidimensional datasets- MRSI can detect metabolic profiles from multiple spatial positions, thereby offering an unbiased characterization of the entire object under investigation.

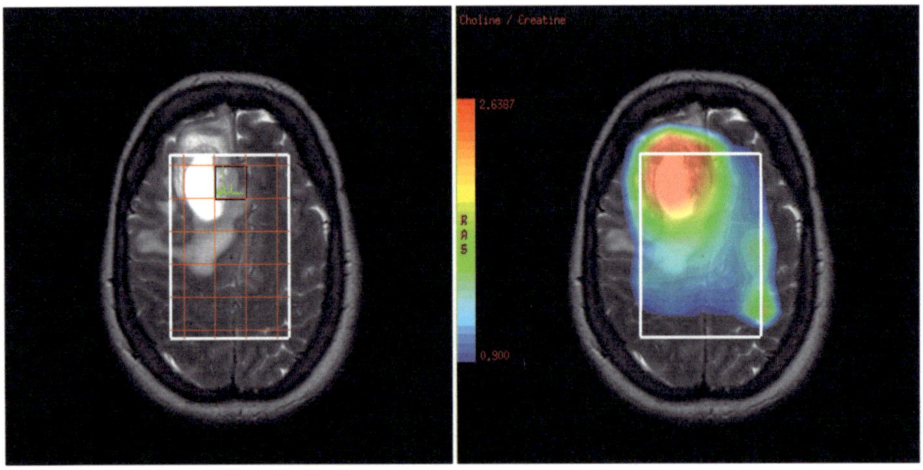

Figure 3. An example of 2D-MRSI of a 50-year old female with a glioblastoma. Simultaneously acquired spectra from multiple regions located at the same plane of the lesion (left). Data are also presented as a metabolic map of Choline/Creatine (right).

4.5. Water and lipid suppression techniques

Water and peri-cranial lipid suppression techniques are of paramount importance in ^{1}H-MRS procedure in order to observe the much less concentrated metabolite signals. The metabolites of interest are usually about a factor of 8,000 less in concentration than water. Therefore, the water suppression efficiency should be robust and should not vary spatially across the field of view (FOV).

The existing water suppression techniques can be divided into three major groups, namely: (1) methods that employ frequency-selective excitation and/or refocusing pulses; or (2) utilize differences in relaxation parameters; and (3) other methods, including software-based water suppression. The most common method of the first group utilizes multiple (typically 3) frequency-selective, 90° pulses (chemical shift selective water suppression (CHESS) pulses [56], prior to localization pulse sequence. Additionally suppression can be achieved by selectively diphase water, while metabolites of interest are rephased using refocusing pulses during the spin echo period [57]. As water and metabolites T1s are sufficiently different, it is possible to suppress the water signal and observe the metabolites in the close proximity to the water resonance [58]. The third method involves the acquisition of two separated scans in which the metabolite resonances are inverted. The large (unsuppressed) water resonance, as well as the water-related sidebands, is not inverted in either scan. The difference between the two scans therefore results in a water-subtracted (suppressed) metabolite spectrum without any interfering water-related sidebands [21].

Lipid suppression can be performed by avoid the excitement of the lipid signal using STEAM or PRESS localization to select a relatively large rectangular volume inside the brain. Since the extracranial lipids are not excited they do not contribute to the detected signal. Opposite to the strategy employed by volume pre-localization, outer volume suppression pulses (OVS) are applied to presaturate the lipid signal [54]. As illustrated in figure 4, rather than avoiding the spatial selection of lipids, OVS excites narrow slices centered the brain's lipid-rich regions. Additionally, the difference in T1s of lipids (250-350 msec) and metabolites (1000-2000msec) allows the application of an inversion pulse (inversion time ~ 200 msec), which will selectively null the lipid signal [59]. By choosing the inversion delay such that the longitudinal lipid magnetization is zero, the lipids are effectively not excited.

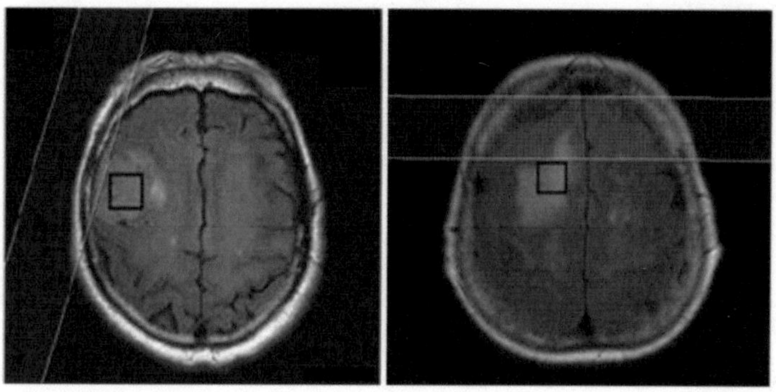

Figure 4. The location and orientation of OVS pulses have been prescribed in order to saturate as much peri-cranial lipid as possible while the signal within the voxel remains unperturbed.

5. Post processing techniques

In MR spectroscopy, post-processing is considered any signal manipulation performed in order to improve the visual appearance of the MR spectrum or the accuracy during metabolite estimation. Therefore, for a reliable analysis of in vivo ^{1}H-MR spectra, an understanding of the principles of post-processing techniques is necessary.

Signal post-processing can be performed either on time domain or after Fourier transformation on frequency domain [60]. Eddy current correction, removal of unwanted spectral components, signal filtering, zero filling, phase correction and baseline correction, consist the most common post-processing techniques for effective signal improvement, and they will be briefly discussed below:

During signal localization RF pulses are applied together with magnetic field gradients. The switching pattern of the gradients applied, can cause eddy current (EC) artifacts that are time and space dependent, causing time dependent phase shifts in the FID and distorted metabolite lineshapes within the spectrum preventing accurate quantification. In a spectrum EC artifacts can be removed by acquiring an additional FID without water suppression. The phase of the water FID is determined in each time point and it is subtracted from the phase of the corrupted FID [24]. The EC artifact correction comprises the first step of the post-processing procedure.

The removal of unwanted signals from the FID which may disturb signals from the resonances of interest is the next step of signal post processing. A typical example of such an unwanted signal in ^{1}H-MRS is that of water. Water suppression during measurement is never perfect and a residual water signal remains in the spectrum which often has a complicated lineshape [24]. Residual water elimination from the FID can be achieved, either by approximating the water signal and subtract it from the FID, or by eliminate it using special filters [61], or by applying baseline correction for the removal of the broad water peak from the spectrum [62].

The existence of a distorted spectral baseline hampers quantitative analysis as the estimation of metabolite peak areas is not reliable. The main sources of the baseline signal are fast decaying components with very short T2* values such as macromolecules, hardware imperfections, signal from the sample and as mentioned above, inefficient water suppression. Thus, for robust data acquisition and quantification methods, baseline correction is of paramount importance. Delayed acquisition (e.g. TE > 80 ms) removes the macromolecules due to their shorter T2 relaxation times (~30 msec), at the expense of loss of information of many scalar-coupled resonances [21] which have been suggested valuable for tumor and stroke characterization [4, 21, 22, 24, 25, 33].

Special functions, called filters, can be subsequently applied at the signal in the time domain. The goal is to enhance or suppress different parts of the FID leading to improved signal quality. The three most commonly used filtering approaches are: sensitivity enhancement, to reduce the noise from the FID; resolution enhancement, to achieve narrower metabolite linewidths; and apodization for signal's ripple (due to signal truncation) reduction [62].

The FID of a spectrum, when acquired, is sampled by the analog-to-digital converter over N points in accordance to the Nyquist sampling frequency. Therefore, if the number of points is not sufficient, the reliable representation of the signal fails. Instead of increasing the acquisition time with the inevitable noise increment, the acquired FID can artificially be extended by adding a string of points with zero amplitude to the FID prior to Fourier Transformation, a process known as zero filling. Zero filling does not increase the information content of the data but it can greatly improve the digital resolution of the spectrum and helps to improve the spectral appearance [21], rendering it an important post-processing step.

After Fourier transformation, the spectrum will be phase corrected. When the zero-phased FID signal shifts to the frequency domain, yields a complex spectrum with absorption (real) and dispersion (imaginary) Lorentz peaks. However, when the initial phase is non-zero, it is not attainable to restore pure absorption or dispersion line shapes and phase correction must be applied [4, 21, 62]. A zero-order phase correction compensates for any mismatch between the quadrature receive channels and the excitation channels to produce the pure absorption spectrum, whereas, a first-order phase correction compensates for the nuclei dephase due to the delay between excitation and the detection of FID [62].

6. ^{1}H-MRS metabolic profiles of brain lesions

The effective differential diagnosis of brain lesions using ^{1}H-MRS depends on the ability of the experienced neuroscientist to interpret and evaluate the metabolic criteria and data underlying each disease. However, similarities in the chemical composition among diseases and/or atypical metabolic characteristics, often burden the diagnosis. Thus, a clinical guide to the main MR spectroscopic findings of cerebral disorders is necessary.

This section focuses on the metabolic patterns of a variety of intra-cranial diseases.

6.1. Multiple Sclerosis (MS)

Multiple Sclerosis (MS) is an auto-immune inflammatory disease of the central nervous system (CNS) in which the myelin sheaths around the axons are damaged leading to demyelination, neuronal affection, inflammation, gliosis and axonal degeneration [14]. ^{1}H-MRS is particularly informative in MS, by providing evidence of the two primary pathologic processes of the disease: active inflammatory demyelination and neuronal injury in both lesional and non-lesional brain tissue [63, 64].

Acute demyelinating lesions reveal increased Cho and Lac resonance intensities due to the release of membrane phospholipids during active myelin breakdown and the impaired metabolism of the inflammatory cells, respectively [63]. Short TE spectra also provide evidence of increased lipids, mI [63, 64] and glutamate levels [34]. Increased glutamate levels in acute MS lesions address a link between the direct axonal injury and glutamate excitotoxicity [65], whereas mI is suggestive of glial proliferation and astrogliosis [63]. The aforementioned changes are accompanied by a substantial decrease in NAA due to axonal injury reflecting metabolic or structural changes [64, 65]. It is important to note that the spectroscopic changes seen in acute MS plaques are often very similar to the spectra observed in brain tumors (high Cho, low NAA, increased Lac, etc.), and therefore this should be kept in mind when evaluating spectra from patients with undiagnosed brain lesions.

After the acute phase transition, Lac, Cho and lipids seem to return to normal levels, whereas NAA may remain decreased or show partial recovery, lasting for several months [64]. The recovery of NAA can be attributed to resolution of edema, diameter increment of the previously shrinked axons, as a result of the re-myelination and reversible metabolic changes in neurons [64, 65]. There are reports of elevated Cho resonance in chronic MS plaque, probably reflecting the associated gliotic process [66]. Cr seems to be a variable metabolite both in chronic and acute, but is also described to be slowly increasing over time, indicative of gliotic reaction or attempts of incomplete re-myelination of the chronic diseased tissue phases [14].

Metabolic abnormalities in MS patients not only concern the lesions, but are found throughout the normal appearing white matter (NAWM) with notably reduced NAA, which is thought to indicate diffuse axonal dysfunction or loss. It must also be stressed out that the presence of intense gliosis may also cause increased levels of mI [67] and Cr [68]. Increased glutamate, lipids and Cho can be also found in regions of the NAWM, which later are going to develop T2-hyperintense focal lesions [64].

6.2. Intracranial abscesses

Brain abscesses are focal, intracerebral infections that begin with a localized region of cerebritis, evolving into a discrete collection of pus surrounded by a well-vascularized capsule. The causative organisms involved in brain abscesses are quite variable, and may consist of mixed cultures: aerobes, anaerobes, facultative anaerobes, and facultative anaerobes in combination with aerobes/anaerobes.

MRS has been proven beneficial in differentiating between brain abscesses and other cystic lesions [69], which can be used to implement the appropriate antimicrobial therapy. Brain abscesses reveal specific metabolic substances, such as succinate, acetate, alanine, valine, pyrouvate, leukine, lipids and lactate [69, 70],which are all present in untreated bacterial abscesses or soon after the initiation of treatment [70]. Increases in lactate, acetate, and succinate presumably may originate from the enhanced glycolysis and fermentation of the infecting microorganisms. Amino acids such as valine and leucine are known to be the end products of proteolysis by enzymes released by neutrophils in pus [14]. However, cerebral abscesses contain no neurons [71], therefore no peaks of NAA and Cr/PCr should be detected. The detection of any NAA and/or Cr/PCr is indicative of either signal contamination or erroneous interpretation of acetate peak as NAA [72]. Similarly no tCho peak is present in an abscesses spectrum because there are no membranous structures in its necrotic core [73]. On the other hand, abscesses of tuberculous origin are characterized by the predominant presence of lipids, moderate increase of tCho resonance and no evidence of cytosolic amino acids [4].

Differential diagnosis of brain abscess versus brain tumor is sometimes difficult on the basis of imaging findings and clinical judgment, especially in the case of a brain tumor with a mainly cystic or necrotic component. However, because the vast majority of the aforementioned amino acids have not been detected in brain neoplasms, their presence strongly differentiates abscesses from highly aggressive tumors [71].

6.3. Ischemia

Most studies of ^{1}H-MRS of the human brain have focused on the signals from NAA and lactate, as potential markers of brain ischemia, respectively, although there are also often changes in the other metabolite signals, such as Cho, Cr, glutamate (Glu) and glutathione (GSH) [74]. The time course of these metabolite changes through time is an important factor for the diagnosis and prognosis of a brain infarct.

In acute stroke the infarct core rapidly shows signs of cell death and a spectrum from this area has the characteristic lactate peak, often with a broad lipid peak too. Lactate could also arise from a shift toward anaerobic glycolysis in potentially viable cells that continue to metabolize glucose under locally hypoxic conditions [75]. Lactate may also be present in smaller concentrations in the ischemic penumbra, the region around the core which if quickly re-perfused may recover its function [75]. Lactate formed in the initial period of ischemia could remain in necrotic tissue and leave the region of injury after cell lysis in a period of weeks or months after the stroke onset.

Unlike to the increase of lactate, NAA is observed to slowly decrease over a time scale of hours after the induction of ischemia [75]. Several studies have described an initial rapid decrease in NAA of about 10% within the first few minutes followed by a slower decrease. It has been suggested that NAA diminish may be due to NAA degradation by enzymes within the injured neurons in the first few days or hours following infarction, or perhaps due to changes in other molecules (e.g. Glu, Gln, GABA etc.) which overlap with the spectral resonance of NAA [74].

tCho has been observed to either increase or decrease both in acute and chronic human ischemia [76]. Increases in Cho in stroke may be the result of gliosis or ischemic damage to myelin, while decreases are probably the result of edema, necrosis and cell loss [4]. Initial reduction in Cr/PCr is identified following infarction and further reductions have been demonstrated up to ten days following the time of onset [74]. Muniz Maniega et al. reported continuous reduction of Cr levels over a period of three months from the stroke onset [76].

A study by Rumpel et al. revealed that mI might also significantly contribute to the understanding of brain tissue response to ischemia, which is in line with a persistent cytotoxic swelling, attributed to the glial population, found in early subacute ischemic infarcts [77]. Acute ischemic also causes changes in the glutathione (GSH) system (decreased GSH in ischemic patients) as stroke is associated with significant oxidative stress [41]. Experimental studies have suggested that ischemic stroke may cause an increment in extracellular level of GABA; however there is very little work on the detection of GABA and glutamate in cerebral ischemia [78].

6.4. Epilepsy

The term epilepsy covers a wide group of syndromes with varied etiology and prognosis. By providing an insight into the biochemical processes related to epileptic seizures, ^{1}H-MRS aids in the localization or lateralization of the epileptogenic foci and in the influence of the metabolites concentration after the administration of antiepileptic drugs and/or after resection of the epileptogenic tissue.

Temporal lobe epilepsy (TLE) associated with hippocampal sclerosis (HS) is the most common refractory focal epilepsy. The localization is performed by the comparison of metabolites on the left and right temporal lobe, especially in the hippocampus and temporal poles, to determine which hemisphere is responsible for the genesis of seizures [79]. The metabolites of interest in epilepsy are NAA, GABA and glutamine/glutamate (Glx) and the less prominent mI and lactate (Figure 5). Most of the studies dealing with mesial TLE, demonstrate decreased levels of NAA in the affected temporal lobe when compared with controls or with the homologous non-epileptic contralateral region, with no changes or mild increases of tCho. Interestingly, not only decrease of NAA content occurs in the epileptogenic foci, but also unilateral presence of lactate in the mesian temporal lobe could potentially be indicative of the side of the epileptogenic zone [16].

Nowadays, a hypothesis exists in which the raise of mitochondrial energy consumption promotes a reduction of neuronal synthesis of NAA, and, therefore, an increase of glutamate (its precursor) [80]. In epileptic patients, it seems to exist a disequilibrium of glutamine/glutamate (Glx) and GABA [81]. Therefore, spectroscopic measurements of Glx complex could yield spatial information on the epileptogenic zone. However, although there is some evidence that Glx is elevated in TLE, its value as a marker for the epileptogenic zone has not been established yet.

Additionally, ^{1}H-MRS studies of TLE have also been focused on mI, however, its role remains controversial. The study of Wellard et al. revealed elevated mI in the epileptogenic temporal lobe of patients with HS [82]. They also reported a difference of mI levels between the seizure focus (temporal lobe) where mI is increased, and areas of seizure spread (frontal lobe) where mI is decreased. Thus, ^{1}H-MRS may aid to the distinction of primary epileptogenic brain damage from seizure secondary effects on adjacent normal brain and help to distinguish drug refractory TLE patients, who will benefit from surgery by predicting postoperative outcome [83].

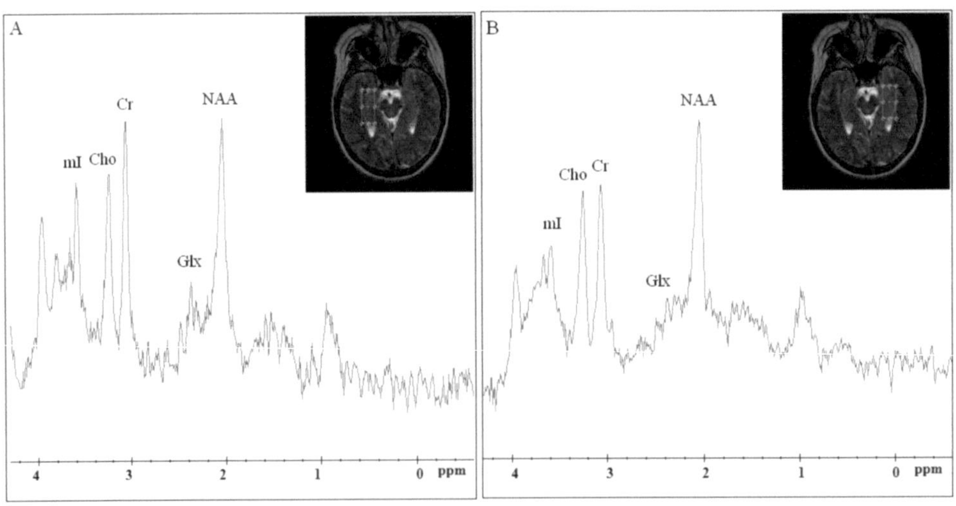

Figure 5. Short TE (35msec) spectra at 3T obtained in the left and right hippocampal formation from a patient with right HS using single-voxel technique. The decreased NAA signal and the increased mI at the affected region (A) are evident when compared with the contralateral normal hippocampal formation (B). Note the mild elevation of the Glx complex at the affected region (B).

6.5. Neurodegenerative diseases (Alzheimer/Parkinson)

Numerous studies have attempted to identify specific metabolic markers for different neurodegenerative diseases, such as Alzheimer's dementia (AD) and Parkinson's disease (PD), which concern loss of structure or function of neurons including death of the neuronal cells. The clinical objective in that cases is to establish a precise and early diagnosis as well as to understand the related brain changes that could help to slow down the course of the disease [60].

^{1}H-MRS has been demonstrated to be highly specific and sensitive to the diagnosis of Alzheimer's dementia (AD) [15]. Reduction in NAA is the most frequent ^{1}H-MRS finding in AD [84, 85]. Single Voxel ^{1}H-MRS studies have consistently found reductions in NAA/Cr ratio in the hippocampal formation [85] as well as other temporal regions [86] and the posterior cingulate gyrus [87]. Findings of reduced NAA have been also detected in the temporoparietal area, and the occipital lobes [85, 87]. There have been conflicting reports regarding Cho levels in patients with AD. Some researchers found elevated Cho and/or Cho/Cr ratios in AD patients, while others not [32, 85, 87]. Increased mI has been also observed, most often, in the temporal-parietal area [85], the posterior cingulate gyrus [32, 86, 87], the parietal white matter 86] and less often in the frontal lobes [86]. Few studies have also reported reduced Glx levels in AD patients compared to control subjects in the posterior cingulated gyrus [88] and lateral temporal cortex [86].

The majority of ^{1}H-MRS studies in Parkinson's Disease (PD) to date have primarily targeted brain levels of NAA, Cr, and Cho [89, 90]. Many researchers disclosed a significant reduction of ratios NAA/Cr and NAA/Cho in the temporoparietal cortex [91], the substantia nigra, the basal ganglia [92], the striatum or the occipital lobe [93]. Griffith et al. have demonstrated lower NAA/Cr ratios in the posterior cingulate gyrus of demented versus non demented subjects with PD [94]. Other investigators, however, have not detected such changes [95] in NAA, Cr, and Cho measurements, and the reasons for these different findings need to be resolved.

6.6. Gliomas

Gliomas are spatially heterogeneous lesions which arise from the 'gluey', or supportive tissue of the brain. The main types of gliomas are astrocytomas, oligodendrogliomas, and ependymomas. ^{1}H-MRS is increasingly used in clinical studies to non-invasively identify regions with metabolic specific characteristics that reflect glioma type and grade.

A common observation in ^{1}H-MRS of all glial tumors is a decreased levels of NAA and increased levels of tCho with a significant overlap among different glioma types [2, 22]. Thus, ^{1}H-MRS is currently used primarily to differentiate glial tumor grade rather than to confirm a histopathological diagnosis [96].

However, the signal intensity of glutamine and glutamate (Glx) may aid the distinction between oligodendrogliomas and astrocytomas. Rijpkema et al. found significantly increased Glx levels for oligodendrogliomas when compared to that of astrocytomas [97] using short TE ^{1}H-MRS. Additionally, in a study by Majos et al, ependymomas differentiated well from the other glial tumors by showing prominent peaks of mI+Gly and Taurine at long TE spectra [98].

Discrimination between tumor grades in gliomas is an important clinical issue, because there is a dispute on the optimum treatment strategy for patients with low-grade tumors. It remains an open question whether ^{1}H-MRS is able to define WHO grade of gliomas. However, a recent study by Porto et al. revealed a more prominent loss of NAA and increase of tCho in WHO III over WHO II astrocytomas [99]. They consequently proposed NAA/tCho ratio as the most accurate index to discriminate between those tumor grades which is in agreement with what it is generally accepted, i.e. NAA/tCho ratios decrease with higher histological grade of gliomas. Law et al. demonstrated a threshold value of 1.6 for tCho/NAA which provided 74.2% sensitivity and 62.5% specificity in predicting the presence of a high-grade glioma [100]. Thus it is obvious that there is a consistent correlation between Cho increase as well as NAA decrease and tumor grade.

A study by Moller-Hartmann et al. revealed that instead of tCho, the amount of lipids proved to be the second-best discriminator between low- and high-grade gliomas, with glioblastomas multiforme (GBM) to exhibit the highest amount of lipids since necrosis is one of their microsopic hallmarks [3]. Although it has been previously proved that lactate also increases with grade, it is not always significantly differentiated between high and low grade gliomas [22]. Poor correlation between tumor grade and lactate is most likely due to the difficulty of accurately quantifying lactate in the presence of high lipid signals.

Short TE studies have also shown that mI levels may aid tumor classification and grading [22, 25]. Specifically, Castillo et al. retrospectively studied 34 patients with astrocytomas and found a trend towards lower mI levels in high-grade compared with low-grade tumors [25].

One of the most interesting results of the study by Server et al. was the elevation in the peritumoral Cho/Cr and Cho/NAA metabolite ratios in relation to glioma grading [101]. Thereby, as gliomas are infiltrating intracerebral tumors, ^{1}H-MRS may allow to readily appreciate their grade in the perifocal region.

6.7. Cerebral metastasis

Cerebral metastases are a common complication of cancer and can affect 20% to 40% of patients [102] who suffer from primary tumors in lung, breast, skin or colon.

When a metastatic brain tumor presents as a solitary lesion, it is usually indistinguishable from a high grade glioma [103]. Their distinction is important because the treatment approach and follow-up are different for these two different tumors.

The potential of in vivo ^{1}H-MRS for differentiating intracerebral metastases from GBMs has been investigated in a number of studies [102, 104]. Older studies [22, 105] have reported that intratumoral ^{1}H-MRS, either on short or long TE, was unable to differentiate between metastases and GBMs, as they share common metabolic features. Those concern increased levels of lipids and tCho and reduced levels of NAA as it is depicted in figure 6.

Nevertheless, a study by Moller-Hartman et al. revealed elevated lipids for metastases, with statistically significant difference from GBMs [3]. Opstad et al. speculated that the differences in lipid profiles may be related to differences of membrane structures of infiltrative versus migratory tumor cells [106]. Significantly higher Cho/Cr ratio for metastases than for GBMs was reported by Server et al. due to GBMs higher levels of necrosis [102]. On the contrary, Law et al. revealed significantly lower Cho/Cr ratio for metastases than for high grade gliomas [105]. These conflicting results may be due to the intrinsic heterogeneity of such tumors.

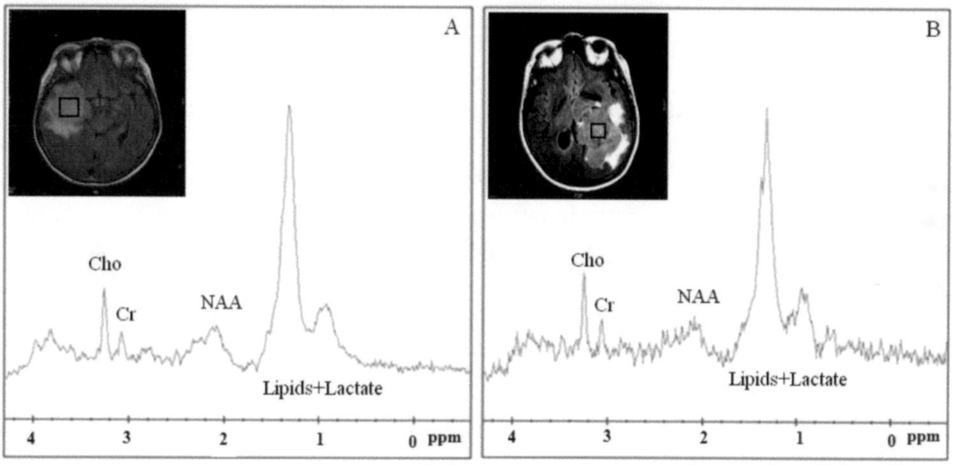

Figure 6. Typical Short TE spectra from glioblastoma multiforme (A) and intracerebral metastases (B).

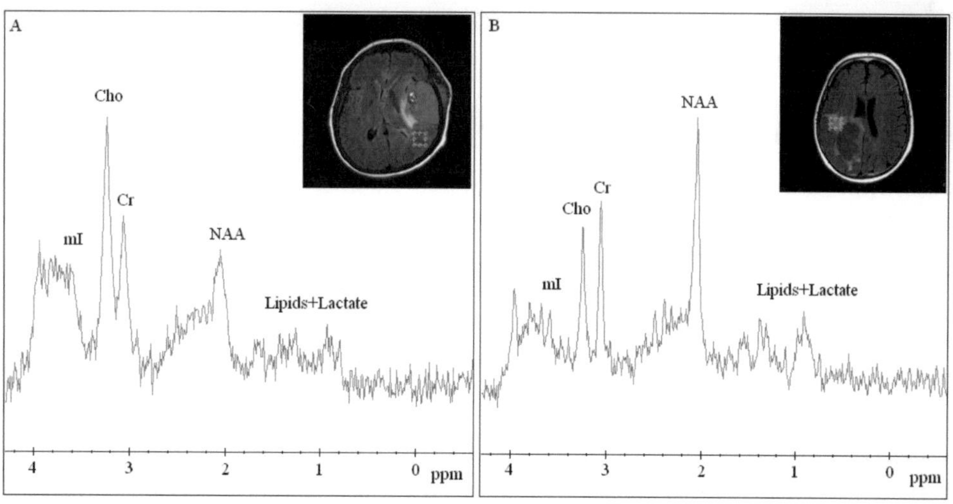

Figure 7. Short TE spectra from peritumoral areas of glioblastoma multiforme (A) and intracerebral metastases (B).

Furthermore, promising results in differentiating between GBMs and metastases by means of the resonances at 3.56 ppm, represented by the sum of mI and Gly, have been previously observed [**36**]. Gly/mI showed a tendency to be higher in GBMs than in metastases.

Measuring the peritumoral metabolites or metabolic ratios is often more useful in differentiating intracranial metastases from high grade gliomas with more reproducible results among different studies. Elevated Cho as well as reduced NAA have been found in the peritumoral region of high-grade gliomas, but not in the peritumoral region of metastases when compared to normal levels as it is illustrated in figure 7.

Those findings support the hypothesis that the edema surrounding metastases is purely vasogenic, while the peritumoral region of GBMs is characterized by extensive infiltration of tumor cells [102, 104-106].

Some patients get their brain metastases detected before the primary cancer. Since GBM case has being withdrawn from the differential diagnosis, identification of metastases type would be important for further treatment. Sjobakk et al. investigated the feasibility of using ^{1}H-MRS to characterize brain metastases originating from different primary cancers. The results presented in their study, demonstrated that lipid signals on both short and long TE spectra are important for metastases characterization. Although non-statistically significant, lung metastases tended to differentiated from breast metastases in respect to their lipid signals, while the melanoma showed no trend [107]. Chernov et al retrospectively studied 25 metastatic brain tumors from lungs, colon, breast, kidney, prostate and cardiac muscle, using ^{1}H-MRS on long TE. The detected metabolic characteristics revealed that metastases of colorectal carcinoma have significantly greater lipid content, expressed as Lipids/Cr ratio, compared to metastatic tumors of other origin. The authors suggested an optimal Lipids/Cr cut off value of 2 for the identification of the colorectal carcinoma [108]. It is obvious that ^{1}H-MRS may aid in the determination of cerebral metastases origin, nevertheless, further research is needed to determine the exact role of proton MR spectroscopy in the identification of the tissue type of metastatic brain tumors.

6.8. Meningiomas

Meningiomas are common intracranial tumors and are generally easily diagnosed by their characteristic radiological imaging appearance of solid mushroom imaging pattern, extracranial location, dura matter conjunction and sinus involvement. However, 15% of meningiomas exhibit rim like enhancement, a prominent cystic component, hemorrhage, or even metaplasia [109], mimicing gliomas or cerebral metastatic tumors. ^{1}H-MRS has been proved useful in differentiating meningiomas with atypical radiologic pattern from other brain tumors [36].

Alanine at 1.47ppm has been considered as the characteristic metabolic marker of meningiomas which differentiates them from other brain tumors [36, 38]. Nevertheless, reported occurrence of Alanine varies among different studies [37, 16] as it can significantly overlap with lactate resonance due to J-coupling effect [37].

In the absence of Alanine, several investigators aimed to correlate other metabolites to meningioma presence. Studying the metabolic profile of different cerebral tumors using short TE ^{1}H-MRS, Howe et al. found that low levels of mI and Cr were characteristic for meningiomas relative to grade II astrocytomas, anaplastic astrocytomas and glioblastomas [22]. In the same study meningiomas revealed the highest Cho/Cr ratio among the other brain tumors, on both short and long TE. Another reported specific finding for meningiomas, is the absence of the neuronal marker NAA. Instead of partial volume effects [3], the peak of NAA at meningioma spectra, may also represent other endogenous NAA compounds (NACs) such as N-acetylaspartylglutamate, N-acetylneuraminic acid and N-acetylgalactosamine [37].

A recent study by Kousi et al. revealed a distinct chemical compound, observed in all meningiomas recruited for that study, which may establish a rather specific marker in their differential diagnosis from high grade gliomas and metastases [6]. This chemical substance, resonated at 3.8ppm using short TE ^{1}H-MRS (Figure 8) and according to the in vitro study of Tugnoli et al. it might receive contribution from phosphoethanolamine (PE) and other amino acids such as Leukine, ALanine, Glutamate, Glutamine, Glutathione, Lysine, Arginine and Serine [110].

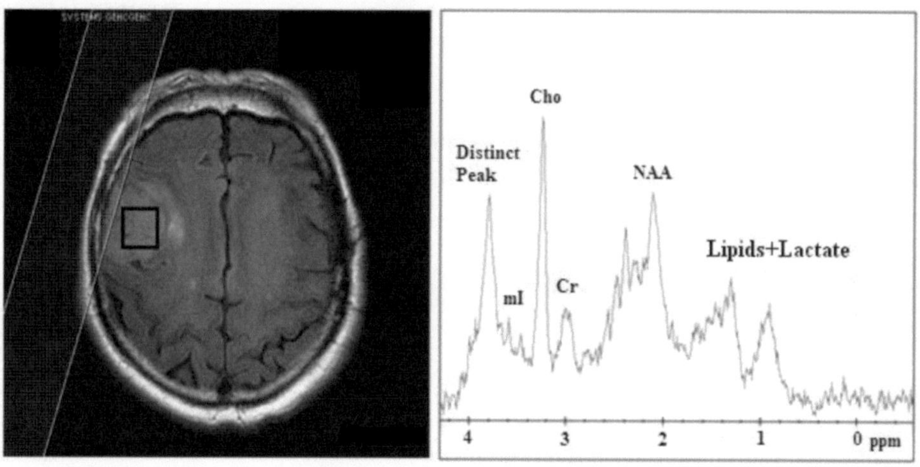

Figure 8. FLAIR T2 images (left) of a meningioma with its corresponding spectrum (right), at short TE (35ms). Elevated Cho and lipid resonances were detected at 3.2ppm and 1.3ppm respectively, as well as a distinct chemical compound resonating at 3.8 ppm [6].

6.9. Primary Central Nervous System Lymphomas (PCNSL)

Primary central nervous system lymphoma (PCNSL) represents 1% of all brain tumors and its incidence has increased in the last 3 decades. Although densely contrast-enhancing lesions, without the presence of necrosis are characteristic imaging features of PCNS lymphoma, it can be difficult, sometimes even impossible, to distinguish PCNSLs from high grade gliomas on conventional MRI [111]. Their differentiation, however, has important diagnostic and therapeutic implications.

For the correct diagnosis of brain lymphomas, ^{1}H-MRS has reported promising results. The most specific finding for PCNSL on MRS is an increase in lipid and Cho resonances (Figure 9). Sometimes, lipid peaks in PCNSL may be more prominent than in high grade gliomas and can help differentiate between the two tumor types [107].

Lipids are typically a signature of cell death; however, a lipid dominated spectrum found in PCNSL does not indicate necrosis. This appears to be due to numerous macrophages and the increased turnover of membrane components in transformed lymphoid cells which contain high concentrations of mobile lipids [112].

Histopathologically, PCNSLs are characterized by a diffusely infiltrative pattern and hence, it is important to survey the peritumoral area also and not just the area of obvious tumor involvement. Like high grade gliomas, the peritumoral area of PCNSLs demonstrates an abnormal metabolite pattern. Chawla et al. reported increased Cho/Cr and Lip+Lac/Cr ratios in the peritumoral area of PCNSLs. They also observed significantly higher Lip+Lac/Cr ratio in the peritumoral area of PCNSLs when compared with that of GBMs, suggesting the presence of infiltrative active lymphocytes and macrophages in areas beyond lymphoma boundaries. Using a threshold value of 7.09 for Lip+Lac/Cr ratio they differentiated PCNSLs from GBMs with 84.6% sensitivity and 75% specificity [107]. Therefore, in the absence of obvious necrosis, increased lipid concentration together with a markedly elevated Cho/Cr ratio for both intratumoral and peritumoral areas can provide important metabolic information which may improve the distinction between PCNSLs and other brain tumors.

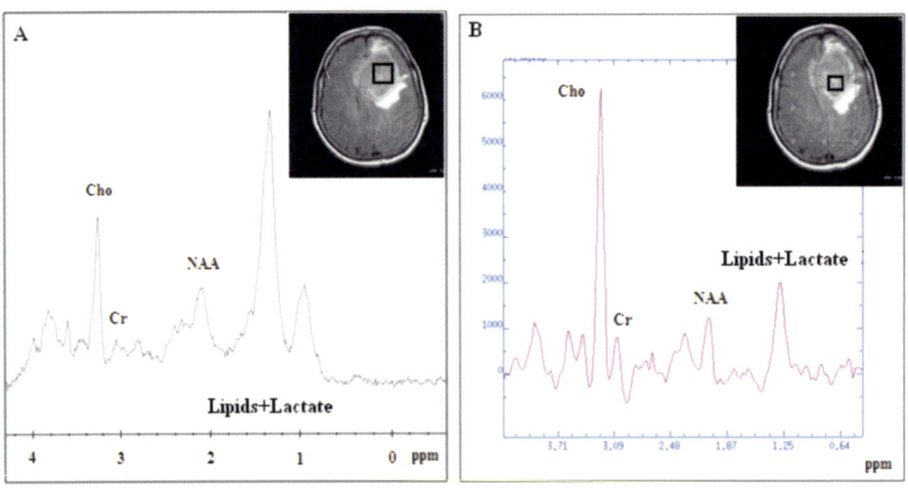

Figure 9. Spectra from an intracerebral lymphoma on both short (A) and long TE (B), demonstrating the characteristic elevation of lipid and Cho resonances.

6.10. Central neurocytomas

Central neurocytomas (CNCs) are a neuronal tumor almost exclusively located in the lateral ventricles that appear in young adults. Most of these tumors do not recur after surgery and are generally considered benign, with a favorable prognosis [28].

Instead of their typical radiological appearance - a well circumscribed lobulated mass in the anterior portion of the lateral ventricles– it may not always be possible to differentiate CNCs from other intraventricular tumors such as oligodendrogliomas and ependymomas [113].

^{1}H-MRS has been proved a valuable tool for the presurgical diagnosis of these neoplasms. Previous studies have reported CNCs to consistently show the tumoral pattern of increased Cho and decreased NAA levels [28, 35]. On the contrary, lactate has not been observed consistently in all studies. Specifically, although Kim et al. reported lactate in all of their patients, Shah et al. observed lactate in only 9% of the CNC cases [114, 115]. A few studies have speculated the rather specific marker of Gly at 3.55ppm on long TE spectra, strongly suggesting CNC occurrence [28, 115].

The presence of Ala in a patient with CNC was first reported by Chuang et al. using a 3T MR system [116]. It was demonstrated as an inverted doublet at 1.5 ppm with a TE of 135 msec. Similarly, Krishnamoorthy et al. also observed Ala in all three CNC cases (100%) studied, whereas in the study of Shah et al. Ala was observed in 64% of the CNCs [35, 115].

Thus, CNCs may show Ala as an inverted doublet at 1.5 ppm in long TE spectra. Although one may observe Ala in other intraventricular tumors such as meningioma, other characteristic peaks such as Gly, high Cho and decreased NAA should help to correclty identify CNC.

6.11. Gliomatosis Cerebri

Gliomatosis Cerebri (GC) is a rare brain tumor characterized by a diffuse neoplastic overgrowth of glial elements of various histological subtypes (astrocytoma, oligodendroglioma, or mixed glioma) and extensive infiltration of at least two lobes [117]. Unlike gliomas, the neuronal architecture is usually preserved [118].

MRI characteristics of GC are non-specific and occasionally it is difficult to differentiate GC from demyelinating diseases or viral encephalitis, and biopsy is often inconclusive [9]. Given the unfavorable prognosis of this tumor type, there is a demand for alternative imaging techniques, such as ^{1}H-MRS, to grade GC and to detect the most anaplastic areas for determining surgical areas and radiotherapeutic targets.

A few studies have looked at the spectral features of such tumors and those are consistent with the spectral features of gliomas discussed above. By studying 8 patients with GC using long TE ^{1}H-MRS, Bendszus et al. found elevated Cho/Cr and Cho/NAA ratios, as well as decreased NAA/Cr ratios of varying degrees in the abnormal areas on T2-weighted images [119]. Similarly, a retrospective analysis by Yu et al. also revealed high Cho/Cr and Cho/NAA ratios and low NAA/Cr ratio within the areas of hyperintensity on T2-weighted images in 8 histopathologically confirmed patients with GC. Anaplastic areas had higher Cho/NAA ratio and the lactate doublet was present [117]. Apart from being beneficial in the grading of GC, ^{1}H-MRS might reflect the true extent of neoplastic infiltration more accurately than MRI. Bendszus et al. found elevated Cho/Cr and Cho/NAA ratios in the tumor margins that appeared normal on T2- weighted images. Tumoral infiltration of the margin of the lesion that appeared normal on T2-weighted images was also confirmed by Yu et al. by observing increased Cho/NAA ratio in those areas [117].

From the aforementioned findings it can be concluded that ^{1}H-MRS when combined to MRI findings may aid to GC diagnosis. Additionally, the determination of highly anaplastic areas and areas of tumoral infiltration may have a great impact in radiotherapy planning.

6.12. Suprasellar tumors

Pituitary adenomas and craniopharyngiomas, are the most frequent suprasellar space occupying lesions and are generally regarded as benign neoplasms of the pituitary gland. Nevertheless, with respect to the differential diagnosis of suprasellar masses, pituitary adenomas, craniopharyngiomas together with gliomas and meningiomas can be considered [120].

To date only a few cases of pituitary adenomas and craniopharyngiomas have been studied by in-vivo ^{1}H-MRS [16, 120, 121], probably because of their relative rarity and the technical difficulties in obtaining in vivo high-quality spectra without artifacts is such a region [120]. In a study by Chernov et al., the vast majority of the 19 pituitary adenomas were characterized by a significant reduction of NAA peak, moderate elevation of Cho, and infrequent presence of small lipid and lactate peaks. This metabolic pattern differentiated them from low grade gliomas which showed a moderate decrease of NAA and Cr peaks. In the same study, craniopharyngiomas were typically characterized by a significant decrease of all metabolites and presence of multiple additional peaks which were possibly resulted from the presence of calcifications and microcysts within the investigated volume of tissue [16]. On the contrary, Sener et al. demonstrated very prominent peaks in the craniopharyngiomas between 0.5 and 1.5 ppm, which probably corresponded to lipid peaks. Histological findings also revealed high amounts of cholesterol, lipids and lactate in the cyst fluid correlating with their spectroscopic findings [120].

7. Conclusion

^{1}H-MRS can provide important in vivo metabolic information, complementing morphological findings from conventional MRI in the clinical setting. This technique is an extremely valuable tool in solving difficult neurological cases and increase confidence in diagnosis; however, it should be always considered a supplementary tool to the patients' clinical history, examination, and conventional MRI when reaching the final diagnosis.

The future would be to combine 1H-MRS with other advanced magnetic resonance techniques such as Diffusion/Diffusion Tensor Imaging and Perfusion-weighted Imaging, which will potentially prove to be useful in both clinical and research settings. Ultimately, these advanced tools may be used in a multiparametric, algorithmic fashion to characterize tissue biology and dramatically improve tumor differential diagnosis.

Author details

Evanthia Kousi and Ioannis Tsougos
Medical Physics Department, School of Medicine, University of Thessaly, Larissa, Greece

Kapsalaki Eftychia
Radiology Department, School of Medicine, University of Thessaly, Larissa, Greece

8. References

[1] Nelson, S. J. Multivoxel magnetic resonance spectroscopy of brain tumors. Mol Cancer Ther 2003;2(5) 497-507.

[2] Soares, D. P. and M. Law. Magnetic resonance spectroscopy of the brain: review of metabolites and clinical applications. Clin Radiol 2009; 64(1) 12-21.

[3] Moller-Hartmann, W., S. Herminghaus, et al. Clinical application of proton magnetic resonance spectroscopy in the diagnosis of intracranial mass lesions. Neuroradiology 2002; 44(5) 371-81.

[4] Jonathan H. Gillard, Adam D. Waldman, Peter B. Barker. Clinical MR Neuroimaging: Diffusion, Perfusion and Spectroscopy. Cambridge University Press; 2004.

[5] Bonekamp, D., M. A. Jacobs, et al. Advancements in MR Imaging of the Prostate: From Diagnosis to Interventions. Radiographics 2011; 31(3) 677-703.

[6] Kousi E, Tsougos I, Vasiou K, et al. Magnetic Resonance Spectroscopy of the Breast at 3T: Pre- and Post-Contrast Evaluation for Breast Lesion Characterization. ScientificWorld Journal. 2012; 2012 754380

[7] Lee, C. W., J. H. Lee, et al. Proton magnetic resonance spectroscopy of musculoskeletal lesions at 3 T with metabolite quantification. Clin Imaging 2010; 34(1) 47-52.

[8] Pinker, K., A. Stadlbauer, et al. Molecular imaging of cancer: MR spectroscopy and beyond. Eur J Radiol.2012;81(3) 566-77

[9] Sibtain, N. A., F. A. Howe, et al. The clinical value of proton magnetic resonance spectroscopy in adult brain tumours. Clin Radiol 2007; 62(2) 109-19.

[10] Doelken MT, Mennecke A, et al. (2009) Multi-voxel magnetic resonance spectroscopy of cerebral metabolites in healthy adults at 3 Tesla. Acad Radiol 2009; 16 (12) 1493-1501.

[11] Tavora DG, Nakayama M, et al. Leukoencephalopathy with brainstem and spinal cord involvement and high brain lactate: report of three Brazilian patients. Arq Neuropsiquiatr 2007;65 (2B) 506-511.

[12] Wattjes MP, Harzheim M, et al. High field MR imaging and 1H-MR spectroscopy in clinically isolated syndromes suggestive of multiple sclerosis: correlation between metabolic alterations and diagnostic MR imaging criteria. J Neurol 2008;255(1) 56-639.

[13] Rosen Y, Lenkinski RE. Recent advances in magnetic resonance neurospectroscopy. Neurotherapeutics. 2007;4(3) 330-45.

[14] Mader I, Rauer S, Gall P, Klose U. (1)H MR spectroscopy of inflammation, infection and ischemia of the brain. Eur J Radiol 2008; 67 (2) 250-257.

[15] Lin A, Ross BD, Harris K, Wong W. Efficacy of proton magnetic resonance spectroscopy in neurological diagnosis and neurotherapeutic decision making. NeuroRx 2005; 2 (2) 197-214

[16] Chernov MF, Ochiai T, et al. Role of proton magnetic resonance spectroscopy in preoperative evaluation of patients with mesial temporal lobe epilepsy. J Neurol Sci 2009; 285 (1-2):212-219.

[17] Wang S, Poptani H, et al. Amyotrophic lateral sclerosis: diffusion-tensor and chemical shift MR imaging at 3.0 T. Radiology 2006; 239 (3) 831-838.

[18] Lai PH, Weng HH, et al. In vivo differentiation of aerobic brain abscesses and necrotic glioblastomas multiforme using proton MR spectroscopic imaging. AJNR Am J Neuroradiol 2008; 29 (8) 1511-1518

[19] Hayashi T, Kumabe T, et al. Inflammatory demyelinating disease mimicking malignant glioma. J Nucl Med 2003; 44 (4) 565-569

[20] Mascalchi M, Brugnoli R, et al. Single-voxel long TE 1H-MR spectroscopy of the normal brainstem and cerebellum. J Magn Reson Imaging 2002; 16(5) 532-537.

[21] Robin A. de Graaf . In vivo nmr spectroscopy: Principles and Techniques.Wiley;2007

[22] Howe FA, Barton SJ, et al.: Metabolic profiles of human brain tumors using quantitative in vivo 1H magnetic resonance spectroscopy. Magn Reson Med 2003; 49(2) 223-232.

[23] Gideon P, Henriksen O, Sperling B, et al. Early time course of N-acetylaspartate, creatine and phosphocreatine, and compounds containing choline in the brain after acute stroke. A proton magnetic resonance spectroscopy study. Stroke 1992; 23(11) 1566-1572, 1992.

[24] van der Graaf M: In vivo magnetic resonance spectroscopy: basic methodology and clinical applications. Eur Biophys J 2010; 39(4) 527-40.

[25] Castillo M, Smith JK and Kwock L. Correlation of myo-inositol levels and grading of cerebral astrocytomas. AJNR Am J Neuroradiol 2000; 21(9) 1645-1649.

[26] Mishra AM, Gupta RK, Jaggi RS, et al. Role of diffusion-weighted imaging and in vivo proton magnetic resonance spectroscopy in the differential diagnosis of ring-enhancing intracranial cystic mass lesions. J Comput Assist Tomogr 2004; 28(4) 540-547.

[27] Kizu O, Yamada K, Nishimura T. Proton chemical shift imaging in normal pressure hydrocephalus. AJNR Am J Neuroradiol 2001;22(9) 1659-64.

[28] Yeh IB, Xu M, Ng WH, et al. Central neurocytoma: typical magnetic resonance spectroscopy findings and atypical ventricular dissemination. Magn Reson Imaging 2008; 26(1) 59-64.

[29] Cecil KM. MR spectroscopy of metabolic disorders. Neuroimaging Clin N Am 2006; 16(1) 87-116

[30] Srinivasan R, Cunningham C, Chen A, et al. TE-averaged two-dimensional proton spectroscopic imaging of glutamate at 3 T. Neuroimage 2006;30(4) 1171-8.

[31] Simister RJ, McLean MA, Barker GJ and Duncan JS: Proton MR spectroscopy of metabolite concentrations in temporal lobe epilepsy and effect of temporal lobe resection. Epilepsy Res 2009; 83(2-3): 168-176.

[32] Kantarci K, Reynolds G, Petersen RC, et al. Proton MR spectroscopy in mild cognitive impairment and Alzheimer disease: comparison of 1.5 and 3 T. AJNR Am J Neuroradiol 2003; 24(5) 843-849.

[33] Ricci R, Bacci A, Tugnoli V, et al. Metabolic findings on 3T 1H-MR spectroscopy in peritumoral brain edema. AJNR Am J Neuroradiol 2007; 28(7): 1287-1291.

[34] Malhotra HS, Jain KK, Agarwal A, et al. Characterization of tumefactive demyelinating lesions using MR imaging and in-vivo proton MR spectroscopy. Mult Scler 2009; 15(2) 193-203.

[35] Krishnamoorthy T, Radhakrishnan VV, Thomas B, et al. Alanine peak in central neurocytomas on proton MR spectroscopy. Neurora- diology 2007;49(7) 551–4.

[36] Majos C, Alonso J, Aguilera C, et al. Proton magnetic resonance spectroscopy ((1)H MRS) of human brain tumours: assessment of differences between tumour types and its applicability in brain tumour categorization. Eur Radiol 2003;13(3) 582-591.

[37] Yue Q, Isobe T, Shibata Y, et al. New observations concerning the interpretation of magnetic resonance spectroscopy of meningioma. Eur Radiol 2008; 18(12) 2901-2911.

[38] Lehnhardt FG, Bock C, Rohn G, Ernestus RI and Hoehn M. Metabolic differences between primary and recurrent human brain tumors: a 1H NMR spectroscopic investigation. NMR Biomed 2005; 18(6): 371-382.

[39] Kinoshita Y and Yokota A. Absolute concentrations of metabolites in human brain tumors using in vitro proton magnetic resonance spectroscopy. NMR Biomed 1997;10(1) 2-12.

[40] Shirayama Y, Obata T, Matsuzawa D, et al.: Specific metabolites in the medial prefrontal cortex are associated with the neurocognitive deficits in schizophrenia: a preliminary study. Neuroimage 2010;49(3) 2783-2790.

[41] An L, Zhang Y, Thomasson DM, et al.: Measurement of glutathione in normal volunteers and stroke patients at 3T using J-difference spectroscopy with minimized subtraction errors. J Magn Reson Imaging 2009; 30(2) 263-270.

[42] Opstad KS, Provencher SW, Bell BA, et al. Detection of elevated glutathione in meningiomas by quantitative in vivo 1H MRS. Magn Reson Med 2003;49(4) 632-637.

[43] Barker PB, Hearshen DO and Boska MD: Single-voxel proton MRS of the human brain at 1.5T and 3.0T. Magn Reson Med 2001;45(5) 765-769.

[44] Stephenson MC, Gunner F, Napolitano A, et al.: Applications of multi-nuclear magnetic resonance spectroscopy at 7T. World J Radiol 2011; 3(4) 105-113.

[45] Di Costanzo A, Trojsi F, Tosetti M, et al. High-field proton MRS of human brain. Eur J Radiol 2003; 48(2) 146-153.

[46] Lange T, Dydak U, Roberts TP, Rowley HA, Bjeljac M and Boesiger P: Pitfalls in lactate measurements at 3T. AJNR Am J Neuroradiol 2006;27(4) 895-901.

[47] Avdievich NI, Pan JW, Baehring JM, Spencer DD, Hetherington HP. Short echo spectroscopic imaging of the human brain at 7T using transceiver arrays. Magn Reson Med 2009;62(1)17-25.

[48] Drost DJ, Riddle WR and Clarke GD. Proton magnetic resonance spectroscopy in the brain: report of AAPM MR Task Group #9. Med Phys 2002;29(9) 2177-2197.

[49] Hetherington HP, Chu WJ, Gonen O, Pan JW. Robust fully automated shimming of the human brain for high-field 1H spectroscopic imaging. Magn Reson Med 2006;56(1)26-33.
[50] Zhang Y, Li S, Shen J. Automatic high-order shimming using parallel columns mapping (PACMAP). Magn Reson Med 2009;62(4)1073-1079.
[51] Donald W. McRobbie , Elizabeth A. Moore , Martin J. Graves , Martin R. Prince From Image to Proton. Cambridge University Press; 2007
[52] Frahm J, Bruhn H, Gyngell ML, et al. Localized high-resolution proton NMR spectroscopy using stimulated echoes: initial applications to human brain in vivo. Magn Reson Med 1989;9(1) 79–93.
[53] Bottomley P. 1984. In U.S. Patent, Vol. 4 480 228 USA.
[54] Duyn JH, Gillen J, Sobering G, van Zijl PCM, Moonen CTW. Multislice proton MR spectroscopic imaging of the brain. Radiology 1993; 188(1) 277– 2 82.
[55] Gruber S, Mlynarik V and Moser E. High-resolution 3D proton spectroscopic imaging of the human brain at 3 T: SNR issues and application for anatomy-matched voxel sizes. Magn Reson Med 2003;49(2) 299-306.
[56] Haase A, Frahm J, Hanicke W, Matthei D. 1H NMR chemical shift selective imaging. 1985; Phys Med Biol 30(4) 341–344.
[57] Mescher M, Tannus A, O'Neil Johnson M, Garwood M. Solvent suppression using selective echo dephasing. J Magn Reson A 1996; 123, 226–229.
[58] Patt SL, Sykes BD. Water eliminated Fourier transform NMR spectroscopy. J Chem Phys 1972; 56, 3182–3184.
[59] Spielman DM, Pauly JM, Macovski A, Glover GH, Enzmann DR.. Lipid-suppressed single- and multisection proton spectroscopic imaging of the human brain. J Magn Reson Imaging 1992; 2(3): 253–262.
[60] Jissendi Tchofo P and Baleriaux D: Brain (1)H-MR spectroscopy in clinical neuroimaging at 3T. J Neuroradiol, 2008; 36(1) 24-40
[61] Coron A,Vanhamme L, Antoine JP,Van Hecke P,Van Huffel S. The filtering approach to solvent peak suppression in MRS: a critical review. J Magn Reson 2001;152(1) 26–40.
[62] Jiru F. Introduction to post-processing techniques. Eur J Radiol 2008;67(2) 202-217, 2008.
[63] Bakshi R, Thompson AJ, Rocca MA, et al. MRI in multiple sclerosis: current status and future prospects. Lancet Neurol 2008;7 (7) 615-625.
[64] De Stefano N and Filippi M. MR spectroscopy in multiple sclerosis. J Neuroimaging 2007; 17 Suppl 1: 31S-35S.
[65] Rovira A, Leon A. MR in the diagnosis and monitoring of multiple sclerosis: an overview. Eur J Radiol 2008; 67 (3):409-414.
[66] Butteriss DJ, Ismail A, Ellison DW, Birchall D.Use of serial proton magnetic resonance spectroscopy to differentiate low grade glioma from tumefactive plaque in a patient with multiple sclerosis. Br J Radiol 2003; 76 (909) 662-665
[67] Fernando KT, McLean MA, Chard DT, et al. Elevated white matter myo-inositol in clinically isolated syndromes suggestive of multiple sclerosis. Brain 2004;127(6) 1361-1369.

[68] Kirov I, Patil V, Babb J, et al. MR Spectroscopy Indicates Diffuse Multiple Sclerosis Activity During Remission. J Neurol Neurosurg Psychiatry 2009; 80(12) 1330-6.
[69] Kimura T, Sako K, Gotoh T, et al. In vivo single-voxel proton MR spectroscopy in brain lesions with ring-like enhancement. NMR Biomed 2001; 14 (6) 339-349.
[70] Lai PH, Ho JT, Chen WL, et al. Brain abscess and necrotic brain tumor: discrimination with proton MR spectroscopy and diffusion weight imaging. Am J Neuroradiol 2002;23(8)1369–77.
[71] Kapsalaki EZ, Gotsis ED, Fountas KN (2008) The role of proton magnetic resonance spectroscopy in the diagnosis and categorization of cerebral abscesses. Neurosurg Focus 2008; 24 (6) E7.
[72] Kadota O, Kohno K, Ohue S, et al: Discrimination of brain abscess and cystic tumor by in vivo proton magnetic resonance spectroscopy. Neuro Med Chir (Tokyo) 2001;41(3) 121–126.
[73] Lai PH, Li KT, Hsu SS, et al: Pyogenic brain abscess: findings from in vivo 1.5-t and 11.7-t in vitro proton MR spectroscopy. AJNR Am J Neuroradiol 2005; 26(2) 279– 288.
[74] Saunders DE. MR spectroscopy in stroke. Br Med Bull 2000; 56 (2):334-345
[75] Graham GD, Blamire AM, Howseman AM, et al. Proton magnetic resonance spectroscopy of cerebral lactate and other metabolites in stroke patients. Stroke 1992; 23(3) 333-340.
[76] Munoz Maniega S, Cvoro V, Armitage PA, et al. Choline and creatine are not reliable denominators for calculating metabolite ratios in acute ischemic stroke. Stroke 2008; 39 (9) 2467-2469.
[77] Rumpel H, Lim WE, Chang HM, et al. Is myo-inositol a measure of glial swelling after stroke? A magnetic resonance study. J Magn Reson Imaging 2003; 17 (1) 11-19.
[78] Glodzik-Sobanska L, Slowik A, Kozub J, et al. GABA in ischemic stroke. Proton magnetic resonance study. Med Sci Monit 2004; 10 Suppl 3:88-93.
[79] Hajek M, Dezortova M, Krsek P. (1)H MR spectroscopy in epilepsy. Eur J Radiol 2008; 67 (2):258-267.
[80] Leite RA, Otaduy MC, Silva GE, et al. Diagnostic methods for extra-temporal neocortical focal epilepsies: present and future. Arq Neuropsiquiatr 2010; 68 (1) 119-126.
[81] Moffett JR, Ross B, Arun P, Madhavarao CN, Namboodiri AMA. N-Acetylaspartate in the CNS: from neurodiagnostics to neurobiology. Prog Neurobiol 2007;81(2) 89-131.
[82] Wellard RM, Briellmann RS, Prichard JW, et al. Myoinositol abnormalities in temporal lobe epilepsy. Epilepsia 2003; 44(6) 815–821.
[83] Doelken MT, Stefan H, Pauli E, et al. (1)H-MRS profile in MRI positive- versus MRI negative patients with temporal lobe epilepsy. Seizure 2008; 17 (6):490-497.
[84] Mueller, S. G., Schuff, N., and Weiner, M. W. Evaluation of treatment effects in Alzheimer's and other neurodegenerative diseases by MRI and MRS. NMR. Biomed. 2006; 19(6), 655–668.
[85] Chantal, S., Braun, C. M., Bouchard, R. W., et al. Similar 1H magnetic resonance spectroscopic metabolic pattern in the medial temporal lobes of patients with mild cognitive impairment and Alzheimer disease. Brain Res. 2004; 1003(1–2), 26–35.

[86] Herminghaus, S., Frolich, L., Gorriz, C., et al. Brain metabolism in Alzheimer disease and vascular dementia assessed by in vivo proton magnetic resonance spectroscopy. Psychiatry. Res. 2003; 123(3), 183–190.

[87] Kantarci K, Jack CR, Xu YC, et al. Regional metabolic patterns in mild cognitive impairment and Alzheimer's disease: a 1H MRS study. Neurology 2000;55(2) 210–217

[88] Hattori, N., Abe, K., Sakoda, S., and Sawada, T. Proton MR spectroscopic study at 3 Tesla on glutamate/glutamine in Alzheimer's disease. Neuroreport 2002; 13(1), 183–186.

[89] Clarke, C.E. & M. Lowry. 2001. Systematic review of proton magnetic resonance spectroscopy of the striatum in parkinsonian syndromes. Eur. J. Neurol. 2001; 8(6) 573–577.

[90] Rango, M. Arighi A, Bonifati C, Bresolin N.Magnetic resonance spectroscopy in Parkinson's disease and parkinsonian syndromes. Funct. Neurol. 2007; 22(2) 75–79.

[91] Hu MT, Taylor-Robinson SD, Chaudhuri KR, et al. Evidence for cortical dysfunction in clinically non-demented patients with Parkinson's disease: a proton MR spectroscopy study. J Neurol Neurosurg Psychiatry 1999;67(1) 20–26.

[92] Choe BY, Park JW, Lee KS, et al. Neuronal laterality in Parkinson's disease with unilateral symptom by in vivo 1H magnetic resonance spectroscopy. Invest Radial 1998; 33(8) 450–455.

[93] Taylor-Robinson SD, Turjanski N, Bhattacharya S, et al. A proton magnetic resonance spectroscopy study of the striatum and cerebral cortex in Parkinson's disease. Metab Brain Dis 1999;14(1) 45–55.

[94] Griffith HR, den Hollander JA, Okonkwo OC et al. Brain N-acetylaspartate is reduced in Parkinson disease with dementia. Alzheimer. Dis. Assoc. Disord. 2008; 22(1) 54–60.

[95] Summerfield, C. et al. 2002. Dementia in Parkinson disease: a proton magnetic resonance spectroscopy study. Arch. Neurol.2002; 59(9) 1415–1420.

[96] Yuh EL, Barkovich AJ, Gupta N. Imaging of ependymomas: MRI and CT. Childs Nerv Syst 2009; 25(10) 1203-13.

[97] Rijpkema, M., J. Schuuring, et al. Characterization of oligodendrogliomas using short echo time 1H MR spectroscopic imaging. NMR Biomed 2003;16(1): 12-8.

[98] Majos, C., C. Aguilera, et al. In vivo proton magnetic resonance spectroscopy of intraventricular tumours of the brain." Eur Radiol 2009;19(8): 2049-59.

[99] Porto, L., M. Kieslich, et al. MR spectroscopy differentiation between high and low grade astrocytomas: a comparison between paediatric and adult tumours. Eur J Paediatr Neurol 2011; 15(3) 214-21.

[100] Law, M., S. Yang, et al. Glioma grading: sensitivity, specificity, and predictive values of perfusion MR imaging and proton MR spectroscopic imaging compared with conventional MR imaging. AJNR Am J Neuroradiol 2003; 24(10) 1989-98.

[101] Server, A., B. Kulle, et al. Measurements of diagnostic examination performance using quantitative apparent diffusion coefficient and proton MR spectroscopic imaging in the preoperative evaluation of tumor grade in cerebral gliomas." Eur J Radiol. 2011 Nov;80(2) 462-70.

[102] Server, A., R. Josefsen, et al. Proton magnetic resonance spectroscopy in the distinction of high-grade cerebral gliomas from single metastatic brain tumors." Acta Radiol 2010; 51(3) 316-25.

[103] Cha, S. Neuroimaging in neuro-oncology. Neurotherapeutics 2009; 6(3): 465-77.

[104] Chawla, S., Y. Zhang, et al. Proton magnetic resonance spectroscopy in differentiating glioblastomas from primary cerebral lymphomas and brain metastases. J Comput Assist Tomogr 2010; 34(6) 836-41.

[105] Law, M., S. Cha, et al. High-grade gliomas and solitary metastases: differentiation by using perfusion and proton spectroscopic MR imaging. Radiology 2002;222(3) 715-21.

[106] Opstad, K. S., M. M. Murphy, et al. Differentiation of metastases from high-grade gliomas using short echo time 1H spectroscopy. J Magn Reson Imaging 2004; 20(2) 187-92.

[107] Sjobakk, T. E., R. Johansen, et al. Metabolic profiling of human brain metastases using in vivo proton MR spectroscopy at 3T. BMC Cancer 2007; 7: 141.

[108] Chernov, M. F., Y. Ono, et al. Comparison of (1)H-MRS-detected metabolic characteristics in single metastatic brain tumors of different origin. Brain Tumor Pathol 2006; 23(1): 35-40.

[109] Hakyemez B, Yildirim N, Erdogan C, et al. Meningiomas with conventional MRI findings resembling intraaxial tumors: can perfusion-weighted MRI be helpful in differentiation? Neuroradiology2006; 48(10) 695-702.

[110] Tugnoli V, Schenetti L, Mucci A, et al. Ex vivo HR-MAS MRS of human meningiomas: a comparison with in vivo 1H MR spectra. Int J Mol Med. 2006;18(5) 859-69.

[111] Weber, M. A., S. Zoubaa, et al. Diagnostic performance of spectroscopic and perfusion MRI for distinction of brain tumors. Neurology 2006; 66(12): 1899-906.

[112] Tang, Y.Z., Booth, T.C., Bhogal, P. et al. Imaging of primary central nervous system lymphoma. Clin Radiol 2011; 66(8) 768-777.

[113] Koeller KK, Sandberg GD. Cerebral intraventricular neoplasms: radiologic–pathologic correlation. Radiographics 2002;22:1473–505.

[114] Kim DG, Choe WJ, Chang KH, et al. In vivo proton magnetic resonance spectroscopy of central neurocytomas. Neurosurgery 2000; 46 (2) 329-333

[115] Shah T, Jayasundar R, Singh VP, Sarkar C. MRS characterization of central neurocytomas using glycine. NMR Biomed 2011; 24 (10) 1408-1413.

[116] Chuang MT, Lin WC, Tsai HY, et al. 3-T proton magnetic resonance spectroscopy of central neurocytoma: 3 case reports and review of the literature. J Comput Assist Tomogr 2005; 29 (5) 683-688.

[117] Yu A, Li K, Li H. Value of diagnosis and differential diagnosis of MRI and MR spectroscopy in gliomatosis cerebri. Eur J Radiol 2006; 59 (2) 216-221.

[118] Arai M, Kashihara K, Kaizaki Y, et al. Gliomatosis cerebri: report of 3 cases and review of recent literatures. No To Shinkei 2003;55(10) 890–7.

[119] Bendszus M, Warmuth-Metz M, Klein R, et al. MR spectroscopy in gliomatosis cerebri. AJNR Am J Neuroradiol 2000; 21 (2) 375-380

[120] Sener RN. Proton MR spectroscopy of craniopharyngiomas. Comput Med Imaging Graph 2001; 25 (5):417-422.

[121] Stadlbauer A, Buchfelder M, Nimsky C, Saeger W, Salomonowitz E, Pinker K, Richter G, Akutsu H, Ganslandt O et al. Proton magnetic resonance spectroscopy in pituitary macroadenomas: preliminary results. J Neurosurg 2008; 109 (2) 306-312.

Chapter 3

Brain Connections – Resting State fMRI Functional Connectivity

Maria de la Iglesia-Vaya, Jose Molina-Mateo, Mª Jose Escarti-Fabra, Ahmad S. Kanaan and Luis Martí-Bonmatí

Additional information is available at the end of the chapter

http://dx.doi.org/10.5772/52273

1. Introduction

With the introduction of electroencephalography (EEG) in 1930, researchers began to explore spontaneous activity in the brain by recording the individual, independently of any task. Subsequently, evoked potential studies, where electrical potentials were recorded at the onset of a stimulus, marked a milestone in brain research. Utilizing such methods coupled with experimental psychology, researchers were able to explore task-related brain activity. These early methods paved the way for new approaches to exploring brain function.

With the advent of blood oxygen-level dependent contrast (BOLD) measurements using MRI, the first fMRI study was published in 1992 by Kwong and colleagues [1]. Within two decades, fMRI has been an indispensable tool in the investigation of cognitive function of brain. Currently fMRI studies comprise 43% of all fMRI publications [2]. At the time, it was believed that when a stimulation paradigm is used to explore brain function (task-based fMRI), only a small percentage of the energy utilized by the brain is actually measured.

The brain represents 2% of our entire body mass. Despite this, studies have shown that the human brain is responsible for approximately 20% of the energy we consume. Additionally, when one performs a specific cognitive task that involves attention or reflection, the brain only uses 5% of its total metabolic expenditure [3, 4]. Yet, how does the brain expend the majority of its energy?

In 1995, Biswal and colleagues observed that regions that are co-activated during a task are correlated in their activity in the absence of a task [5]. This observation led to the conclusion that intrinsic activity in the brain is a major source of energy expenditure. Up to that point of time, spontaneous low frequency BOLD fluctuations were discarded as noise in task based fMRI studies. These signals were considered to be crucial to understanding the intrinsic activity of the brain.

Resting state fMRI relies on the assumption that spontaneous low frequency BOLD fluctuations are a measure of intrinsic activity in the brain. Furthermore, the robustness of functional connectivity analysis as a tool that reflects fundamental aspects of brain organization through various cognitive states is another assumption that underlies this methodology. Early methods of clinical observation and measurement were essential to the development of the neurosciences. With the emergence of these techniques in the 19th century, their application to the investigation of certain diseases and syndromes led the conclusion that certain areas of the brain are correlated with specific higher executive function, such as language and memory [6].

However, it is currently understood that higher cognitive functions are not localized to specific areas of the brain, nor are they organized in a topographic fashion. Higher mental processes are based on the cohesive and dynamic interplay of a complex set of functional systems and cortical networks. To explore these dynamic and cohesive networks, the utility of fMRI in linking a specific task with a specific pattern of brain activation (a set of co-activated areas) is indispensable. For example, studies that sought to demarcate cortical regions of face recognition and mathematical computation demonstrated that such higher mental functions require the integration of distributed cortical regions. Thus, cognitive activities of higher mental order are not region specific, but are the result of the dynamic interplay of a diffuse set of cortical areas and their underlying anatomical connectivity. Consolidating the knowledge gleaned from various studies that focus on patterns of neural Activation is a serious challenge that the neuro-scientific community faces today. Studies of neurological and neuropsychiatric diseases [7] have substantiated that dysfunction in the brain is not due to a focal lesion or the alteration of a single brain area, but due to the failure of more widespread and diffuse systems. Schizophrenia and autism, for example, are currently regarded as complex disorders of connectivity between components of large-scale brain networks. The human brain is composed of approximately one billion neurons that establish a complex underlying network of structurally and functionally interconnected regions. Complex cognitive processes are possible as a result of the transmission of information between different functional areas of the brain [8]. By exploring the neuroanatomy of the brain and the underlying connectivity of different functional areas, we can afford new insights on the organization of the human brain.

2. Brain connectivity: Basic concepts

To better understand the concept of functional connectivity, it is necessary to differentiate between functional connectivity and structural connectivity. We define the two concepts in the sections below.

2.1. Structural connectivity

Structural connectivity is defined as the set of physical connections between neural units. Physically, anatomical connections are relatively stable over short time scales (seconds or minutes), however, on larger time scales (days) they are subject to significant morphological changes due to neuroplasticity. Nonetheless, the acquisition of these 'static' images of the microstructure underlying the brain has wide implications on neuroscientific and clinical questions. Currently, structural connectivity is investigated via methods that span axonal tracing, histology and MRI. Technical progress in high-resolution MR has paved the road for the examination the human cortex in vivo at resolutions of up to 300 microns. These scales are approaching the resolutions obtained by histological analysis, which allow for the verification of information obtained with cytoarchitectural maps for better division of the images obtained by MR. [9]

Early work by Hahn [10] focusing on the effects of molecular diffusion on the magnetic resonance signal marked a landmark in nuclear magnetic resonance research. Within a decade, pulsed magnetic field gradients for the measurement of molecular diffusion were introduced by Stejskal and Tanner [11]. Later, Le Bihan was able to incorporate diffusion sensitizing magnetic field gradients into MRI [12]. This led to a novel method that had wide applications in the analysis of the microstructure of the brain (Diffusion MRI). Diffusion MRI is based on the simple idea of tracking the random walk of water molecules in the anisotropic and confined space of axonal fibers. In 1994, Basser proposed a simple method to quantify the Brownian motion of water molecules using tensor models (Diffusion Tensor Imaging) [13]. While others models of quantifying diffusion were proposed, Basser`s single tensor model is the most popular. Further research on the application of the tensor model led to the introduction of tractography techniques (DTT, Diffusion Tensor Tractography). By tracking the path of the principal eigenvector in a single voxel, researchers were now able to reconstruct various white matter tracts noninvasively. However, the Diffusion Tensor models introduced had a limited number of degrees of freedom and assumed that the probability density function was Gaussian. As a result, single tensor diffusion imaging is intrinsically limited in the analysis of voxels with multiple fiber populations, which could be crossing, fanning or kissing [14]. Although multi-tensor models (high angular resolution diffusion) and Diffusion Spectrum Imaging methods were introduced to overcome these limitations, assumptions persist in these methods, making it difficult to explore neuroanatomy to a high degree of accuracy.

To investigate the accuracy of these methods, several groups have attempted to compare noninvasive fiber tracking with gold standard methods [15,16]. Lawes performed a direct comparison between atlas based reconstruction methods and postmortem classical dissection methods [17]. Tracts reconstructed using the Diffusion Tensor model are accurate to some degree, as they have been applied to the clinical setting.

Nonetheless, although it may provide important information about the structural connectivity between different brain areas, diffusion MRI does not provide a direct measure of functional connectivity in the brain. While diffusion imaging can provide information about the spatial relationship between two areas, it does not provide any information about their temporal correlation. Such information has vast implications for cognitive neuroscience research.

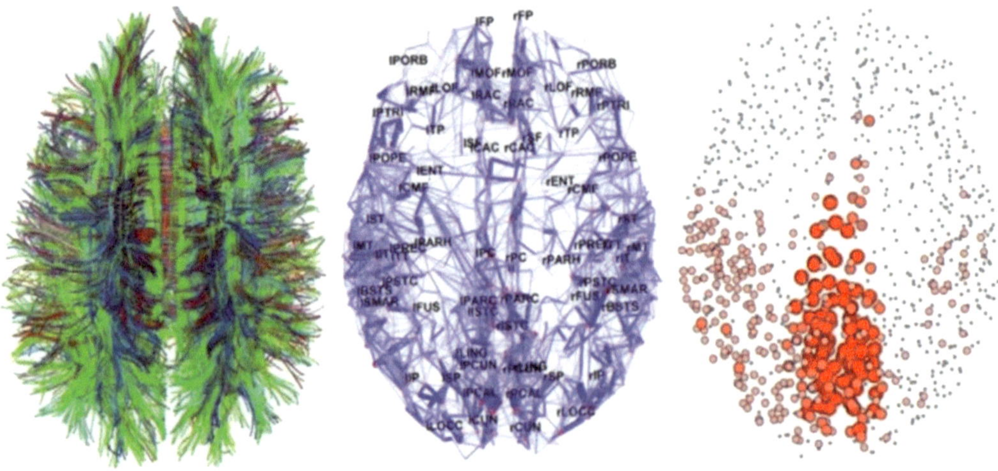

Figure 1. Diffusion Tensor Tractography (left), graph of connectivity (center), functional connectivity (right). Modified from Hagmann P, Cammoun L, Gigandet X, Meuli R, Honey CJ, Wedeen VJ, Sporns O (2008) Mapping the structural core of human cerebral cortex. PLoS Biology.

2.2. Functional connectivity

Functional connectivity (FC) can be investigated through various analytic methods that include electroencephalogram (EEG), infrared light spectroscopy, task-based and resting state fMRI. By extracting correlation measurements from time series, functional connectivity information can be acquired. Functional connectivity is essentially a statistical concept [18]. Unlike anatomical connectivity, which describes physical pathways of information exchange, functional connectivity describes the correlation of spatially remote areas in the temporal domain. Dependence is calculated between all elements of a system, whether these elements are connected by direct or indirect structural links. Functional connectivity relies primarily on traditional fMRI techniques, but takes advantage of low BOLD frequency fluctuations to examine intrinsic activity in the brain. Functional networks generated using this method have been termed 'resting-state networks'. Approximately 60-80% of brain metabolic consumption is due to the intrinsic activity of these networks.

2.3. Linking structure and function

In order to link structure to functions, one must consider the mechanism by which two spatially remote areas are coactivated at any given time. It is currently unclear how many of the networks detected at rest consist of direct anatomical links between cortical regions. Can areas that do not have direct anatomical links exhibit functional connectivity? White matter tracts can be considered as information highways that allow the exchange of functional information between spatially remote regions. In this context, a high temporal correlation between spatially remote areas must reflect a path of communication. Temporal correlation between two regions implies that there are underlying anatomical links that facilitate information transfer. Recently, studies that utilized both diffusion weighted MRI and resting state fMRI, have suggested that there is a direct association between functional connectivity and structural connectivity in the human brain [15, 19]. Having a clearer picture of anatomical structure is critical for the analysis of functional dynamics. However, structural connectivity does not provide any information about the temporal organization of information exchange between regions. Therefore, it is important to note that while functional connectivity implies structural connectivity, it does not imply that two areas a directly connected. For example, the primary visual cortex has been shown to have strong functional connections between its left and the right cerebral hemispheres, although underlying white matter links are lacking between those regions [20].

It is observed that the functional interactions and their expression in behavior of the whole organism can profoundly influence the structural patterns through a variety of mechanisms of plasticity so that shows how the structural and functional connectivity are reciprocally linked.

Studies that utilized EEG methods to examine spontaneous neuronal activity have shown similar patterns of correlations exhibited by resting state fMRI. The nature of spontaneous neuronal dynamics is a potential indicator of the presence of a "critical state", similar to a dynamic regime that is characterized by a diverse set of intrinsic neuronal states that provide answers to extrinsic disturbances. These consistent patterns of activation and deactivation of brain regions during the transition from the task and resting state, led to the discovery of a default mode state called default mode network (DMN) that is consistent across multiple studies of rs-fMRI and/or EEG [21-25].

3. Functional connectivity: Resting state fMRI methods

In the following sections, we review several commonly used techniques for investigating functional connectivity using resting state fMRI data. While these methods range across numerous mathematical fields, and are based in various different assumptions about how to understand underlying brain organization, they can fundamentally be grouped into two categories: model-based and model-free methods. In any case all methodologies can lead us to define a brain network as we will see in the following sections.

3.1. Model-based functional connectivity methods

Seed-based analysis is a hypothesis-driven method that is based on a priori decision regarding the region-of-interest (ROI). Functional connectivity is then calculated using the signal from this ROI as the model in subsequent voxelwise analysis.

Another common method used to establish ROIs for seed-based functional connectivity analysis is meta-analysis. This technique is used to summarize the results across several neuroimaging studies in order to establish common regions of activation. Such results then serve to establish a consensus on the location of functional regions and to develop hypotheses for further investigation.

The goal of this analysis is to locate regions consistently activated (if any) on a set of diverse and independent studies, which are related to the same psychological state [26]. This method works basically by counting the number of peaks of activation in the studies presented, comparing the number of peaks observed with a distribution of null to set a criterion of significance. The two most representative approaches to perform such an analysis are kernel density analysis (KDA) and activation likelihood estimation (ALE) [27].

3.2. Model-free functional connectivity methods

By definition, hypothesis independent methods lack a priori assumptions. These methods are especially useful in the analysis of spatially distributed functional connectivity networks, as they are not reliant of localized assumptions [15, 28-36].

The first analysis to study the functional integration used **Principal Component Analysis** (PCA) [15, 37] to decompose fMRI data into a set of mutually uncorrelated components in either space or time. More recently, **Independent Component Analysis** (ICA) has been used to identify components that describe the activity in a widely dispersed network [28-35]. ICA is an extension of the classical methods of Blind Source Separation (BSS). This technique decomposes the time series in order to identify statistically independent components that define functional networks. This technique has the advantage of extracting independent components that may consist of noise signal, such as physiological or movement-related noise. Although this analysis has many advantages and its applicability has opened doors to new possibilities in the study design, the maps generated with this method are usually more difficult to explain in comparison with those generated with the seed voxel analysis, therefore, its applicability has some restrictions and limitations. Different authors have analyzed the methodology of this technique and there are different variations of the method [38, 39]. ICA has been used to explain a better way the large-scale structures that have been detected in several independent studies [15, 36].

Clustering techniques aim to subdivide the data by means of a mathematical algorithm, so that the observations assigned to the same group are more similar to each other than the observations assigned to other groups. In the context of the study of functional connectivity analysis in rs-fMRI, clustering algorithms have been used to perform brain parcellation in groups of voxels or regions that are functionally connected to other regions. It should be noted that clustering techniques applied to fMRI data are having a good acceptance both in the detection of functional connectivity networks and in the architectural (anatomical) subdivision of the brain [36].

The first application of clustering techniques to resting state functional data was performed by Cordes et al [40]. Firsts attempts to employ this technique were limited due to the computational complexity [41, 42]. Recently, more sophisticated studies have been performed [43, 44] that have enabled identification of large-scale networks that agree with those found in other studies [44].

Still, we should take into account some limitations to the technique. The most important is that most clustering techniques require a priori selection of the number of clusters (K), which will partition the data [36]. Since this value clustering (K) is unknown, multiple solutions are usually calculated using a metric that predicts the "goodness" to determine the optimal number of groups for that data set.

There is no single measure or an optimized solution, so different methods are used. Ultimately, it is unlikely that the clustering is entirely independent of the initial partition decision (K) determined by the subjectivity of the user, since it must evaluate the appropriateness of pooling the results compared with networks of functional connectivity well known. It can be concluded, therefore, that this technique also depends on the subjectivity of the observer when describing the goodness of a grouping, as well as ICA.

3.3. Brain networks and graph theory

In 1998 Watts and Strogatz introduced the concept of small-world network [45]. There are certain reasons, both empirical and theoretical, to understand the brain as a small-world network [46] because the brain supports both distributed and modular processing (linked to the concepts of functional segregation and functional integration). Considering the cognitive processes under the network architecture, it is more efficient when exchanging information at various scales: a high clustering allows a modular processing, while further distances allow for distributed processing. Thus, small-world networks maximize the efficiency of parallel processing and minimize the cost of communication between modules of nodes, as well as being tolerant to failures.

Graph theory is the field of mathematics that is used to characterize various aspects of network structure. In functional connectivity analysis, the application of graph theory aims to ascribe nodes to various regions of interest, and generates links or arcs between them. This approach makes it possible to explore functional connectivity networks using tools that characterize typical properties of networks, for example the study of efficiency and modularity.

Applying graph theory to resting state fMRI data involves assigning nodes to various regions of interest. A functional connectivity graph is generated once edges are assigned to connect nodes that have correlation values above a certain threshold. An important feature is to study "the path", which is defined as a sequence of connected nodes. Path length between two nodes is defined as the number of edges passing through node i to a node j. The distance between two nodes of a graph is the minimum length among all possible paths connecting these nodes. Degree of a node is defined as the number edges that are connected to it.

Two types of metrics are used to characterize graphs: local and global metrics. In local metrics, values are assigned to each node individually, while in global metrics, values characterize the graph as a whole.

A very important metric is the degree of distribution of a graph P(k). This metric provides information on the number of nodes that offer a high degree of centrality. Various studies have shown that the scarcity of these nodes can be related to cognitive decline as observed in Alzheimer's patients.

A complex network can be represented mathematically by edges and nodes [47]. Mathematically, nodes represent different parts of a system, and the relationship between two nodes is represented by an edge. Applying these mathematical concepts to the brain, nodes represent different areas of the brain, while edges represent anatomical, functional or effective connectivity's between these nodes. Utilizing such tools, we can construct (i) anatomically based networks of white matter tracts; (ii) functional connectivity maps representing patterns of correlation between BOLD signals; and (iii) effective networks representing causal interaction patterns between brain areas. All three methods of network depiction can be represented by adjacency matrices. In these matrices, rows and columns represent nodes, while each array element (i, j) represents the interaction between two nodes i, j.

Criteria for the selection of nodes and edges to represent cortical networks often combine methods from anatomical parcellation schemes and connectivity measures. Nodes must represent brain regions with consistent patterns of connectivity, since only similar patterns of fragmentations can be compared. Weighting of edges is interpreted differently in different connectivity models. In anatomical connectivity modelling, weighting is interpreted as a measure of the density of the anatomical tracts. While in functional connectivity models, weighting indicates the magnitude of a correlation between brain areas. And in effective connectivity models, weights may indicate causal interactions. By thresholding weights of connections, networks could be trimmed to establish the topology of significant links. The possibility of directionality in the edges makes it possible to represent anatomical and effective models, while functional models can be perfectly modelled by non-directional arcs.

Functional segregation refers to the involvement of specialized regions or networks in specific functions. Segregation measures are important as they seek to quantify clusters in given network. A basic strategy is to divide a network into subgroups, minimizing the number of edges within a group and maximizing the number of edges outside of a group. Utilizing such means, we can divide a network to be able to analyse a networks modular structure.

Certain areas of the brain that act as hubs are crucial to the functionality of given networks. In order to quantify this importance there are measures of centrality for the network. The degree of a node can be used as a simple measure of the centrality of a node. Other more sophisticated measures can also be used to quantify centrality. Many centrality measures are based on important hubs that play a role in various networks. Measures of centrality have different interpretations depending on type of network under study. A central node in an anatomical network allows the assignment of structure to function between distant regions. Such central anatomic nodes decrease values of centrality in functional networks.

Here we conclude that the analysis of complex networks has equipped use with necessary tools to examine anatomical and functional networks of the brain, paving the way for the possibility of quantifying many of their parameters.

4. RS-fMRI in cognitive neuroscience

It was in 1995 when Biswal and colleagues observed that a significant fraction of supposed noise showed organized patterns consistent with known brain systems [5]. Biswal's work aimed to examine patterns of neural activity of the motor system, and for that, experimental subjects were asked for a standard task of finger opposition and then compared to a rs-fMRI without asking them to do something. As Biswal initially demonstrated, the left and right primary motor networks are correlated. This suggested that these areas are functionally connected and that the process of information transfer between them is on-going [7, 39]. Later, groups were able to replicate these results and further demonstrate correlations between primary visual networks, auditory networks and higher order cognitive networks [3,7, 48-51].

4.1. Adquisition

Advantages of employing resting state functional connectivity analysis in cognitive neuroscience studies include:

1. **A brief period of time of acquisition** (minutes) provides an expanded application to the clinical setting. One of the most frequently cited motivations for using resting state functional connectivity in clinical studies, is that it allows for increased sampling of patient populations, since (i) it requires a brief acquisition period and (ii) has no specific stimulation paradigm. This allows the patient to remain rest, or asleep or under the influence of anesthesia. The absence of a stimulation paradigm in this case, is especially important to the sampling of patient populations with neuropsychiatric disorders.
2. **Computation**: Several resting state functional connectivity methods are available for analysis of neural circuitry in vivo. In contrast, using task-based fMRI, we are only afforded connectivity information about the activated regions only.
3. **Simple design**: (baseline acquisition). Resting state studies may offer a better signal to noise ratio than conventional task-based approaches.

4.2. Networks identified using resting state functional connectivity

A resting state network of particular interest is the **default mode network (DMN).** This group of brain regions is active during rest and deactivates during most externally oriented tasks [7, 52]. This component has been studied in different ways, the main interest of past studies that implemented model-dependent method (seed voxel techniques) [5, 52] as well as independent component analysis (ICA) [29].

Compared with other networks, the DMN is unique in the direction of its response to task performance, which probably relates to its baseline level of neuronal and metabolic activity and its role in brain function. The DMN is not unique, however, in demonstrating correlated intrinsic activity; multiple networks exhibit coherent resting state activity that persists across different states. The default mode network is one of the most robustly identified and extensively investigated resting state networks that involves a set of regions that routinely decrease their activity with tasks that demand attention [3, 7, 52]. Interestingly, this network has also been found to be negatively correlated with regions that tend to increase their activity during attention demanding tasks. Other identified networks include a self-referential system engaging the medial prefrontal regions; a posterior network involved in visual processing; an attention network engaging superior frontal and parietal cortex; a superior temporal system; and a network-engaging precentral and postcentral cortex [3, 7]. The most consistently reported resting state networks include the primary sensorimotor network; the primary visual and extra-striate visual network consisting of bilateral temporal/insular and anterior cingulate cortex regions; left and right lateralized networks consisting of superior parietal and superior frontal regions; and the default mode network consisting of precuneus, medial frontal, inferior parietal cortical regions and medial temporal lobe [53].

Given the success of resting state functional connectivity for probing the brain's functional architecture in normal subjects, it is a great benefit to employ this technique towards the investigation of dysfunction in the brain. A review by Fox and Greicius [8] highlights advantages of examining the resting state signal for clinical applications and discusses methodological issues that need to be resolved to facilitate translational applications of rs-fMRI. A number of clinical applications are already emerging as emphasized by the studies of functional connectivity in premature children [54], adolescents with schizotypal traits [55], major depression, and aging [56]. Two recent reviews detail the large number of studies that have utilized resting state fcMRI to study various neurological and psychiatric conditions [4, 57].

4.3. Networks involved in neurological and psychiatric diseases

The functional connectivity of the DMN has been linked to core process of human cognition such as the integration of cognitive and emotional processing [7], monitoring [58] and mind-wandering. As a result, analysis of the connectivity patterns of the DMN is especially important in examining cognitive dysfunction in neurological and neuropsychiatric brain disorders [57, 59]. DMN alterations have been reported in a number of neuropsychiatric diseases.

It has been shown that the DMN exhibits decreased connectivity patters in patients with **Alzheimer disease** [60], decreased correlations within the DMN including hippocampi, decreased anticorrelations with the DMN, and reduced local connectivity as reflected in clustering coefficients, in which parts of this network have been clearly implicated.

Schizophrenia has been marked as a potential disconnection disease [61]. Widespread functional disconnectivity between brain regions has been suggested to underlie these symptoms [62, 63]. Schizophrenia is known to have aberrant effects on frontal and parietal regions involved with the DMN. Resting state fMRI studies have reported a decrease in the functional connectivity between medial frontal cortex and precuneus in schizophrenic patients [64]. Additionally, diffusion tensor imaging studies have reported diminished white matter integrity in patients with schizophrenia [65]. Specifically, a decrease in white matter integrity was observed in the cingulum tract, which is known to be interconnected with DMN regions MFC and PCC [50, 57]. Therefore, symptoms of patients with schizophrenia can be attributed to alterations of the functional connectivity of the DMN. Moreover, studies have also marked spatial differences in the default mode network in schizophrenia patients together with significant higher frequency fluctuations in default mode regions, as well as hyperactivity and hyperconnectivity of the default mode network in patients in the early phase of schizophrenia [64]. These studies suggest an important role for the default mode network in the pathophysiology of schizophrenia.

Altered functional connectivity patterns have been reported in other neurological disorders. For example, in **multiple sclerosis (MS)** a decreased functional connectivity in the primary motor has been established. This has substantiated studies that showed decreased microstructural integrity of the callosal white matter tracts [66]. Additionally, in patients with amyotrophic lateral sclerosis (ALS), ICA analysis has suggested a decrease in functional connectivity [67].

5. Global initiatives and the Human Connectome Project

There has been a long standing interest in the unrestricted sharing and access of functional neuroimaging data within the neuroimaging community. Inherent within the methodology of task based fMRI, the complexity of conforming task paradigms across different acquisition sites limited the potential of having such an open access platform. However, with the introduction of the unique methodological approach of resting state fMRI, a new era in open access data sharing was ushered. Most notably, a data sharing consortium - the 1000 Functional Connectomes project (fcon_1000.projects.nitrc.org) - composed of various groups from all around began this initiative in 2009. The fcon1000 project aggregated and publicly released over 1200 resting state and anatomical MRI datasets acquired at 33 sites around the world. Within the first six months, the release generated over 9000 download from 78 countries. The benefit of unrestricted data sharing on the advancement of neuroimaging is self-evident. Researchers with the resources to acquire data can ensure that their resources are most widely used, while those researchers who prefer to focus on data analysis can do so. Such initiatives had wide implications on the neuroimaging community. Since large sets of data are now freely accessible, the valued commodity of the imaging community is no longer the data itself, but the analytic tools and approaches of interpretation and analysis. This new paradigm of unrestricted data access will be an integral part of the future of brain research. The human brain is usually divided into several hundred areas that exhibit highly specialized function. Cortical and subcortical regions of divergent function exhibit distinct cytoarchitecture when viewed under a microscope. As the human brain develops, mechanisms of axonal guidance allow the projection of millions of axonal fibbers to target destinations. In the process, a complex network of information processing pathways is formed.

The Human Connectome Project (HCP) [68] is an ambitious five year initiative that was launched in 2010. Its main objective is to build a network map of the human brain to shed light on its structural and functional connectivity. HCP leans on the general facet that the function of a system is determined by its structure. By elucidating the complete underlying structure of white matter pathways, we will be able to glean significant information about the function of this composite organ.

The term *Connectome* was introduced by Olaf Sporns in analogy to the human genome. An approach that is more elaborate than mapping Connectomes, is mapping Synaptomes of the brain. Such an effort would require imaging synaptic clefts at ultra-structural levels of resolution. This endeavour is currently out of reach of the methods we possess today, as it necessitates acquiring images of proteins and neurochemicals that govern the various biochemical pathways of all synapses. Nonetheless, by relying on simple models systems such as *Caenorhabditis elegans* – which has a total number of 302 neurons – we can examine the feasibility of such a project.

Such mapping undertakings would provide considerable information to solve mysteries of brain function. Connectivity in the brain can be studies at three levels of analysis. Combining information from macroscopic, microscopic and nanoscopic levels of analysis, would have wide implications on appreciating the full structural map of the brain.

Author details

Maria de la Iglesia-Vaya
Centre of Excelence in Biomedical Image (CEIB-CIPF), Medical Bioimage Unit, Bioinformatics & Genomics Department. Prince Felipe Research Centre (CIPF). Eduardo Primo Yúfera (Científic), Valencia,Spain
CIBERSAM, ISC III, Valencia, Spain

Jose Molina-Mateo
Centre for Biomaterials and Tissue Engineering, Universitat Politècnica de València, (Spain)

Jose Escarti-Fabra
CIBERSAM, ISC III, Valencia, Spain
Psychiatric Unit, Clinic Hospital, Valencia, Spain

Ahmad S. Kanaan
Max Planck Institute for Human Cognitive and Brain Sciences, Leipzig,Germany

Luis Martí-Bonmatí
Centre of Excelence in Biomedical Image (CEIB-CIPF), Medical Bioimage Unit, Bioinformatics & Genomics Department. Prince Felipe Research Centre (CIPF). Eduardo Primo Yúfera (Científic), Valencia,Spain
Radiology. Faculty of Medicine, Universitat de Valencia, Spain

Acknowledgement

The authors wish to thank Erika Proal, Xavier Castellanosand Daniel Margulies for their helpful discussion. This study was supported by Spanish grants from Ministry of Science and Innovation (ISCIII: FIS P.I. 02/0018, P.I. 05/2332.), Spanish Mental Health Network: CIBERSAM.

6. References

[1] Kwong KK, Belliveau JW, Chesler DA, Goldberg IE, Weisskoff RM, Poncelet BP, et al. (1992) Dynamic magnetic resonance Imaging of human brain activity during primary sensory stimulation. Proc Natl Acad Sci U S A. 89: 5675-5679.

[2] Logothetis NK (2008) What we can do and what we cannot do with fMRI. Nature. 453: 869-878.

[3] Fox MD, Raichle ME (2007) Spontaneous fluctuations in brain activity observed with functional magnetic resonance imaging. Nat Rev Neurosci. 8: 700-711.

[4] Zhang D, Raichle ME (2010) Disease and the brain's dark energy. Nat Rev Neurol. 6: 15-28.

[5] Biswal B, Yetkin FZ, Haughton VM, Hyde JS (1995) Functional connectivity in the motor cortex of resting human brain using echo-planar MRI. Magn Reson Med. 34: 537-541.

[6] Fair DA, Dosenbach NU, Church JA, Cohen AL, Brahmbhatt S, Miezin FM, et al. (2007) Development of distinct control networks through segregation and integration. Proc Natl Acad Sci U S A. 104: 13507-13512.

[7] Greicius M (2008) Resting-state functional connectivity in neuropsychiatric disorders. Curr Opin Neurol. 21: 424-430.

[8] Fox MD, Greicius M (2010) Clinical applications of resting state functional connectivity. Front Syst Neurosci. 4: 19.

[9] Walters NB, Eickhoff SB, Schleicher A, Zilles K, Amunts K, Egan G, et al. (2007) Observer-Independent Analysis of High-Resolution MR Images of the Human Cerebral Cortex: In Vivo Delineation of Cortical Areas. Human Brain Mapping. 28: 1-8.

[10] Hahn EL. (1950) Phys. Rev. 80: 580-594.

[11] Stejskal EO, Tanner JE (1965) Spin Diffusion Measurements: Spin Echoes in the Presence of a Time-Dependent Field Gradient. The Journal of Chemical Physics 42: 288-292.

[12] Le Bihan D, Breton E, Lallemand D, Grenier P, Cabanis E, Laval-Jeantet M (1986) MR imaging of intravoxel incoherent motions: application to diffusion and perfusion in neurologic disorders. Radiology. 161: 401–407.

[13] Basser PJ, Mattiello J, LeBihan D (1994) MR diffusion tensor spectroscopy and imaging. Biophys J. 66: 259-267.

[14] Basser PJ, Pajevic S, Pierpaoli C, Duda J, Aldroubi A (2000) In vivo fiber tractography using DT-MRI data. Magn Reson Med. 44: 625-632.

[15] De la Iglesia-Vaya M, Molina-Mateo J, Escarti-Fabra MJ, Martí-Bonmatí L, Robles M, Meneu T, et al. (2011) Magnetic resonance imaging postprocessing techniques in the study of brain connectivity. Radiologia. 53: 236-245.

[16] Ellison-Wright I, Bullmore E (2009) Meta-analysis of diffusion tensor imaging studies in schizophrenia. Schizophr. Res. 108: 3-10.

[17] Lawes IN, Barrica TR, Murugam V, Clark CA (2007) Atlas based segmentation of white matter tracts of the human brain using diffusion tensor tractography and comparison

with classical dissection. In: International Society of Magnetic Resonance in Medicine 15th Annual Meeting. Berlin: Abstract #229.

[18] Friston KJ (1994) Functional and effective connectivity in neuroimaging: a synthesis. *Hum. Brain Mapp.* 2: 56-78.

[19] Proal E, Álvarez-Segura M, de la Iglesia-Vaya M, Martí-Bonmatí L, Castellanos FX (2011) Actividad funcional cerebral en estado de reposo: redes en conexión. Rev Neurol 52: S3-S10.

[20] Damoiseaux JS, Rombouts SA, Barkhof F, Scheltens P, Stam CJ, Smith SM, et al. (2006) Consistent resting-state networks across healthy subjects. Proc Natl Acad Sci U S A. 103: 13848-13853.

[21] Andrews-Hanna JR, Reidler JS, Sepulcre J, Poulin R, Buckner RL (2010) Functional-anatomic fractionation of the brain's default network. Neuron. 65: 550-562.

[22] Buckner RL, Andrews-Hanna JR, Schacter DL (2008) The brain's default network: anatomy, function, and relevance to disease. Ann N Y Acad Sci. 1124: 1-38.

[23] Garrity A, Pearlson GD, McKiernan K, Lloyd D, Kiehl KA, Calhoun, VD (2007) Aberrant 'default mode' functional connectivity in schizophrenia. Am. J. Psychiatry. 164: 450–457.

[24] Pomarol-Clotet E, Salvador R, Sarró S, Gomar J, Vila F, Martínez A, et al. (2008) Failure to deactivate in the prefrontal cortex in schizophrenia: dysfunction of the default-mode network? Psychol. Med. 38: 1185–1193.

[25] Thermenos HW, Milanovic S, Tsuang MT, Faraone SV, McCarley RW, Shenton ME, et al. (2009) Hyperactivity and hyperconnectivity of the default network in schizophrenia and in first-degree relatives of persons with schizophrenia. Proc. Natl. Acad. Sci. *U.S.A.* 106: 1279–1284.

[26] Wager TD, Lindquist M, Kaplan L (2007) Meta-analysis of functional neuroimaging data: current and future directions. SCAN. 2: 150-158.

[27] Wager TD, Lindquist M, Kaplan L (2007) Meta-analysis of functional neuroimaging data: current and future directions. Soc Cogn Affect Neurosci. 2: 150-158.

[28] Beckmann CF, Smith SM (2004) Probabilistic independent component analysis for functional magnetic resonance imaging. IEEE Trans. Med. Imaging. 23: 137–152

[29] Beckmann CF, De Luca M, Devlin JT, Smith SM (2005) Investigations into resting-state connectivity using independent component analysis. Philos. Trans. R. Soc. Lond., B, Biol. Sci. 360: 1001–1013.

[30] Bell AJ, Sejnowski TJ (1995) An information maximisation approach to blind separation and blind deconvolution. *Neural Comput.* 7: 1129–1159.

[31] Calhoun VD, Adali T, Giuliani N, Pekar JJ, Pearlson GD, Kiehl KA (2006) A method for multimodal analysis of independent source differences in schizophrenia: combining gray matter structural and auditory oddball functional data. Hum. Brain Mapp. 27: 47–62.

[32] Calhoun VD, Adali T, Pearlson GD, Pekar JJ (2001) A Method for making group inferences from functional MRI data using independent component analysis. Hum. Brain Mapp. 14: 140–151.

[33] Calhoun VD, Adali T, Pearlson GD, Pekar JJ (2001) Spatial and temporal independent component analysis of functional MRI data containing a pair of task-related waveforms. Hum. Brain Mapp. 13: 43–53.

[34] Calhoun VD, Adali T, McGinty V, Pekar JJ, Watson T, Pearlson GD (2001) fMRI Activation In A Visual-Perception Task: Network Of Areas Detected Using The General Linear Model And Independent Component Analysis. NeuroImage. 14: 1080-1088.

[35] Calhoun VD, Kiehl KA, Pearlson GD (2008) Modulation of temporally coherent brain networks estimated using ICA at rest and during cognitive tasks. Hum. Brain Mapp. 29: 828–838.

[36] Margulies DS, Boettger J, Long X, Lv Y, Kelly C, Schäfer A, et al. (2010) Resting developments: A review of fMRI post-processing methodologies for spontaneous brain activity. Magnetic Resonance Materials in Physics, Biology and Medicine. 23: 289-307.

[37] Liu J, Xu L, Calhoun VD (2008) Extracting Principle Components for Discriminant Analysis of FMRI Images. ICASSP IEEE, Las Vegas: 449–452.

[38] Liu J, Demirci O, Calhoun VD (2008) A Parallel Independent Component Analysis Approach to Investigate Genomic Influence on Brain Function. IEEE Signal Proc. Letters. 15: 413-416,

[39] Liu, Pearlson JGD, Windemuth A, Ruano G, Perrone-Bizzozero NI, Calhoun VD (2009) Combining fMRI and SNP data to investigate connections between brain function and genetics using parallel ICA. Hum. Brain Map 30: 241-255.

[40] Cordes D, Haughton V, Carew JD, Arfanakis K, Maravilla K (2002) Hierarchical clustering to measure connectivity in fMRI resting-state data. Magn Reson Imaging. 20: 305–317.

[41] Salvador R, Suckling J, Coleman MR, Pickard JD, Menon D, Bullmore E (2005) Neurophysiological architecture of functional magnetic resonance images of human brain. Cereb Cortex. 15: 1332–1342.

[42] Thirion B, Dodel S, Poline JB (2006) Detection of signal synchronizations in resting-state fMRI datasets. Neuroimage. 29: 321–327.

[43] Van den Heuvel M, Mandl R, Hulshoff Pol H (2008) Normalized cut group clustering of resting-state fMRI data. PLoS One. 3: e2001.

[44] Bellec P, Rosa-Neto P, Lyttelton OC, Benali H, Evans AC (2010) Multi-level bootstrap analysis of stable clusters in resting- state fmri. Neuroimage. 51: 1126–1139.

[45] Watts DJ, Strogatz SH (1998) Collective dynamics of "smallworld" networks. Nature 393: 440-442.

[46] Bassett DS, Bullmore E (2006) Small-world brain networks. Neuroscientist. 12: 512–523.

[47] Rubinov M, Sporns O. (2010) Complex network measures of brain connectivity: uses and interpretations. Neuroimage. 52: 1059-1069.

[48] Biswal BB, Van Kylen J, Hyde JS (1997) Simultaneous assessment of flow and BOLD signals in resting-state functional connectivity maps. NMR Biomed. 10: 165–170.

[49] Damoiseaux JS, Rombouts SA, Barkhof F, Scheltens P, Stam CJ, Smith SM, et al. (2006) Consistent resting-state networks across healthy subjects. Proc Natl Acad Sci USA. 103: 13848-13853.

[50] van den Heuvel MP, Mandl RC, Kahn RS, Hulshoff Pol HE. (2009) Functionally linked resting-state networks reflect the underlying structural connectivity architecture of the human brain. Hum Brain Mapp. 30: 3127-3141.

[51] Deco G, Jirsa VK, McIntosh AR. (2011) Emerging concepts for the dynamical organization of resting-state activity in the brain. Nat Rev Neurosci. 12: 43-56.

[52] Raichle ME, MacLeod AM, Snyder AZ, Powers WJ, Gusnard DA, Shulman GL (2001) A default mode of brain function. Proc Natl Acad Sci USA. 98: 676-682.
[53] Van den Heuvel MP, Hulshoff Pol HE (2010) Exploring the brain network: a review on resting-state fMRI functional connectivity. Eur Neuropsychopharmacol. 20: 519-534.
[54] Damaraju E, Phillips JR, Lowe JR, Ohls R, Calhoun VD, Caprihan A (2010) Resting-state functional connectivity differences in premature children. Front Syst Neurosci. 4: 23.
[55] Lagioia A, Eliez S, Schneider M, Simons JS, Van der Linden M, Debbané M. (2011) Neural correlates of reality monitoring during adolescence. Neuroimage. 55: 1393-1400.
[56] Langan J, Peltier SJ, Bo J, Fling BW, Welsh RC, Seidler RD (2010) Functional implications of age differences in motor system connectivity. Front Syst Neurosci. 4: 17.
[57] Greicius M (2008) Resting-state functional connectivity in neuropsychiatric disorders. Curr Opin Neurol. 21: 424-430.
[58] Gusnard DA, Raichle ME (2001) Searching for a baseline: functional imaging and the resting human brain. Nat Rev Neurosci. 2: 685-694.
[59] Bullmore E, Sporns O (2009) Complex brain networks: graph theoretical analysis of structural and functional systems. Nat Rev Neurosci. 10: 186-198.
[60] Greicius M, Srivastava G, Reiss A, Menon V. (2004) Default-mode network activity distinguishes Alzheimer's disease from healthy aging: Evidence from functional MRI. Proc Natl Acad Sci USA 101: 4637-4642.
[61] Bleuler E (1911) Dementia Praecox or the Group of Schizophrenias. English Translation 1961. New York: International Universities Press.
[62] Andreasen NC, Nopoulos P, O'Leary DS, Miller DD, Wassink T, Flaum M (1999) Defining the phenotype of schizophrenia: cognitive dysmetria and its neural mechanisms. Biol. Psychiatry. 46: 908–920.
[63] Friston KJ, Frith CD (1995) Schizophrenia: a disconnection syndrome? Clin. Neurosci. 3: 89–97.
[64] Whitfield-Gabrieli S, Thermenos HW, Milanovic S, Tsuang MT, Faraone SV, McCarley RW, et al. (2009) Hyperactivity and hyperconnectivity of the default network in schizophrenia and in first-degree relatives of persons with schizophrenia. Proc Natl Acad Sci USA. 106: 1279-1284.
[65] Ellison-Wright I, Bullmore E (2009) Meta-analysis of diffusion tensor imaging studies in schizophrenia. Schizophr Res. 108: 3-10.
[66] Lowe MJ, Beall EB, Sakaie KE, Koenig KA, Stone L, Marrie RA, et al. (2008) Resting state sensorimotor functional connectivity in multiple sclerosis inversely correlates with transcallosal motor pathway transverse diffusivity. Hum Brain Mapp. 29: 818-827.
[67] Mohammadi B, Kollewe K, Samii A, Krampfl K, Dengler R, Münte TF (2009) Changes of resting state brain networks in amyotrophic lateral sclerosis. Exp Neurol. 217: 147-153.
[68] Sporns O, Tononi G, Kötter R. (2005) The human connectome: A structural description of the human brain. PLoS Comput Biol. 1: 245-251.

Chapter 4

Activation of Brain Sensorimotor Network by Somatosensory Input in Patients with Hemiparetic Stroke: A Functional MRI Study

Hiroyuki Kato and Masahiro Izumiyama

Additional information is available at the end of the chapter

http://dx.doi.org/10.5772/51693

1. Introduction

Stroke is one of the leading causes of disability in the elderly in many countries. Residual motor impairment, especially hemiparesis, is one of the most common sequelae after stroke. Motor recovery after stroke exhibits a wide range of difference among patients, and is dependent on the location and amount of brain damage, degree of impairment, and nature of deficit (Duncan et al., 1992). Full recovery of motor function is often observed when initial impairment is mild, but recovery is limited when there were severe deficits at stroke onset. The motor recovery after stroke may be caused by the effects of medical therapy against acute stroke, producing a resolution of brain edema and an increase in cerebral blood flow in the penumbra and remote areas displaying diaschisis. However, functional improvements may be seen past the period of acute tissue response and its resolution. The role of rehabilitation in facilitating motor recovery is considered to be produced by promoting brain plasticity.

Non-invasive neuroimaging techniques, including functional magnetic resonance imaging (fMRI) and positron emission tomography (PET), enable us to measure task-related brain activity with excellent spatial resolution (Herholz & Heiss, 2000; Calautti & Baron, 2003; Rossini et al., 2003). The functional neuroimaging studies usually employ active motor tasks, such as hand grip and finger tapping, and require that the patients are able to move their hand. Neuroimaging studies in stroke patients have reported considerable amounts of data that suggest the mechanisms of motor functional recovery after stroke. Initial cross-sectional studies at chronic stages of stroke have demonstrated that the pattern of brain activation is different between paretic and normal hand movements, and suggested that long-term recovery is facilitated by compensation, recruitment and reorganization of cortical motor function in both damaged and non-damaged hemispheres (Chollet et al., 1991; Weiller et al., 1992; Cramer et al., 1997; Cao et al., 1998; Ward et al., 2003a). Subsequent longitudinal studies from subacute to chronic stages (before and after rehabilitation) have revealed a dynamic, bihemispheric reorganization of motor network, and emphasized the necessity of successive studies (Marshall et al., 2000; Calautti et al., 2001; Feydy et al., 2002; Ward et al, 2003b).

When the stroke patients are unable to move their hand, alternative paradigms are necessary to study their brain function. Passive, instead of active, hand movement has been employed for this purpose, and increases in brain activities are found not only in sensory but also motor cortices (Nelles et al., 1999; Loubinoux et al., 2003; Tombari et al., 2004). Functional neuroimaging studies suggest that a change in processing of somatosensory information in the sensorimotor cortex may play an important role in motor recovery after stroke (Schaechter et al., 2006).

Most significant recovery of motor function takes place within the first weeks after stroke and an early introduction of rehabilitation is crucial for a good outcome. Rehabilitation at the early stages of stroke uses physiotherapy, such as massage and passive movement of the paretic hand, as an initial step of rehabilitation, especially in patients with severe motor impairment. However, it is difficult to assess the effects of physiotherapy in patients with severe impairment early after stroke. In this fMRI study, we investigated the effects of somatosensory input on the activity of brain sensorimotor network in stroke patients. Since somatosensory feedback is essential for the exact execution of hand movement, the result can provide a scientific basis for the establishment of rehabilitation strategies.

2. Materials and methods

2.1. Subjects

We selected 6 stroke patients with pure motor hemiparesis (4 men and 2 women, 63-85 years old). Three of them received fMRI during a task of unilateral palm brushing (stimulation of tactile sensation using a plastic hairbrush at approximately 1 Hz), and three other patients received fMRI during a task of unilateral passive hand movement (stimulation of proprioceptive sensation by passive flexion-extension of fingers at approximately 1 Hz). The fMRI studies were performed 5 days to 2 months after stroke onset.

The patients presented with neurological deficits including moderate to severe hemiparesis, and were admitted to our hospital. They received standard medical therapy for stroke and rehabilitation. All of them were right-handed. All the cerebral infarcts were evidenced by MRI, and were located in various regions of the cerebrum. They could hardly move their hands when the fMRI was performed. Clinical data are summarized in Table 1. Three right-handed, normal subjects (59-68 years of age; 2 men and 1 woman) served as controls for a comparison to show normal brain activation during a unilateral hand grip task. This study was approved by the ethics committee of our hospital and informed consent was obtained from all subjects in accordance with the Declaration of Helsinki.

	Age Sex	H	Stroke location	PMH	day	fMRI activation
Palm brushing						
1	68M	L	R corona radiata	HT DM	28	N: L S1M1, L SMA, R Cbll P: R S1M1, R SMA
2	75M	L	R internal capsule	DM	39	N: L S1M1, L SMA P: R S1M1, R SMA, Blt IPC
3	63F	R	L corona radiata	HT DM HL	5	N: R S1M1 P: L S1M1, Blt SPC, R IPC
Passive movement						
4	85F	L	R internal capsule	HT HL	72	N: L S1M1 P: R S1M1
5	79M	R	L MCA cortex	HT HL af	13	N: L S1M1, R Cbll P: R S1M1
6	76M	L	R pons	DM HT	21	N: L S1M1, L SMA, R Cbll P: R S1M1

M = male; F = female; H = hemiparesis; R = right; L = left; MCA = middle cerebral artery; PMH = past medical history; HT = hypertension; DM = diabetes mellitus; HL = hyperlipidemia;af = atrial fibrillation; N = non-affected hand, P = paretic hand; S1M1 = primary sensorimotor cortex; SMA = supplementary motor areas: Cbll = cerebellum; Blt = bilateral; SPC = superior parietal cortex; IPC = inferior parietal cortex;

Table 1. Patient characteristics

2.2. Functional MRI

The fMRI studies were performed using a 1.5 T Siemens Magnetom Symphony MRI scanner as described previously (Kato et al., 2002). Briefly, blood oxygenation level-dependent (BOLD) images were obtained continuously in a transverse orientation using a gradient-echo, single shot echo planar imaging pulse sequence. The acquisition parameters were as follows: repetition time 3 s, time of echo 50 ms, flip angle 90°, 3-mm slice thickness, 30 slices through the entire brain, field of view 192 x 192 mm, and 128 x 128 matrix. During the fMRI scan, the patients and normal controls received or performed a task as mentioned above. This task performance occurred in periods of 30 s, interspaced with 30 s rest periods. The cycle of rest and task was repeated 5 times during each hand study. Therefore, the fMRI scan of each hand study took 5 min to complete, producing 3,000 images. A staff member monitored the patient directly throughout the study, and gave the sensory stimulations or the start and stop signals of hand grip by tapping gently on the knee.

Data analysis was performed using Statistical Parametric Mapping (SPM) 2 (Wellcome Department of Cognitive Neurology, London, UK, http://www.fil.ion.ucl.ac.uk/spm/) implemented in MATLAB (The MathWorks Inc., Natick, MA, USA). After realignment and smoothing, the general linear model was employed for the detection of activated voxels. The voxels were considered as significantly activated if $p<0.05$ using the FWE analysis. All the measurements were performed with this same statistical threshold. The activation images were overlaid on corresponding T1-weighted anatomic images.

3. Results

Both tactile and proprioceptive inputs via the unaffected hand activated contralateral primary sensorimotor cortex (S1M1) in all the patients, and the supplementary motor areas (SMA) and the ipsilateral cerebellum in part of the patients (Table, Figs. 1 &2). This activation pattern is similar to that activated during active hand movement (Fig. 3), although the activation was less extensive. Both tactile and proprioceptive inputs via the paretic hand also activated the contralateral S1M1 in all the patients, and in SMA and superior and inferior parietal cortices in part of the patients (Table, Figs. 1 & 2), although to a lesser extent as compared with unaffected hand. No cerebellar activation was observed when paretic hand was stimulated.

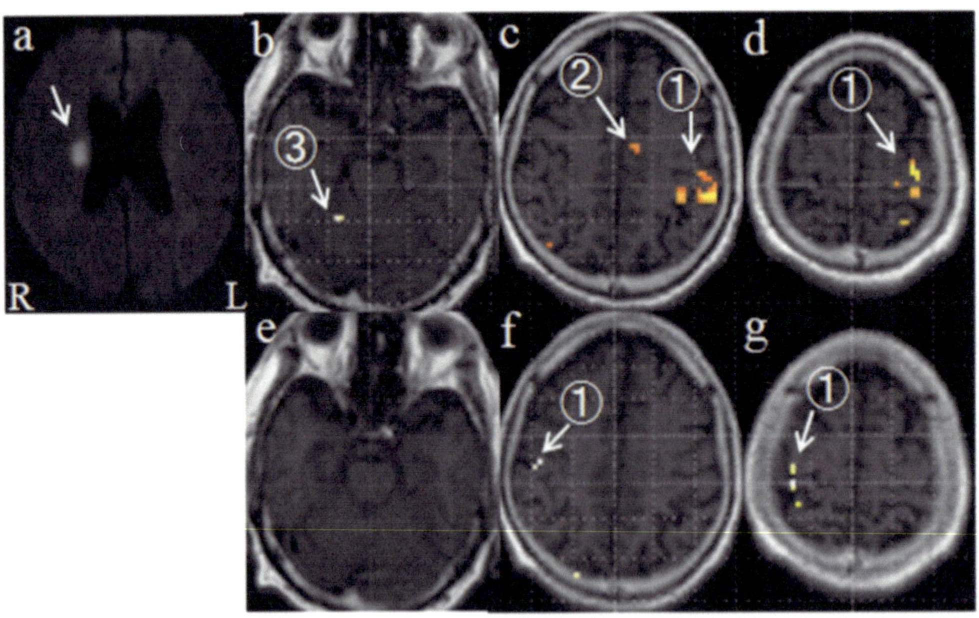

Figure 1. fMRI of a 68-year old man (patient 1) who had a cerebral infarct in the right corona radiata (arrow in a, diffusion-weighted MRI) . After 28 days of stroke onset, palm brushing of the right (unaffected) hand (b-d) induced activation in the left primary sensorimotor cortex (1), the supplementary motor area (2), and right cerebellum (3). During palm brushing of the left (paretic) hand (e-g), activation in contralateral primary sensorimotor cortex (1) was seen, although less extensive, and no activation was seen in the supplementary motor areas and the cerebellum.

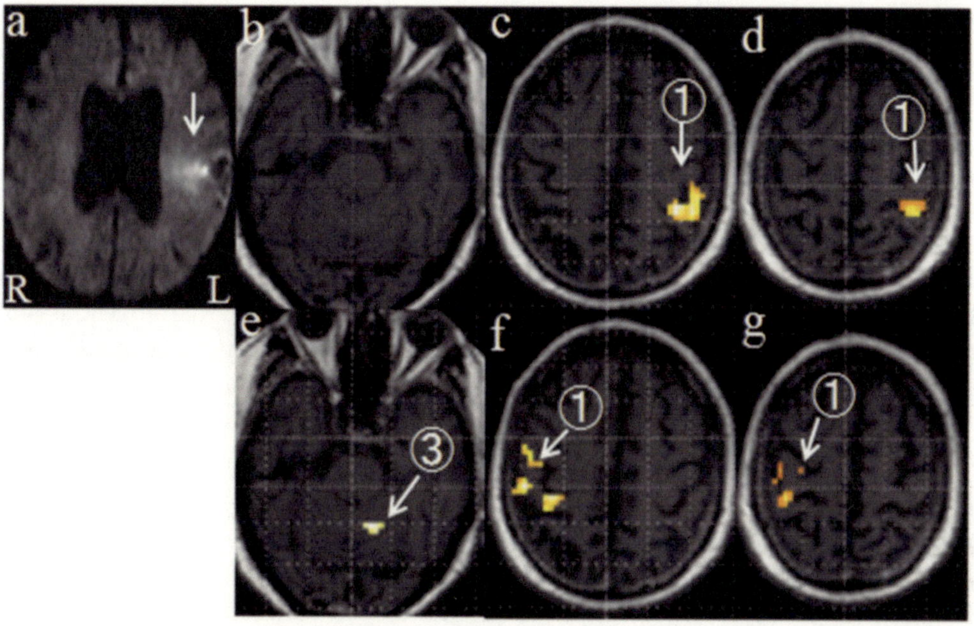

Figure 2. fMRI of a 79-year old man (patient 5) who had a cerebral infarct in part of the right middle cerebral artery territory (arrow in a, diffusion-weighted MRI). After 13 days of stroke onset, passive movement of the left (unaffected) hand (e-g) induced activation in the right primary sensorimotor cortex (1) and left cerebellum (3). During passive movement of the right (paretic) hand (b-d), activation in contralateral primary sensorimotor cortex (1) was observed.

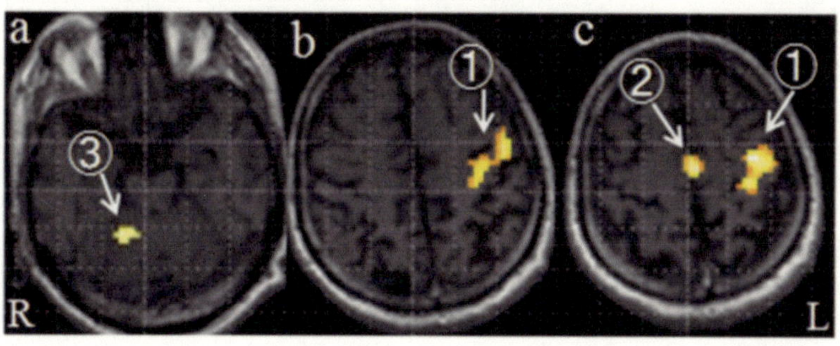

Figure 3. fMRI of a 61-year old man (control). Active right hand movement (a-c) induced a normal activation pattern in the left primary sensorimotor cortex (1), supplementary motor areas (2) and right cerebellum (3).

4. Discussion

4.1. Activation of sensorimotor network by somatosensory input

The results demonstrated that somatosensory stimulation of the unaffected hand, both tactile and proprioceptive input, activated sensorimotor network in the brain, and that the activation pattern was similar to that induced by active hand movement. Somatosensory input to the paretic hand also activated the sensorimotor network in the brain, although to a lesser degree. Of importance was that the activation involved not only postcentral S1 but also precentral M1, as observed in previous reports employing somatosensory stimulation as a task.

Passive movement studies have shown that brain activation during passive movement is seen in regions such as the contralateral sensorimotor cortex, the bilateral premotor cortex, supplementary motor areas, and inferior parietal cortex (Nelles et al., 1999; Loubinoux et al., 2003; Tombari et al., 2004). The similarity of activation patterns between passive and active hand movements highlights the contribution of afferent synaptic activity for central motor control, and suggests that the sensory systems play an important role in central motor control. Additional explanation may be that the repetitive sensory input induces motor imagery in the patients. Imagery of movement activates largely the same brain areas that are activated when movements are actually executed (Decety, 1996; Grezes & Decety 2001).

The brain activation during paretic hand sensory stimulation in this study was reduced as compared to that during unaffected hand sensory stimulation. This reduction may reflect the sensorimotor network damage caused by stroke, although the fMRI BOLD response could be reduced in the cerebral hemisphere of the lesion side (Murata et al., 2006; Mazzetto-Betti et al., 2010). Nevertheless, the result confirms the possibility of inducing sensorimotor transformations even in severely impaired stroke patients.

The observation of S1 and M1 activation during sensory input as well as active movement suggests that the sensorimotor network is functionally connected with each other. Actually, human motor and sensory hand cortices overlap, and are not divided in a simple manner by the central sulcus (McGlone et al., 2002; Morre et al.; 2000; Nii et al., 1996). Furthermore, S1 and M1 are heavily interconnected (Jones et al., 1978) and both are the sites of origin of pyramidal tract neurons in the monkey (Fromm & Evarts, 1982). Proprioceptive afferents from the muscle spindles (fibers IA, II), along with the projections from other articular and cutaneous receptors (fibers I to IV), gain access not only to S1 but also to M1 in the monkey (Lemon, 1999; Lemon & Porter, 1976).

Previous studies have also demonstrated the activation of secondary sensorimotor areas induced by passive hand movements, as seen in our study. SMA has rich anatomical connections with many areas in the central nervous system, such as thalamus, dorsal premotor cortex (PMd), spinal cord, and contralateral hemisphere (Juergens, 1984; Rouiller et al., 1994; Dum & Strick, 1996; Dum & Strick, 2005), and may be an important source of descending commands for the generation and control of distal movements in the monkey (He et al., 1995). SMA is also involved in motor learning in man (Halsband & Lange, 2006). Therefore, SMA has been suggested to play a crucial role in the early processes of recovery after lesions of primary motor pathways (Loubinoux et al., 2003).

Ventral premotor cortex (PMv) receives strong projections from S1 (Stepniewska et al., 2006), and PMv neurons project onto cervical and thoracic motoneurons in the monkey (He et al., 1993; Rouiller et al., 1994). The PMv corticospinal neurons supply part of the hand function after M1 lesion in the monkey (Liu & Rouiller, 1999). Nudo and colleagues demonstrated rewiring from M1 to PMv after ischemic brain injury, with substantial enlargements of the hand representation in the remote PMv that are proportional to the amount of hand representation destroyed in M1 (Frost et al., 2003; Dancause et al., 2005). Nelles et al. (2001) pointed out the crucial role of a network including the lower part of BA40 and PMv, bilaterally, in task-oriented passive training aimed at improving motor recovery in severely impaired stroke patients. These areas could also be crucial for promoting reorganization in the rest of the brain.

4.2. Activation of sensorimotor network by active motor task

Previous functional neuroimaging studies on poststroke cerebral reorganization from acute to chronic stages revealed several activation patterns during active paretic hand movement (Ward & Cohen, 2004; Jang, 2007; Kato & Izumiyama, 2010). These include (1) a posterior shift of contralateral S1M1 activation (Pineiro et al., 2001; Calautti et al., 2003) , (2) peri-infarct reorganization after infarction involving M1 (Cramer et al., 1997; Jang et al., 2005a), (3) a shift of M1 activation to the ipsilateral (contralesional) cortex (Chollet et al., 1991; Marshall et al., 2000; Feydy et al., 2002), (4) contribution of the secondary motor areas (Cramer et al., 1997; Carey et al., 2002; Ward et al., 2006), and (5) higher contralateral activity in the cerebellar hemisphere (Small et al., 2002).

These studies have also shown that the expanded activations may later decrease with functional improvements, indicating that best recovery is obtained when there is restitution of activation toward the physiological network over time. The contralesional shift of activation may return to ipsilesional S1M1 activation with functional gains (Feydy et al., 2002; Takeda et al., 2007), but worse outcome may correlate with a shift in the balance of activation toward the contralesional S1M1 (Calautti et al., 2001; Feydy et al., 2002; Zemke et al., 2003). Thus, the patterns of cerebral activation evoked by active hand movement show impaired organization and reorganization of brain sensorimotor network, and best recovery may depend on how much original motor system is reusable. The patterns of activation may also be dependent on the patient's ability to recruit residual portions of the bilateral motor network (Silvestrini et al., 1998).

Early involvement of secondary sensorimotor areas after M1 lesion may temporarily substitute for the original sensorimotor network involving M1. This step may be a prerequisite to M1 functional reconnection through indirect pathways and to its efficacy in processing motor signals. The previous data suggest that different motor areas operate in parallel rather than in a hierarchical manner, and they are able to substitute for each other (Traversa et al., 1997; Loubinoux et al., 2003). Thus, remodeling of activation within a pre-existing network may be an important process for recovery.

4.3. Implication of somatosensory input as a rehabilitation strategy

There is consensus on the efficacy of physiotherapy. Active training is more efficient than passive training, but active training cannot be applied to very impaired patients. We need to consider other approaches for patients who cannot move the paretic limbs at the early phase of recovery. Physiotherapists apply sensory stimulation and passive movement daily to acute stroke patients and only these approaches are possible when the patients have complete paralysis. A few studies have validated the efficacy of sensory or proprioceptive stimulation on motor recovery.

Carel et al. (2000) have shown that proprioceptive training induces a reorganization of sensorimotor representation in healthy subjects, and that the anatomical substrates are SMA and S1M1 contralateral to the stimulation. Subsequently, Dechaumont-Palacin et al. (2008) showed that paretic wrist proprioceptive training produced change in SMA, premotor cortex, and a contralesional network including inferior parietal cortex (lower part of BA 40), secondary sensory cortex, and PMv. Thus, increased contralateral activity in secondary sensorimotor areas may facilitate control of recovered motor function by simple proprioceptive integration in severely impaired patients. Brain activation during passive movement increase with time after stroke (Nelles et al., 1999; Loubinoux et al., 2003; Tombari et al., 2004). Nelles et al. (2001) tested a mixed, task-oriented rehabilitative program that is at first passive, then active as recovery permits, and observed hyperactivation of the bilateral low parietal cortex and premotor cortex and a smaller hyperactivation of the ipsilateral M1. Thus, the changes might represent increased processing of sensory information relevant to motor output.

Somatosensory input to the motor cortex, via corticocortical connections with the somatosensory cortex, is important for learning new motor skills (Sakamoto et al., 1989; Pavlides et al., 1993; Vidoni et al., 2010). Somatosensory input may also play a critical role in motor relearning after hemiparetic stroke (Dechaumont-Palacin et al., 2008; Conforto at al. 2007; Vidoni et al., 2009). Schaechter et al. (2012) showed that increased responsiveness of the ipsilesional S1M1 to tactile stimulation over the subacute posrstroke period correlated with concurrent motor recovery and predicted motor recovery experienced over the year. This finding suggests that a strong link between change in processing of somatosensory information in the S1M1 during the early poststroke period and motor recovery in hemiparetic patients.

Muscular and peripheral nerve electrical stimulation increases motor output after stroke (Conforto et al., 2002; Kimberley et al., 2004; Wu et al., 2006; Conforto et al., 2010). Peripheral nerve stimulation increases corticomotoneuronal excitability (Kaelin-Lang et al., 2002; Ridding et al., 2000), and activation of S1M1 and PMd in healthy subjects (Wu et al., 2005). If applied to paretic hand of stroke patients paired with motor training, electrical nerve stimulation may enhance training effects on corticomotoneuronal plasticity in stroke patients (Sawaki et al, 2006; Yozbatiran et al., 2006; Celnik et al., 2007).

Thus, increased activity in brain sensorimotor network by somatosensory input may facilitate control of recovered motor function by operating not only at a high-order processing level but also at a low level of simple sensory integration. Therefore, early post-stroke fMRI studies using sensory stimulation as a task may be of great clinically importance and somatosensory stimulation over the poststroke recovery period may form a basis for improving motor recovery in stroke patients.

Another merit of massage or touch therapy may be the psychological effects produced by tactile stimulation, such as relaxation, alleviation of anxiety and depression. These effects may be evoked by stimulation of dopamine and serotonin secretion since increased levels of dopamine and serotonin have been shown in the urine following tactile skin stimulation (Field et al., 2005). Tactile stimulation in the rat evokes an increased dopamine release in the nucleus accumbens of the brain, which is thought to play a key role in motivational and reward processes (Maruyaka et al.; 2012). Relieving anxiety and depression seems important in the early steps of rehabilitation for patients with acute stroke.

5. Conclusion

The findings of this study demonstrate that the somatosensory inputs via the normal hand can activate brain sensorimotor network to a comparable extent with the areas that are activated during active hand movement, and that the somatosensory inputs via the paretic hand at the early stages of stroke before clinical motor recovery can also induce activities to some of the brain sensorimotor network. The result suggests that physiotherapy that employs somatosensory input via the paretic hand may be used as a first step to activate rehabilitation-dependent changes in the motor network in the brain toward restoration of motor function. The result may provide new insight into the establishment of rehabilitation strategies after stroke.

Author details

Hiroyuki Kato
Department of Neurology, International University of Health and Welfare Hospital, Nasushiobara, Japan

Masahiro Izumiyama
Department of Neurology, Sendai Nakae Hospital, Sendai, Japan

Acknowledgement

We thank the staff members of the MRI section of Sendai Nakae Hospital, Ms. Fumi Kozuka, Ms. Satsuki Ohi, Mr. Takeru Ohmukai, Ms. Yoko Sato, Ms. Aya Kanai, and Mr. Katsuhiro Aki, for their help to perform fMRI studies. We also thank Dr. Naohiro Saito, Department of Physiology, Tohoku University School of Medicine, Sendai, Japan, for his expert assistance on the fMRI-spm analysis. This study was supported by Grant-in-Aid for Scientific Research (22500473), Japan Society for the Promotion of Science.

6. References

Cao, Y.; D'Olhaberriague, L.; Vikingstad, E.M.; Levine, S.R. & Welch, K.M.A. (1998). Pilot study of functional MRI to assess cerebral activation of motor function after poststroke hemiparesis. *Stroke*, 29, 112-122.

Calautti, C. & Baron, J.-C. (2003). Functional neuroimaging studies of motor recovery after stroke in adults. A review. *Stroke,* 34, 1553-1566

Calautti, C.; Leroy, F.; Guincestre, J.Y. & Baron, J.-C. (2001). Dynamics of motor network overactivation after striatocapsular stroke: a longitudinal PET study using a fixed-performance paradigm. *Stroke,* 32, 2534-2542

Carel, C.; Loubinoux, I.; Boulanouar, K.; Manelfe, C.; Rascol, O.; Celsis, P. & Chollet, F. (2000). Neural substrate for the effects of passive training on sensorimotor cortical representation: a study with functional magnetic resonance imaging in healthy subjects. *J. Cereb. Blood Flow Metab.,* 20, 478-484

Carey, J.R.; Kimberley, T.J.; Lewis, S.M.; Auerbach, E.J.; Dorsey, L.; Rundquist, P. & Ugurbil, K. (2002). Analysis of fMRI and finger tracking training in subjects with chronic stroke. *Brain,* 125, 773-788

Celnik, P.; Hummel, F.; Harris-Love, M.; Wolk, R. & Cohen, L.G. (2007). Somatosensory stimulation enhances the effects of training functional hand tasks in patients with chronic stroke. *Arch. Phys. Med. Rehabil.,* 88, 1369-1376

Chollet, F.; DiPiero, V.; Wise, R.J.S.; Brooks, D.J.; Dolan, R.J. & Fracowiak, R.S.J. (1991). The functional anatomy of motor recovery after stroke in humans: a study with positron emission tomography. *Ann. Neurol.,* 29, 63-71

Conforto, A.B.; Cohen, L.G.; dos Santos, R.L.; Scaff, M. & Marie, S.K. (2007). Effects of somatosensory stimulation on motor function in chronic cortico-subcortical strokes. *J. Neurol.,* 254, 333-339

Conforto, A.B.; Ferreiro, K.N.; Tomasi, C.; dos Santos, R.L.; Moreira, V.L.; Marie, S.K.; Baltieri, S.C.; Scaff, M. & Cohen, L.G. (2010). Effects of somatosensory stimulation on motor function after subacute stroke. *Neurorehabil. Neural Repair,* 24, 263-272

Conforto, A.B.; Kaelin-Lang, A. & Cohen, L.G. (2002). Increase in hand muscle strength of stroke patients after somatosensory stimulation. *Ann. Neurol.,* 51, 122-125

Cramer, S.C.; Nelles, G.; Benson, R.R.; Kaplan, J.D.; Parker, R.A.; Kwong, K.K.; Kennedy, D.N.; Finklestein, S.P. & Rosen, B.R. (1997). A functional MRI study of subjects recovered from hemiparetic stroke. *Stroke,* 28, 2518-2527

Dancause, N.; Barbay, S.; Frost, S.B.; Plautz, E.J.; Chen, D.; Zoubina, E.V.; Stowe, A.M. & Nudo, R.J. (2005). Extensive cortical rewiring after brain injury. *J. Neurosci.,* 25, 10167-10179

Decety, J. (1996). The neurophysiological basis of motor imagery. *Behav. Brain Res.,* 77, 45-52

Dechaumont-Palacin, S.; Marque, P.; De Boissezon, X.; Castel-Lacanal, E.; Carel, C.; Berry, I.; Pastorm, J.; Albucher, J.F.; Chollet, F. & Loubinoux, I. (2008). Neural correlates of proprioceptive integration in the contralesional hemisphere of very impaired patients shortly after a subcortical stroke: an fMRI study. *Neurorihab. Neural Repair,* 22, 154-165

Dum, R.P. & Strick, P.L. (1996). Spinal cord terminations of the medial wall motor areas in macaque monkeys. *J. Neurosci.,* 16, 6513-6525

Dum, R.P. & Strick, P.L. (2005). Frontal lobe inputs to the digit representations of the motor areas on the lateral surface of the hemisphere. *J. Neurosci.,* 25, 1375-1386

Duncan, P.W.; Goldstein, L.B.; Matchar, D.; Divine, G.W. & Feussner, J. (1992). Measurement of motor recovery after stroke: outcome measures and sample size requirements. *Stroke*, 23, 1084-1089

Feydy, A.; Carlier, R.; Rody-Brami, A.; Bussel, B.; Cazalis, F.; Pierot, L.; Burnod, Y. & Maier, M.A. (2002). Longitudinal study of motor recovery after stroke: recruitment and focusing of brain activation. *Stroke*, 33, 1610-1617

Field, T.; Hernandez-Reif, M.; Diego, M.; Schanberg, S. & Kuhn, C. (2005). Cortisol decreases and serotonin and dopamine increase following massage therapy. *Int. J. Neurosci.*, 115, 1397-1413

Fromm, C. & Evarts, E.V. (1982). Pyramidal tract neurons in somatosensory cortex: central and peripheral inputs during voluntary movement. *Brain Res.*, 238, 186-191

Frost, S.B.; Barbay, S.; Friel, K.M.; Plautz, E.J. & Nudo, R.J. (2003). Reorganization of remote cortical regions after ischemic brain injury: a potential substrate for stroke recovery. *J. Neurophysiol.*, 89, 3205-3214

Grezes, J. & Decety, J. (2001). Functional anatomy of execution, mental simulation, observation, and verb generation of actions: a meta-analysis. *Hum. Brain Mapp.*, 12, 1-19

Halsband, U. & Lange, R.K. (2006). Motor learning in man: a review of functional and clinical studies. *J. Physiol. Paris*, 99, 414-424

He, S.Q.; Dum, R.P. & Strick, P.L. (1995). Topographic organization of corticospinal projections from the frontal lobe: motor areas on the medial surface of the hemisphere. *J. Neurosci.*, 15, 1284-3306

Herholz, A. & Heiss, W.-D. (2000). Functional imaging correlates of recovery after stroke in humans. *J. Cereb. Blood Flow Metab.*, 20, 1619-1631

Jang, S.H. (2007). A review of motor recovery mechanisms in patients with stroke. *Neurorehabilitation*, 22, 253-259

Jang, S.H.; Ahn, S.H.; Yang, D.S.; Lee, D.K.; Kim, D.K. & Son, S.M. (2005). Cortical reorganization of hand motor function to primary sensory cortex in hemiparetic patients with a primary motor cortex infarct. *Arch. Phys. Med. Rehabil.*, 86, 1706-1708

Jones, E.G.; Coulter, J.D. & Hendry, S.H. (1978). Intracortical connectivity of architectonic fields in the somatic sensory, motor and parietal cortex of monkeys. *J. Comp. Neurol.*, 181, 291-347

Juergens, U. (1984). The efferent and afferent connections of the supplementary motor area. *Brain Res.*, 300, 63-81

Kaelin-Lang, A.; Luft, A.R.; Sawaki, L.; Burstein, A.H.; Sohn, Y.H. & Cohen, L.G. (2002). Modulation of human corticomotor excitability by somatosensory input. *J. Physiol.*, 540(Pt 2), 623-633

Kato, H. & Izumiyama, M. (2010). Restorative and compensatory changes in the brain during early motor recovery from hemiparetic stroke: a functional MRI study, Neuroimaging, Cristina Marta Del-Ben (Ed.), ISBN: 978-953-307-127-5, Sciyo, Available from: http://sciyo.com/articles/show/title/restorative-and-compensatory-changes-in-the-brain-during-early-motor-recovery-from-hemiparetic-strok

Kato, H.; Izumiyama, M.; Koizumi, H.; Takahashi, A. & Itoyama, Y. (2002). Near-infrared spectroscopic topography as a tool to monitor motor reorganization after hemiparetic stroke. A comparison with functional MRI. *Stroke,* 33, 2032-2036

Kimberley, T.J.; Lewis, S.M.; Auerbach, E.J.; Dorsey, L.L.; Lojovich, J.M. & Carey, J.R. (2004). Electrical stimulation driving functional improvements and cortical changes in subjects with stroke. *Exp. Brain Res.,* 154, 450-460

Lemon, R.N. (1999). Neural control of dexterity: what has been achieved? *Exp.Brain Res.,* 128, 6-12

Lemon, R.N. & Porter, R. (1976). Afferent input to movement-related precentral neurons in conscious monkeys. *Proc. R. Soc. Lond. B. Biol. Sci.,* 194, 313-339

Liu, Y. & Rouiller, E.M. (1999). Mechanisms of recovery of dexterity following unilateral lesion of the sensorimotor cortex in adult monkeys. *Exp. Brain Res.,* 128, 149-159

Loubinoux, I.; Carel, C.; Pariente, J.; Dechaumont, S.; Albucher, J.-F.; Marque, C. & Chollet, F. (2003). Correlation between cerebral reorganization and motor recovery after subcortical infarcts. *Neuroimage,* 20, 2166-2180

McGlone, F.; Kelly, E.F.; Trusson, M.; Francis, S.T.; Westling, G. & Bowtell, R. (2002). Functional neuroimaging studies of human somatosensory cortex. *Behav. Brain Res.,* 135, 147-158

Marshall, R.S.; Perera, G.M.; Lazar, R.M.; Krakauer, J.W.; Constantine, R.C. & DeLaPaz, R.L. (2000). Evolution of cortical activation during recovery from corticospinal tract infarction. *Stroke,* 31, 656-661

Maruyama, K.; Shimojo, R.; Ohkubo, M.; Maruyama, H. & Kurosawa, M. (2012). Tactile skin stimulation increases dopamine release in the nucleus accumbens in rats. *J. Physiol. Sci.,* 62, 259-266

Mazzetto-Betti, K.C.; Leoni, R.F.; Pontes-Neto, O.M.; Santos, A.C.; Leite, J.P.; Silva, A.C. & de Araujo, D.B. (2010). The stability of the BOLD fMRI response to motor tasks is altered in patients with chronic ischemic stroke. *Stroke,* 41, 1921-1926

Moore, C.I.; Stern, C.E.; Corkin, S.; Fischi, B.; Gray, A.C.; Rosen, B.R. & Dale, A.M. (2000). Segregation of somatosensory activation in the human rolandic cortex using fMRI. *J. Neurophysiol.,* 84, 558-569

Murata, Y.; Sakatani, K.; Hoshino, T.; Fujiwara, N.; Kano, T.; Nakamura, S. & Katayama, Y. (2006). Effects of cerebral ischemia on evoked cerebral blood oxygenation responses and BOLD contrast functional MRI in stroke patients. *Stroke,* 37, 2514-2520

Nelles, G.; Jentzen, W.; Jueptner, M.; Mueller, S. & Diener, H.C. (2001). Arm training induced brain plasticity in stroke studied with serial positron emission tomography. *Neuroimage,* 13, 1146-1154

Nelles, G.; Spiekermann, G.; Jueptner, M.; Leonhardt, G.; Mueller, S.; Gerhard, H. & Diener, C. (1999). Reorganization of sensory and motor systems in hemiplegic stroke patients. A positron emission tomography study. *Stroke,* 30, 1510-1516

Nii, Y.; Uematsu, S.; Lesser, R.P. & Gordon, B. (1996). Does the central sulcus divide motor and sensory functions? Cortical mapping of human hand areas as revealed by electrical stimulation through subdural grid electrodes. *Neurology,* 46, 360-367

Pavlides, C.; Miyashita, E. & Asanuma, H. (1993). Projection from the sensory to the motor cortex is important in learning motor skills in the monkey. *J. Neurophysiol.*, 70, 733-741

Pineiro, R.; Pendlebury, S.; Johansen-Berg, H. & Matthews, P.M. (2001). Functional MRI detects posterior shifts in primary sensorimotor cortex activation after stroke. Evidence of local adaptive reorganization? *Stroke*, 32, 1134-1139

Ridding, M.C.; Brouwer, B.; Miles, T.S.; Pitcher, J.B. & Thompson, P.D. (2000). Changes in muscle responses to stimulation of the motor cortex induced by peripheral nerve stimulation in human subjects. *Exp. Brain Res.*, 131,135-143

Rossini, P.M.; Calautti, C.; Pauri, F. & Baron, J.C. (2003). Post-stroke plastic reorganization in the adult brain. *Lancet Neurol.*, 2, 493-502

Rouiller, E.M.; Babalian, A.; Kazennikov, O.; Moret, V.; Yu, X.H. & Wiesendanger, M. (1994). Transcallosal connections of the distal forelimb representations of the primary and supplementary motor cortical areas in macaque monkeys. *Exp. Brain Res.*, 102, 227-243

Sakamoto, T. ; Arissian, K. & Asanuma, H. (1989). Functional role of the sensory cortex in learning motor skills in cats. *Brain Res.*, 503, 258-264

Sawaki, L.; Wu, C.W.; Kaelin-Lang, A. & Cohen, L.G. (2006). Effects of somatosensory stimulation on use-dependent plasticity in chronic stroke. *Stroke*, 37, 246-247

Schaechter, J.D.; van Oers, C.A.; Groisser, B.N.; Salles, S.S.; Vangel, M.G.; Moore, C.I. & Dijkhuizen, R.M. (2012). Increase in sensorimotor cortex response to somatosensory stimulation over subacute poststroke period correlates with motor recovery in himipareric patients. *Neurorehabil. Neural Repair*, 26, 325-334

Silvestrini, M.; Cupini, L.M.; Placidi, F.; Diomedi, M. & Bernardi, G. (1998). Bilateral hemispheric activation in the early recovery of motor function after stroke. *Stroke*, 29, 1305-1310

Small, A.L.; Hlustik, P.; Noll, D.C.; Genovese, C. & Solodkin, A. (2002). Cerebellar hemispheric activation ipsilateral to the paretic hand correlates with functional recovery after stroke. *Brain*, 125, 1544-1557

Stepniewska, I.; Preuss, TM. & Kaas, J.H. (2006). Ipsilateral cortical connections of dorsal and ventral premotor areas in New World owl monkeys. *J. Comp. Neurol.*, 495, 691-708

Takeda, K.; Gomi, Y.; Imai, I.; Shimoda, N.; Hiwatari, M. & Kato, H. (2007). Shift of motor activation areas during recovery from hemiparesis after cerebral infarction: a longitudinal study with near-infrared spectroscopy. *Neurosci. Res.*, 59, 136-144

Tombari, D.; Loubinoux, I.; Pariente, J.; Gerdelat, A.; Albucher, J.-F.; Tardy, J.; Cassol, E. & Chollet, F. (2004). A longitudinal fMRI study: in recovering and then in clinically stable subcortical stroke patients. *Neuroimage*, 23, 827-839

Traversa, R.; Cicinelli, P.; Bassi, A.; Rossini, P.M. & Bernardi, G. (1997). Mapping of motor cortical reorganization after stroke. A brain stimulation study with focal magnetic pulses. *Stroke*, 28,110-117

Vidoni, E.D.; Acerra, N.E.; Dao, E.; Meehan, S.K. & Boyd, L.A. (2010). Role of the primary somatosensory cortex in motor learning: An rTMS study. *Neurobiol. Learn. Mem.*, 93, 532-539

Vidoni, E.D. & Boyd, L.A. (2009). Preserved motor learning after stroke is related to the degree of proprioceptive deficit. *Behav. Brain Funct.*, 5,36

Ward, N.S.; Brown, M.M.; Thompson, A.J. & Frackowiak, R.S.J. (2003a). Neural correlates of outcome after stroke: a cross-sectional fMRI study. *Brain,* 126, 1430-1448

Ward, N.S.; Brown, M.M.; Thompson, A.J. & Frackowiak, R.S.J. (2003b). Neural correlates of motor recovery after stroke: a longitudinal fMRI study. *Brain,* 126, 2476-2496

Ward, N.S. & Cohen, L.G. (2004). Mechanisms underlying recovery of motor function after stroke. *Arch. Neurol.*. 61, 1844-1848

Ward, N.S.; Newton, J.M.; Swayne, O.B.; Lee, L.; Thompson, A.J.; Greenwood, R.J.; Rothwell, J.C. & Frackowiak, R.S. (2006). Motor system activation after subcortical stroke depends on corticospinal system integrity. *Brain,* 129(Pt. 3), 809-819

Weiller, C.; Chollet, F.; Fristo, K.J.; Wise, R.J. & Frackowiak, R.S. (1992). Functional reorganization of the brain in recovery from striatocapsular infarction in man. *Ann. Neurol.,* 315, 463-472

Wu, C.W.; Seo, H.J. & Cohen, L.G. (2006). Influence of electric somatosensory stimulation on paretic-hand function in chronic stroke. *Arch. Phys. Med. Rehabil.,* 87, 351-357

Wu, C.W.; van Gelderen, P.; Hanakawa, T.; Yaseen, Z. & Cohen, L.G. (2005). Enduring representational plasticity after somatosensory stimulation. *Neuroimage,* 27, 872-884

Yozbtiran, N.; Donmez, B.; Kayak, N. & Bozan, O. (2006). Electrical stimulation of wrist and fingers for sensory and functional recovery in acute hemiplegia. *Clin. Rehabil.,* 20, 4-11

Zemke, A.C.; Heagerty, P.J.; Lee, C. & Cramer, S.C. (2003). Motor cortex organization after stroke is related to side of stroke and level of recovery. *Stroke,* 34, e23-28

Section 2

Novel Frontiers of Neuroimaging

Chapter 5

Intraoperative Computed Tomography/Angiography Guided Resection of Skull Base Lesions

Hoan Tran and Howard Yonas

Additional information is available at the end of the chapter

http://dx.doi.org/10.5772/50895

1. Introduction

It can be said that the history of neurosurgery has been interdependent with the history of concurrent technology, making it one of the more avante garde fields of medicine. Since the advent of monopolar cautery more than one hundred years ago, neurosurgeons have been rapid to apply the most recent technological advances to intraoperative uses to make surgery safer and less invasive. Since the first brain computed tomography was done in October 1971, neurosurgeons have quickly started adapting commercially available computed tomography machines for uses in the operating room to access some of the most formidable problems in neurosurgery: skull base lesions. In fact it was only 7 years later that computed tomography was adapted for intraoperative use with neuronavigation of intracranial lesions. Early publications of CT guided surgery already demonstrated benefits of real time data integration: navigation of eloquent areas of the brain, lesion localization, maximal lesion resection, immediate recognition of intraoperative hemorrhage, improved confidence for post operative care. Much of the work done was with cortical and subcortical lesions. Early CT scanners were very large, and competed with precious limited operating space; often scanners were placed near and operating suit and not necessarily within the operating suite. This necessitated transferring patients from the actually operating suite to the CT scanner prior to the completion of the case, in essence moving patients with open surgical wounds, on full mechanical ventilation, and other calculated risks. With improved computing, CT scanners increased in resolution and decreased in size, making it possible to obtain true intraoperative computed tomography, without exposing patients to all the risks of transferring a patient.

Neuronavigation is an invaluable tool to the modern skull base surgeon. Its ubiquity allows for safer and more effective treatment of lesions in difficult regions of the skull and brain. However because of brain shift once the calvarium is open, its ubiquity has its limitations.

Several modalities of imaging have developed into intraoperative uses, each with their own advantages and disadvantages. When used correctly, these tools provide powerful real time data needed to guide decision making, direct surgical approaches, and reveal lesional remnants. For skull base lesions, soft tissue discrimination and boney anatomy are both integral and necessary to execute resection of the most formidable lesions, while preserving the brain and its cranial nerves. We illustrate the feasibility of intraoperative computed tomography (CT) and CT angiography (CTA) in the resection of different skull base lesions with the following examples.

2. Methods/Results

After the patient have undergone general anesthesia, a DORO head holder (ProMed Instruments, Freiburg, Germany) is used for head fixation, which is like the Mayfield except for radiolucent arms. The radiolucent arms are variable to fit the length of an individual's neck and are designed to fix the cranium but extend the fixation capability towards the shoulders. (Figure 1a). The shoulders are supported by the operating table, but the head and neck are suspended using the DORO head holding system to allow entrance into the CT gantry. Once a CT is warranted, the surgical field is draped with a large C-arm cover and the CT gantry is translated around the head. CT images are obtained, and reviewed within a few minutes as needed for integration into clinical management (Figure 1b).

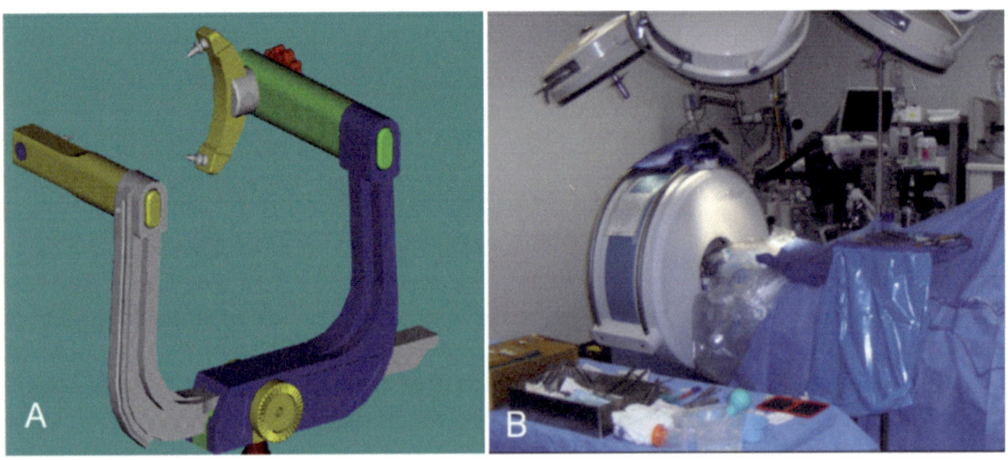

Figure 1. A. The DORO head holder is a Mayfield-type holder but with extensions that are radiolucent. **B.** Ceretom is translated over the patients head during surgery without moving patients.

Case 1

This patient is a 39 year old female who had noticed for at least eight years a growing hard prominence on the left side of her face. She also noted proptosis that had been getting worse for the last year accompanied by headaches that were increasing in frequency and intensity. Routine CT brain and MRI brain was consistent with an interosseous meningioma and a superficial biopsy confirmed the diagnosis. The tumor involved the left middle fossa and

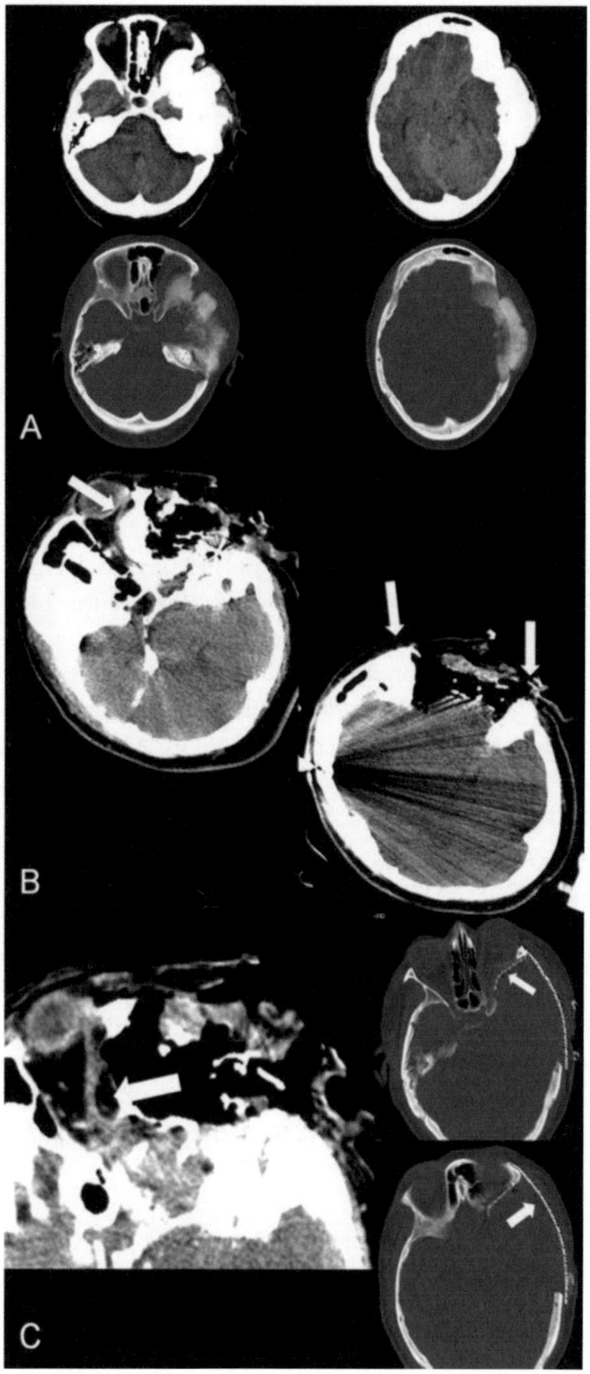

Figure 2. **A**. Interosseus meningioma invading the petrous temporal bone, squamous temporal bone, and lateral orbital wall. **B**. Intraoperative CT showing residual tumor along the lateral orbital wall and petrous apex (arrows). **C**. Repeat CT shows complete removal and reconstruction of lateral orbital wall and calvarium (arrows).

hyperostosis of the squamous temporal bone, the petrous temporal bone, sphenoid wing, the zygomatic process, and the lateral orbital wall.

The patient was placed in a supine position, with the head held in radiolucent arms. The interosseous meningioma in the middle fossa with 3 centimeters of extracranial extension and 2 centimeters of intracranial soft dural based tumor was directly attached (Figure 2a). A CT taken during surgery showed residual tumor along the petrous apex and it provided exact guidance on how extensively to decompress the orbital contents (Figure 2b). Once an adequate tumor removal was accomplished and validated by a second CT, the lateral orbital wall and cranial vault was reconstructed, again confirmed by CT prior to closing (figure 2c). For tumors that surgery is the primary modality of treatment and surgery can provide a cure, image guidance for total resection instead of debulking offer the best prognosis for treatment, rather than subtotal resection followed by radiation or chemotherapy. Intraoperative ct provided excellent soft tissue and bone discrimination.

Case 2

This patient is a 55 year old male with dizziness and balance problems for a year. A CT angiogram, followed by magnetic resonance imaging (MRI) of the brain, showed a left superior cerebellar arteriovenous malformation. Preoperative angiogram confirmed the lesion was a left cerebellar AVM that had multiple feeding vessels but primarily from the left superior cerebellar artery (figure 3a). The patient had undergone preoperative embolization. The next day, the patient was taken to the operating room for a left suboccipital craniectomy and resection of the AVM through a infratentorial supracerebellar approach. During surgery, a CT angiogram was obtained, which showed residual AVM just medial to the operative field (Figure 3b). The surgical approach was modified to resect the remaining lesion. Postoperative angiogram confirmed complete resection of the AVM (Figure 3c). For vascular lesions such as arteriovenous malformation, incomplete resection can lead to a delayed hemorrhage within the first 24 hours after surgery, often when the patient is in the intensive care unit leading to catastrophic results. Traditionally intraoperative angiograms are performed for these vascular lesions to ensure complete resection, however this case illustrates the technical difficulties of a prone angiogram; the femoral artery is not available to the interventionalist. Bringing a portable ct scanner provides the same information and does not require awkward positioning and technical difficulties of performing an angiogram in the prone position.

Case 3

This patient is a 63 year old male with worsening pressure-like headaches, loss of smell for six months. He was treated for frontal sinusitis but was refractory of antibiotic treatment. A CT positron emission tomography (PET) scan shows an anterior skull base tumor with invasion into the frontal sinus, through the anterior and middle ethmoidal air cells and down to the middle nasal concha.

The patient had a transnasal endoscopic biopsy which showed poorly differentiated invasive sinonasal adenocarcinoma. The patient underwent a combined transfacial and transcranial approach for tumor resection. The tumor had extended into the subfrontal

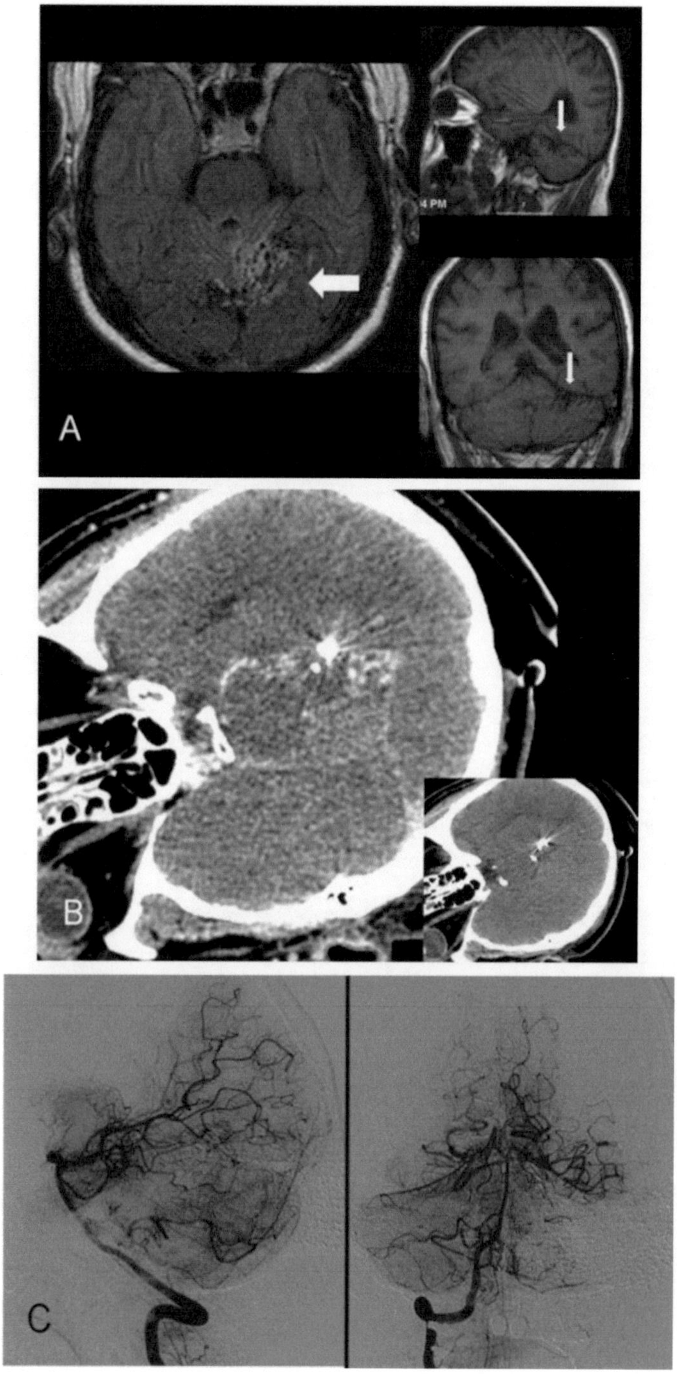

Figure 3. **A**. Left superior cerebellar AVM seen on T1 weighted MRI axial (left), sagittal (upper insert), and coronal view (lower insert). **B**. Intraoperative CT of partially resected AVM juxtaposed to preoperative embolization not visualized under microscope. **C.** Post operative cerebral angiogram confirms complete resection of AVM.

cortex and extended back past the middle ethmoid cells (figure 4a). After a bifrontal craniotomy, the frontal sinus was cranialized. Resection of the tumor from below allowed access to the bilateral medial orbital walls. A CT taken during surgery revealed tumor adherent to the right medial orbital wall (Figure 4b). Once the resection was

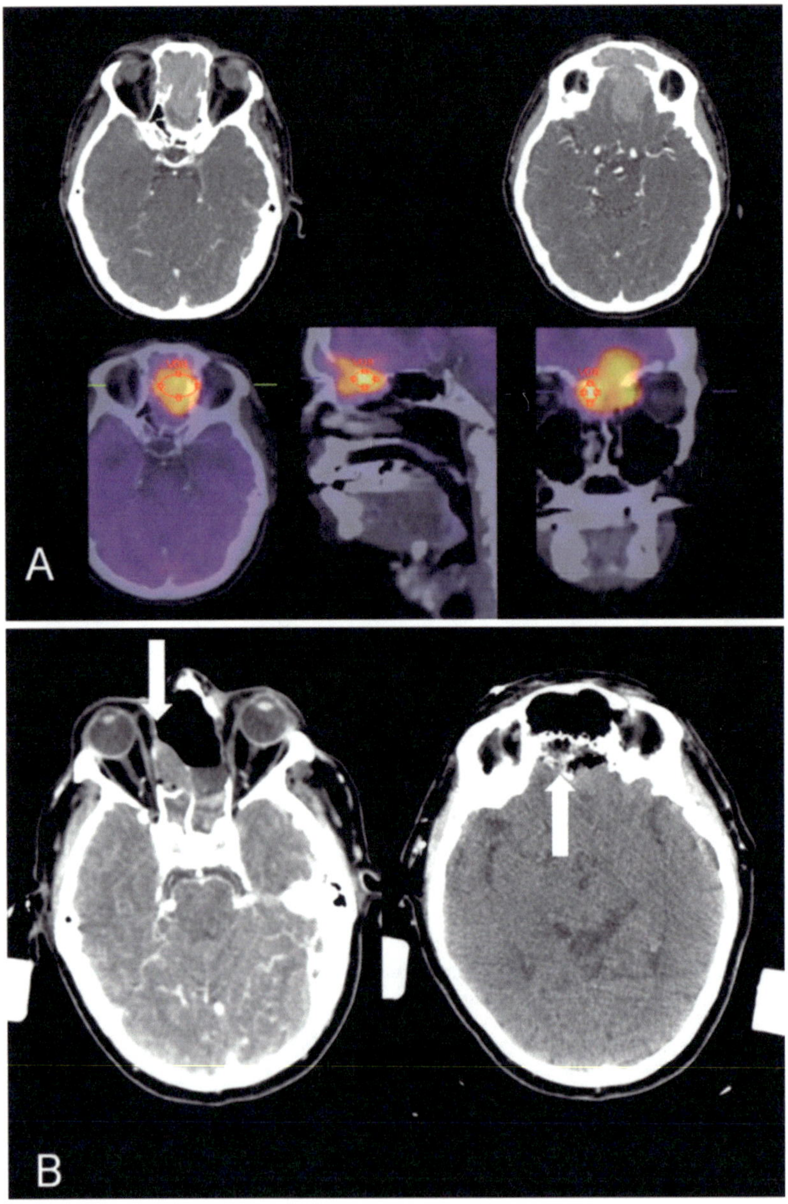

Figure 4. **A** Preoperative CT PET study shows tumor of anterior skull base extending down into middle nasal concha, back to posterior ethmoidal air cells, and into inferior frontal lobes. **B**. Intraoperative CT shows residual tumor adherent to right medial orbital wall (left), and reconstruction of anterior fossa floor with titanium mesh (right).

completed, reconstruction of the anterior fossa ensued with titanium mesh, fascia lata, and duraplasty. An aggressive resection of tumor and structural integrity of the anterior fossa reconstruction was confirmed by CT prior to closing the skin. For pathology of the skull base, reconstruction of the skull base is often technically challenging due to migration of prosthesis and brain shift. Confirming that the skull base is adequately reconstructed can prevent cerebral spinal fluid leaks leading to meningitis and devastating consequences.

The time required for obtaining intraoperative CT scans was less than 15 minutes with the data being immediately available for clinical integration. There were no complications from bring the portable CT scanner into the surgical field in each of these cases.

3. Discussion

Advancements in neuronavigation have mirrored advancements in microsurgical techniques, leading to less intraoperative and postoperative complications (1,2). This has led to smaller surgical exposures with increase accessibility to difficult regions of the head and neck. Since the early 1980's, neuronavigation systems have become ubiquitous and commonplace in the practice of neurosurgeons, ENT surgeons, and maxillofacial surgeons alike, all vying for use in the operating room (3). Many computer assisted neuronavigation systems require prescanned images, done the night before surgery, uploaded into the navigational computer at the time of surgery, and used for planning the skin incision and craniotomy. The problem with preoperative image guidance systems is that the static images become invalid once the cranium is open, CSF is lost and or a portion of the tumor mass is removed. Ultimately, the limitations with these neuronavigational systems is that they cannot adjust to brain shifts and lead to gross errors in anatomical localization, in addition to the inherent error that already exists in fiducial registration. Hence, the need for intraoperative imaging for real time evaluation becomes paramount.

Intraoperative MRI has the advantage of obtaining real time data, providing excellent soft tissue discrimination and allows the surgeon to accommodate to brain shift during surgery. However the feasibility of intraoperative MRI is still being determined with increasing medical costs (4). Existing surgical suites have to be retrofitted to accommodate the intraoperative MRI; specialized nonferromagnetic instruments must be used, and accessibility to the patient is limited by the MRI machine itself. For large intraoperative MRI, patient has to be moved in and out of the scanner during surgery (5). Smaller machines directly translate over the patient, restricting surgeon access to the surgical field.

Intraoperative 3D ultrasound technology has also found its use in the operating room. Ultrasound imaging allows for real time data requisition and does not require special instruments, but traditionally low quality images and cumbersome equipment has limited its uses. Recently, high quality ultrasound has made the image quality better but it is still cumbersome to use, requiring complete hemostasis of the field, distortion of the image the further away you are from the wand, and requires a high learning curve for correlating surgical anatomy and ultrasound images (6).

Intraoperative CT technology was initially used in the 1980's but its reluctant use was due to radiation exposure, long scan time, and maneuverability in the operating room (Lunsford). For skull base pathology, the localization and removal of bone elements is vital to the success of the operation in order to minimize retraction of delicate neural structures. It is then critical that neuronavigation for these lesions include not only show soft tissue and vascular discrimination but also boney elements as well. This is the advantage of CT over MRI and Ultrasound.

The CereTom portable CT scanner (Neurologica, Danvers, Mass) has many advantages. It is small, compact, and can move freely in and out of operating suites. It does not require specialized equipment to use with the exception of a radiolucent arms and head holder and does not require retrofitting into existing OR suites. It has scanning capabilities that allow for multiple windowing, high resolution contrasted study for soft tissue discrimination, CT angiography, and 3-D rendering capabilities. Opponent of this technology point out the risk of radiation exposure, but Butler et al showed that actual risk is quite low (7). Radiation dose report for our institutional 64 slice CT scanner is approximately 68 mGY per routine 5 mm slice head CT. Radiation report from our portable scanner is 41mGY for low dose 5 mm slice head CT, and 117 mGY for high resolution 1mm slice head CT. Most of the intraoperative scanning required for even the deepest lesions is the lower resolution scan, a 27 mGY less than our traditional CT scanner. The higher dose/resolution scans are used for intraoperative CT angiography, reserved for vascular lesions, judicially used because the cost of untreated vascular lesion is dire. Although no study has been done to assess the amount of total radiation exposure for any given patient with a skull base lesion, we have not increased the amount of CT scans obtained postoperatively since the use of the portable CT scanner. It would seem that the benefits of accomplishing what was intended in the operating room outweigh any theoretical and relatively small risk of radiation.

The risk of intraoperative CT cannot be weighed against the potential risk of injuring delicate neural structures along the complex skull base, leaving tumor/AVM residual leading to postoperative bleeding, or morbidity and cost of repeat surgery to the patient and the instituition. Although no cost analysis has been performed specifically for intraoperative CT guidance, we know that intraoperative guidance with MRI reduces length of stay by 55% for patients with initial surgery versus traditional surgery, repeat surgery rates were much lower with intraoperative guidance and, and total overall hospital costs was a 46% lower for initial surgery versus traditional surgery and 44% lower for repeat surgery (8); it is possible that intraoperative CT can do the same. We have used the portable CT scanner for imaging convexity tumors, gliomas, intraventricular tumors, confirmation of ommaya reservoirs and shunt placement. Prior to closing the surgical wound, a CT is done for final confirmation; this obviates the need to perform post operative CT imaging, saving a transport of the patient to the traditional CT scanner and minimizing risk to the patient, especially for critically ill patients and those needing mechanical ventilation.

4. Conclusion

These cases illustrate the feasibility of using intraoperative CT scanner during resection of skull base lesions. Windowing of already familiar CT images provide excellent soft tissue and bone discrimination. It can also provide CT angiogram data for evaluation of vascular lesions without the inherent risks of a conventional angiogram. Valuable real-time information is available without the need to move patients during surgery, guide decision-making for gross total resection and avoid reoperation for the removal of tumor remnants.

Author details

Hoan Tran* and Howard Yonas
Department of Neurosurgery/University of New Mexico, Mexico

5. References

[1] Paleologos TS, Wadley JP, Kitchen ND, et al. Clinical Utility and Cost-effectiveness of Interactive Image-guided Craniotomy: Clinical Comparison between Conventional and Image-guided Meningioma Surgery. Neurosurgery 2000 July; 47(1):40-48

[2] Slavin KV. Neuronavigation in neurosurgery: current state of affairs. Expert Rev Med Devices. 2008 Jan; 5(1):1-3

[3] Lunsford LD, Martinez AJ. Stereotactic exploration of the brain in the era of computed tomography. Surg Neurol. 1984 Sep; 22(3):222-30

[4] Steinmeier R , Fahlbusch R, Ganslandt O, et al. Intraoperative Magnetic Resonance Imaging with the Magnetom Open Scanner: Concepts, Neurosurgical Indications, and Procedures: A Preliminary Report. Neurosurgery 1998 October; 43(4): 739-747

[5] Hall WA, Truwit CL. Intraoperative MR-guided neurosurgery. J Magn Reson Imaging 2008 Feb;27(2):368-75

[6] Unsgaard G, Ommedal S, Muller T, Gronningsaeter A, Nagelhus Hernes TA. Neuronavigation by intraoperative three-dimensional ultrasound: initial experience during brain tumor resection. Neurosurgery 2002 Apr; 50(4):804-12

[7] Butler WE, Piaggio CM, Constantinou C, et al. A mobile computed tomographic scanner with intraoperative and intensive care unit applications. Neurosurgery. 1998 Jun;42(6):1304-10

* Corresponding Author

[8] Hall WA, Kowalik K, Liu H, Truwit CL, et al. Costs and benefits of intraoperative MR-guides brain tumor resection. Acta Neurochir Suppl 2003; 85:137-142.

Chapter 6

Neuroimaging Helps to Clarify Brain Affective Processing Without Necessarily Clarifying Emotions

Peter Walla and Jaak Panksepp

Additional information is available at the end of the chapter

http://dx.doi.org/10.5772/51761

1. Introduction

Literally, Neuroimaging gives us deeper insight into the brain's function. But, what actually is its function? The brain is an organ, almost just as our lungs and hearts. The big difference is that we can see the imprints of evolutionary progressions in its organization. Although the stamp of evolution is clearly imprinted in the genes that govern the functions of all the other organs, that stamp is special within the brain: Brain functions that evolved earlier are concentrated in more caudal and medial regions of the brain while those that emerged later (e.g., neocortex) are concentrated more rostrally and laterally. Thus, although our brain is an organ like no other in the body, we should envision the mind as largely the product of this bodily organ, although mind is surely not disconnected from other bodily functions.

Our heart pumps blood to provide all body parts with essential chemicals. The blood pumping is the function (or the mechanism) and the delivery of chemicals the goal. Likewise, the brain has various intrinsic functions and evolutionary goals (the "what for" evolutionary issue, in Dan Dennett's terms, as contrasted to the scientifically more workable "how come" dimensions of brain mechanisms). The brain's overall function is to process external information, as referenced to internal survival issues that are often coded as affective states, and the goal is to produce behaviours that sustain existence. Thinking of Darwin's (1859) idea that fitter organisms are better survivors the brain must have evolved to adapt the behaviour of its carrier organism to an ever-changing environment, however the adaptive behaviours also need to be referenced to internal survival issues. Sensory input representing the outer world is processed and forms an important basis for decisions to be made, which need to be related to internal survival issues, which in turn form the basis for actual behaviour in terms of movement (any form of muscle contraction). Sensory input, information processing and motor output, these are the well-accepted major steps of the brain's function (see Walla, 2011). However, the internal "set-points"—the within brain value referencing of behaviour—is often left out of the equation. Here we also seek to bring that dimension, as reflected in the affective lives of organisms (Panksepp, 1998; Panksepp & Biven, 2012), back into the discussion more explicitly, in scientifically testable ways.

This chapter focuses specifically on the affective side of information processing, especially taking into account findings from neuroimaging studies. In addition, the issue is raised that the term "emotion" is at times confusingly and interchangeably used between and even within disciplines that study the brain and mind, which is itself delaying advances in our understanding of the brain. Without conceptual agreement on key terms such as affect, emotion and motivation, along with the recognition that each has undergone multi-tiered evolutionary progressions, the likelihood of talking past each other increases, as with the perennial debates between basic emotion theory and constructivist approaches to similar problems (e.g., Lindquist, et al., 2012; Zachar & Ellis, 2012).

Despite the rather confusing existing terminologies, it must be admitted that neuroimaging technologies have shed considerable light on functions underlying emotions. These mainly include cognitively preconscious and unconscious aspects (Berlin, 2011), which are not easily accessible by questionnaire-based investigations (although they may be mentalized with depth-psychoanalytic interviews (see Kaplan-Solms & Solms, 2000), giving neuroimaging technologies one of their most attractive feature. The brain knows (and maybe experiences) more than it admits at the cognitive tertiary-process level (Solms & Panksepp, 2012), and among the objective tools, only neuroimaging (and startle reflex modulation; see Walla et al. 2011) has access to this knowledge. In fact, the advent of sophisticated brain imaging methods has facilitated demonstration of the existence of various apparently non-conscious brain processes that guide human behaviour within both affective and the cognitive domains, even as certain aspects like affective changes often reflect brain changes that are not easily measured with fMRI (functional Magnet Resonance Imaging) approaches which require precise timing, but can be dramatically envisioned with PET (Positron Emission Tomography) scans that are not subject to rigid temporal constrains (Damasio, et al., 2000). In any event, there is more to emotion than subjective feelings, with many unconscious underpinnings, and it is important to better understand all levels. For many issues we simply need to look inside the box that processes all the information, for only a fraction of this turns into responses that can be measured via self report. Also, since it is well-established that cognitive and affective processes are often in a see-saw balance (Liotti & Panksepp, 2004), in fMRI environments that use discrete emotional-cognitive stimuli (e.g., facially expressive pictures), it is often best to instruct subjects to experience their feelings in the scanner without reporting on their internals states, and then to harvest subjective reports after the brain-imaging session is completed; through such procedures, it is clear that affective changes are typically directly related more to subcortical arousals, and inversely correlated with cortical ones (Northoff, et al., 2009).

Our goal here is to share relevant research to highlight some of the points already made. Besides introducing some of the key findings of various neuroimaging methods and proposing a clear and distinct use of the terms "emotion" and "affective processing", we also entertain clear ways to separate cognitions from affective processing and emotion (although a lot of interaction occurs). Mauss and Robinson (2009) finished their abstract by concluding that experiential, physiological, and behavioural measures are all relevant to understanding emotion and that they cannot be assumed to be interchangeable. We agree and add that a full-blown emotion is the result of physiological activity—both of brain and body--which we call **affective processing**, but that affective processing alone does not yet qualify for an emotion. In animals, emotions are evident in distinct behavioural displays, along with complex changes, in which all relevant components are already organized at subcortical levels, along with some form of primal affective states as monitored by the rewarding and punishing properties of those circuits (Panksepp, 1998). However, those low levels of the brain do not elaborate the many cognitive processes that always accompany emotional arousal in humans. The distinction between affective processing and emotion shall be the most important basis of the proposed emotion model (see final section of paper). Here affect is seen as the raw valenced aspect of emotional arousals, while the concept of emotion remains more indeterminated. Although it has traditionally included everything, from diverse cognitive, behavioural and autonomic associates to very subtle and diverse feeling states, we suspect that it is time to re-simplify this term, so it does not cause as much mischief as it has, ever since Darwin brought it to the scientific table.

2. Further background

The idea that the primary purpose of the brain is to produce some sort of movement fits the notion of the evolutionary process called cephalisation, the creation of a separate specialised head enclosing a central brain. As organisms developed limbs for locomotion, their body shape also began to change. The body took on a longitudinal forward-facing position and the sensory organs began to move to the front and/or develop at the front of the body, where first contact with new environmental stimuli would be made. Since a major attribute of the brain's overall functioning is to process sensory input, it seems obvious that having sensory organs at the front of the body and the brain close by is a big advantage. Thus, by simply observing the stages of evolution it can be said that the movements allowed our brain to produce complex action patterns that reflect various within-brain processes, including both unconscious and phenomenally experienced ones. It is always hard to imagine such major evolutionary steps, but doing so tremendously facilitates our understanding of how the brain works. It also affords discourse sufficient complexity to reduce the likelihood that investigators working at different evolutionary levels indulge in seemingly substantive but often empty controversies.

An example may help here: In trying to understand both unconscious and phenomenally experienced action tendencies, it is critical to recognize that an ancestral urge to move forward and approach resources—e.g., a reward SEEKING system—has both unconscious and experienced brain functions. This urge was built into the brain early in brain evolution (i.e., it is a primary-process) shared in basic form—as "a major brain reward system"--by all vertebrates; it is experienced as a diffuse positive enthusiasm to pursue resources (the felt component is inferred from the rewarding property of this system, even in the absence of higher brain functions as in decorticate animals), but it is one that has remained linked to the emergence and refinement of sophisticated action routines permitted by cephalization and hence ever more sophisticated cognitive capacities to guide behaviour (Panksepp, 1998; Panksepp & Moskal, 2008). It looks like a series of such fundamental affective systems govern the basic "secondary process" learning and memory functions of the brain that, to the best of our knowledge, operate totally unconsciously (affective memory). The harvesting of memories about the world (semantic and episodic memory) provides opportunities for the highest regions of the brain, whose functions are best visualized with modern brain imaging—from fMRI to MEG (Magnetoencephalography) procedures—to generate diverse higher mental functions, many of which reflect subconscious processing while some appear as experienced thoughts within our minds (conscious processing).

Now, let's take a closer look at our brain's function. We will especially focus on the processing of external information entering the brain via sensory organs. Put simply, there are two major aspects of any sensory input that update our brain with the conditions of the world outside in order to adapt behavior. One aspect refers to detailed semantic information, i.e. "What is it that I see through my eyes, hear through my ears, or detect with any of my other sensory systems?" That aspect reflects the rationale or cognitive domain. The other aspect is not detailed at all and refers to rather abstract information, i.e. "Is what I see through my eyes, hear through my ears, or detect through any of my other sensory systems supporting my life or is it detrimental?" That aspect reflects the affective domain, which is pre-cognitive in the sense that internal neuro-affective emotional states intrinsically guide action tendencies since they arise from the neural circuitries of instinctual emotional action tendencies. By the way, the sense of olfaction might be the modality that first delivered the mammalian brain (or maybe even the brains of all vertebrates) with external information leading to strong affective processing (see Walla , 2008; Walla & Deecke, 2010). In general, affective state processing appears to be more primitive than cognitive information processing and might have evolved as a first "evaluation system" guiding behavior on the basis of more precise external information processing, slightly above the unconscious behaviors that reflect reflexes and other completely automatic processes (e.g., cardiac dynamics) that proceed without any obligatory mental contents.

However, we do not wish to suggest that automatic processes are always unconscious since at the foundational level we have "instinctual" systems that are more than reflexive in that there are large-scale systems that guide dynamic instinctual behavioral routines that already *evaluate* the environment for conditions that support or detract from survival. They may exist without any sophisticated cognitive mind, but may already have developed the capacity for affective experiential capacities as a primal way to steer behavior and guide learning based on incoming sensory inputs—such arousals feel good and bad in various ways, and promote basic learning mechanisms (e.g., operant conditioning; affective memory). If certain life events lead to bad sensory feelings such as pain, some of these systems promote various escape and avoidance behaviors that reduce those feelings (by withdrawal from negative affects). If life events lead to good feelings, there are intrinsic systems that are well positioned to increase those feelings (via various approach behaviors).

These low-level instinctual-integrative systems are the ones we call intrinsic primary-processes. Thus, we already have distinct sensory-affects and emotional affects at the very foundations of the mind and brain (Panksepp & Biven, 2012; Solms & Panksepp, 2012). Further, both of these types of primal affects are modulated by bodily state—e.g., hunger and thirst. The way we can determine such affective states of mind in animals is by direct evaluation of the rewarding and punishing properties of artificial arousal of emotional action systems as with direct electrical deep brain stimulation (DBS) (Panksepp, 1998, 2005).

The topmost, tertiary-process, levels of our brain's function can thus be extended to conjoint *affective* and *cognitive* processing. Panksepp's Affective Neuroscience (1998) framework states that the affective aspects of a stimulus are processed before and independently of any cognitive aspects, given their more ancient role in decision-making. This makes sense given that key structures engaged in the generation of primal emotions are found to be mainly subcortical (see later)—caudo-rostrally areas such as periaqueductal gray, hypothalamus, ventral striatum, bed nucleus of the stria terminalis, dorsomedial thalamus, septum and amygdala, as well as at higher levels in regions such as cingulate cortex, insula, and orbitofrontal cortex. Although some have posited that the amygdala lies at the heart of affective life (LeDoux, 1996), while others have bestowed a primary role on the insula (Craig, 2009), it is quite clear that humans with both of these brain regions completely burned out by brain diseases have vibrantly rich affective lives (for most compelling case study and relevant literature, see Damasio, et al., 2012).

In contrast, most explicit cognitive processing is heavily neo-cortical. Additionally, subcortical structures are evolutionarily older than cortical structures, meaning that the first elements of decision-making must have involved basic affective processing. Thus, older and faster are two distinctive features of affective processing versus cognitive processing. This has important consequences for the relationship between locomotion and cephalization. Moving forward means to continuously face different environments and it is of utmost importance to evaluate all new stimuli with respect to their survival value. Much of the psychomotor energy for this persistent urge of the nervous system is due to arousal of the mesolimbic SEEKING system (Ikemoto & Panksepp, 1999; Alcaro, et al., 2007, 2011; Panksepp & Moskal, 2008). At the primary process level (see Panksepp, 2011), it is more important to evaluate the survival value of external stimuli as well as internal states than to know what they actually are, giving affective information processing a more primary survival role than cognitive information processing. Further, affective processing needs to be sub-categorized into at least three levels of analysis: sensory affects (such as taste and olfaction), homeostatic affects (such as hunger and thirst mediated by bodily interoceptors), and emotional affects (the most subtle, and most important for psychiatric issues, which seem to arise from the intrinsic affective action schema of the brain).

3. Subcortical structures process non-conscious affective information

Most neuroimaging studies find that various subcortical and some cortical structures are involved in affective information processing. According to Tracy and Randles (2011), four key investigators in emotion research agree that "basic emotions" arise from activities in subcortical structures. In particular, Panksepp and colleagues (see Panksepp & Biven, 2012; Panksepp & Watt, 2011) assert that only subcortical structures house genetically determined, fixed emotional networks whose activities generate various rewarding and punishing states, while neocortex provides the necessary cognitive space to think about them. While all four scholars discussed by Tracy and Randles come up with slightly different sets of basic emotions, indicating there are still abundant ambiguities in the field, only one of the above is based on rigorous neuroscientific analysis of the underlying brain systems with DBS (e.g. Panksepp, 1992). In any event, all agree that emotions start with some kind of subcortical processing.

By far the most frequently noted subcortical structure is the well-known amygdala (one in each hemisphere). This structure is the size of a hazelnut and it has become the star in affective processing (to cite just a few key investigators: Halgren et al., 1978; LeDoux, 1993; Bechara et al., 1995; Adolphs et al., 1995; Calder et al., 1996). Many others also report that this structure is critically involved in affective information processing, although it does not seem to be essential for experienced affective feelings (Damasio, et al., 2012). While it seems obvious that increased activity in the amygdala is important for the learning of fear, it is wrong to assume that amygdala activity alone is enough for generating feelings of fear. In fact, it is more involved in the learned information processing related to fearful arousals, and much of that secondary-processing can be unconscious. In fact, it has been shown that amygdala activity as a consequence of visual negatively valenced stimulation occurs and changes behaviour even in the absence of conscious visual perception (e.g. Öhman, 2002). Morris et al. (1999) nicely demonstrated in an fMRI study that amygdala activity is also increased in case of unseen negative emotional information content (not consciously perceived visual stimuli). Another team of investigators titled their paper "Affective blindsight" (Hamm et al., 2003). They found startle reflex enhancement as a consequence of visual fear conditioning in a cortically blind patient. Their data suggest that visual subcortical pathways including the amygdala are sufficient to activate negatively valenced affective information processing in humans in the total absence of visual awareness.

From the idea that subcortical structures are the ones that process basic emotion-related information it is not far to the idea that affective processing happens outside of cognitive awareness. Some investigators have elaborate ideas about "unconscious emotion". Zajonc (2000) addressed the issue of non-conscious (or unconscious) emotions. For instance, in a book titled "The Nature of Emotion: Fundamental Questions" (edited by Ekman and Davison in 1994) he wrote an essay with the title "Evidence for non-conscious emotion". In 2003, Berridge and Winkielman report about evidence supporting the idea of genuinely unconscious emotion (particularly unconscious liking). The authors report about their findings that despite the absence of detectable subjective shifts in affective experiences, subliminally induced unconscious liking can influence concurrent consumption of a sweetened drink. After all that, we also believe that much unconscious processing occurs related to "emotion", but what's unconscious here should be labeled "affective information processing" and not "emotion", because emotion is not information processing, it is the output of it as we propose (see final section of this paper).

In 2000, Zajonc also proposed in an article provocatively entitled "Closing the debate over the independence of affect" that the separation of affective and cognitive neuroscience exists and makes sense. This gives Panksepp's "Affective Neuroscience" (1998) a stand-alone character and it might also support the notion to exclude any intrinsic cognitive aspects in an emotion definition. Cognition is a separate, parallel function, which of course can and does synergize with as well as interfere with affective information processing, but it adds little to see cognition as an intrinsic aspect of primary-process emotionality, while at a tertiary-process level, it clearly has a role. In any event, affective information processing can and certainly does influence cognition. Cognitive influences on affective processing are top-down, whereas affective influences on cognition are rather bottom-up. In some neuroimaging studies about "emotion" neural structures that have been shown to be involved in some sort of cognition have commonly been found to be active (Lindquist, et al., 2012). Unfortunately, such findings have been commonly interpreted as "cognitive aspects of emotion" it may be wiser to see them as distinct associated processes. It may well be that at some point in information processing, perhaps shortly before a decision is made, affective information merges with cognitive information. In this combination, both initially separate processes subserve decision-making. However, a clear distinction should be made and a clear line drawn.

4. Emotion through facial expression

Much of the human basic-emotion literature has focused on emotions elicited through facial expressions (e.g. Ekman et al., 1987; Izard, 1971; Tracy & Robins, 2008). There is considerable evidence showing that, for instance, a facial expression of disgust elicits brain activity in the observer's brains other than that evoked by a disgusting non-facial picture (Faces versus scenes; e.g. Sabatinelli et al., 2011). Unpublished electroencephalography (EEG) data of a diploma student supervised by Peter Walla show that pictures of natural scenes of different emotional categories elicit larger deviating event-related potentials (ERPs) between emotion categories than facial expressions of the same emotion categories. This is the case for early (below 200 ms) and for later (200 ms to 800 ms) time windows.

Narumoto et al. (2001) wrote a paper entitled "Attention to emotion modulates fMRI activity in the right superior temporal sulcus (STS). However, it is clear that they scanned their study participants while exposing them to facially expressive stimuli. Their finding was that the right STS, a structure that they found involved in face processing alone turned out to be more active in case of emotion attention. The point here is that a facial expression is an emotion of the person the face belongs to. The image of a facial expression is not necessarily in itself a matching affective stimulus such as the scene that elicited affect in the person demonstrating the facial expression. Again, imagine a disgusting scene versus a disgusted face. Let us call the difference "direct versus indirect affective information" (or first- and second-hand affective information). It instantly becomes clear that indirect affective information as communicated via facial expression can be misinterpreted and actually lead to different affective processing and a different emotion in the observer of a facial expression. Second-hand affective information is influenced (or biased) by all sorts of context-dependent information. For example, an angry facial expression can be the result of true primary-process anger, but it can equally likely be the result of tertiary-process victory ("DAMN IT, I WON!", see figure 1) and would thus be the result of positive affective information. It seems that context plays a crucial role in the higher-order perception of emotion as in human facial expressions, and much of the existing literature has never attempted to ferret out levels of control within the brain or mind that may reflect synergistic or distinct affective processes. That failure could have led to enormous and persistent controversies in human emotion research, especially when it comes to perennial debates between advocates of basic emotion theory, e.g., Paul Ekman and Cal Izard, and those who pursue constructivist agendas such as Lisa Feldman Barrett and Jim Russell (for a thorough discussion, see Lindquist, et al., 2012, and associated commentaries). On the other hand, in scenes context is always present eliciting affective processing and emotions more directly.

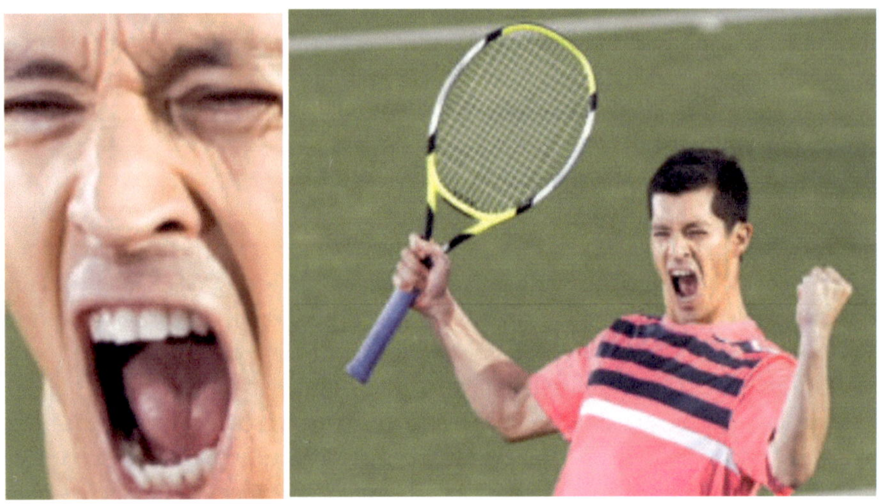

Figure 1. Left: facial expression alone looks like "anger" or "pain". Right: with context it turns into a quite positive and rewarding emotion communication (Game – Set – Match). iStockphoto.

5. Affective processing and self-reference

Self-reference might be critically involved in some specific emotion-related brain processes (Northoff et al., 2006; Garrett and Maddoc, 2006). The insular cortex has been suggested to be involved in processing self-referential information in a magnetoencephalography (MEG) (Walla et al., 2007) and an electroencephalography (EEG) study (Walla et al., 2008). In these studies, pairs of possessive pronouns and nouns (e.g. my pencil; his pencil) were used to provide controlled independent variables reflecting varying conditions of ownership. These were compared with a neutral condition (e.g. a pencil) with no personal reference. Two temporal time windows were found to demonstrate interesting effects. In an early time window, the investigators found brain activity elicited by both referenced conditions "my pencil" and "his pencil" to differ from the unreferenced, neutral condition (a pencil). Figure 2 shows MEG data reflecting this finding. In a later time window though, "my pencil" elicited different brain activity compared to "his pencil", a clear sign of self-referential information processing (Figure 3). Figure 4 provides localisation results leading to the insular cortex hypothesis.

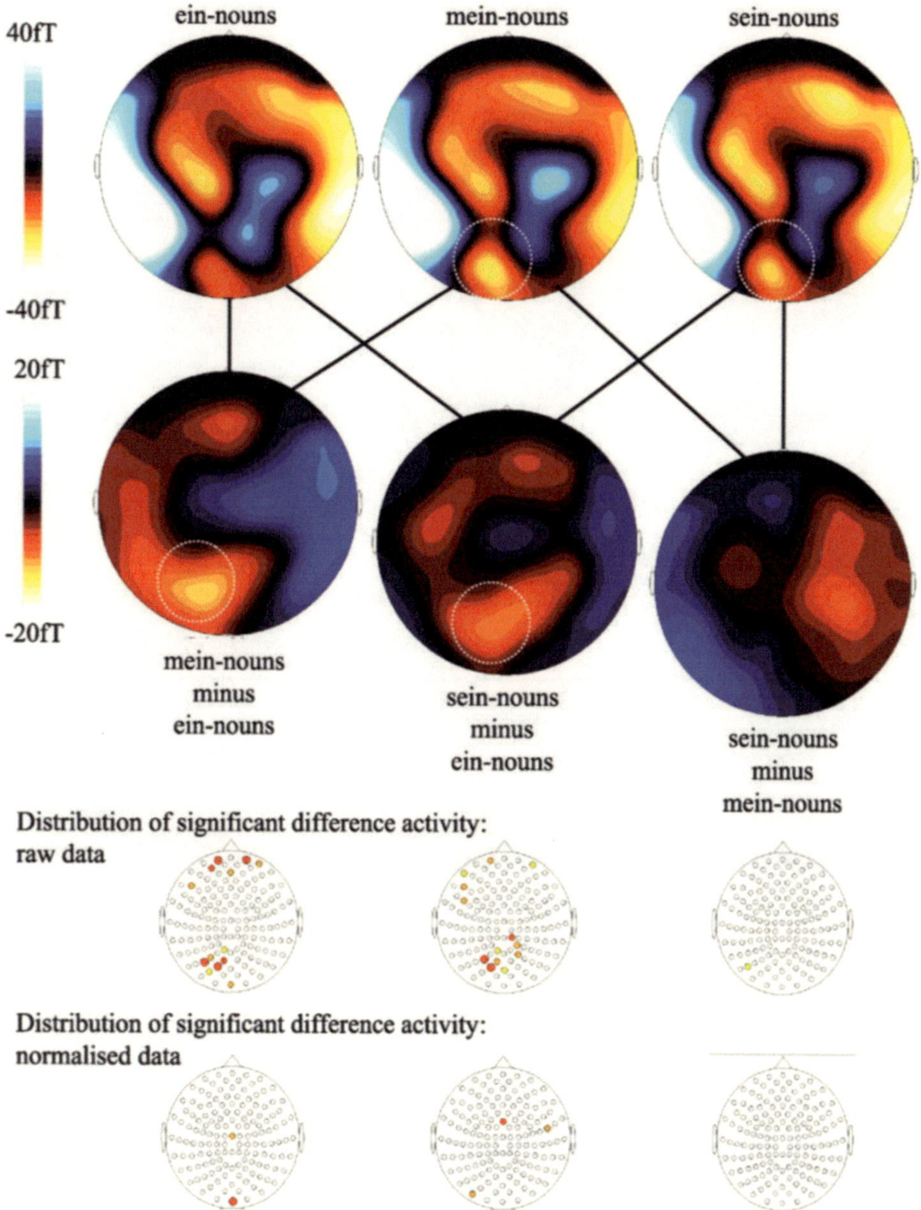

Figure 2. MEG maps. Early neurophysiological effect: MEG maps (magnetic field distributions) averaged across depth of word processing and across all study participants for the time interval from 200 to 300 ms after stimulus onset. First line: one map for each of the three conditions of pronoun ("ein" ("a"), "mein" ("my"), "sein" ("his")). Second line: difference magnetic field distributions related to comparisons (subtractions) between each possible pair of pronoun condition ("mein" vs. "ein", "sein" vs. "ein", "sein" vs. "mein"). Sensor areas where t-tests resulted in significant differences are marked

with a white dotted circle. Third line: t-maps showing the distribution of significant differences for each of the above-mentioned comparisons (raw data). Note that "mein" vs. "ein" and "sein" vs. "ein" both resulted in significant differences, whereas no differences occurred for the comparison "sein" vs. "mein". Fourth line: t-maps showing the distribution of significant differences for each of the above-mentioned comparisons (amplitude-normalized data). Note that hardly any differences occurred (adapted from Walla et al., 2007 with permission).

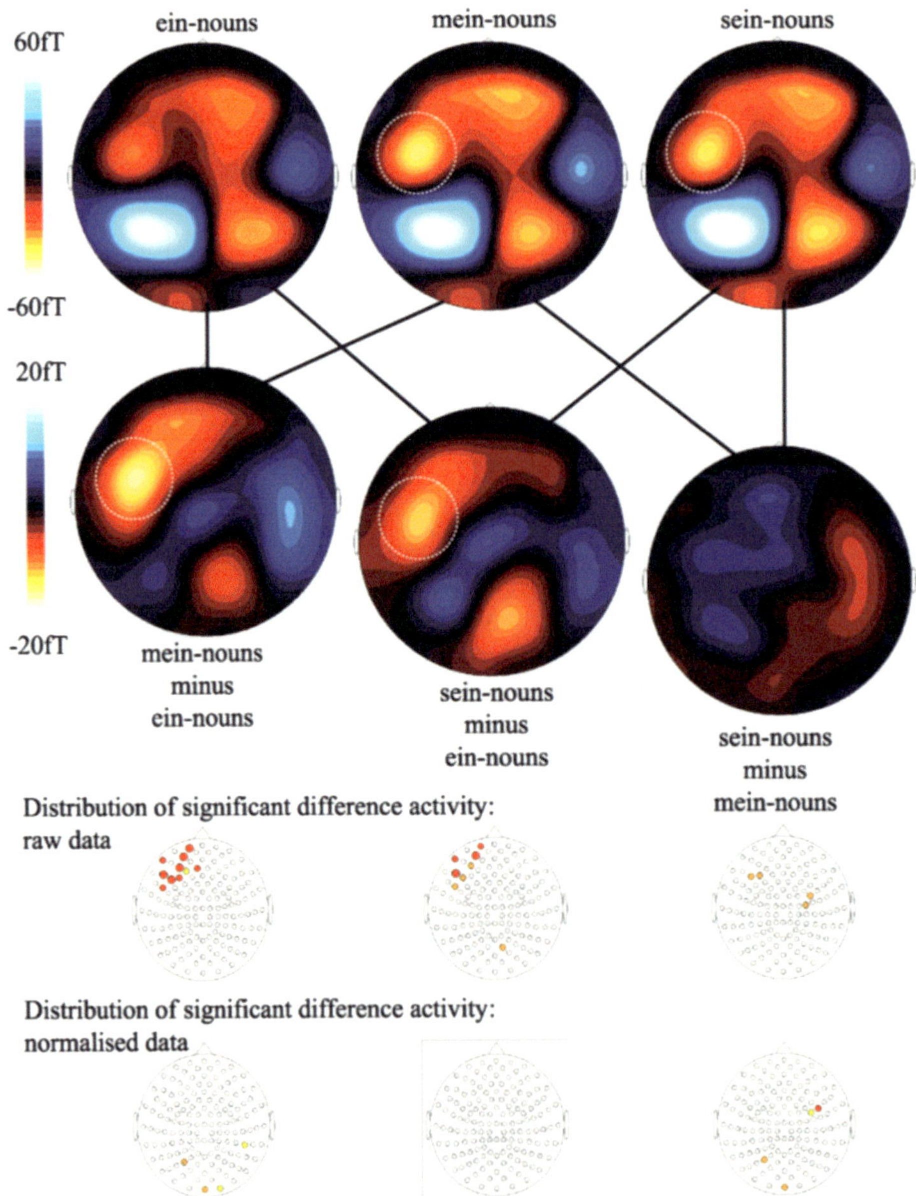

Figure 3. MEG maps. Later neurophysiological effect: MEG maps (magnetic field distributions) averaged across depth of word processing and across all study participants for the time interval from

500 to 800 ms after stimulus onset. First line: one map for each of the three conditions of pronoun ("ein" ("a"), "mein" ("my"), "sein" ("his")). Second line: difference magnetic field distributions related to comparisons (subtractions) between each possible pair of pronoun condition ("mein" vs. "ein", "sein" vs. "ein", "sein" vs. "mein"). Sensor areas where t-tests resulted in significant differences are marked with a white dotted circle. Third line: t-maps showing the distribution of significant differences for each of the above-mentioned comparisons (raw data). Note that "mein" vs. "ein" and "sein" vs. "ein" both resulted in significant differences. In addition, the comparison between "sein" and "mein" also resulted in significant differences at some of the sensor sites (no such differences were found during the early period of time). Fourth line: t-maps showing the distribution of significant differences for each of the above-mentioned comparisons (normalized data) (adapted from Walla et al., 2007 with permission).

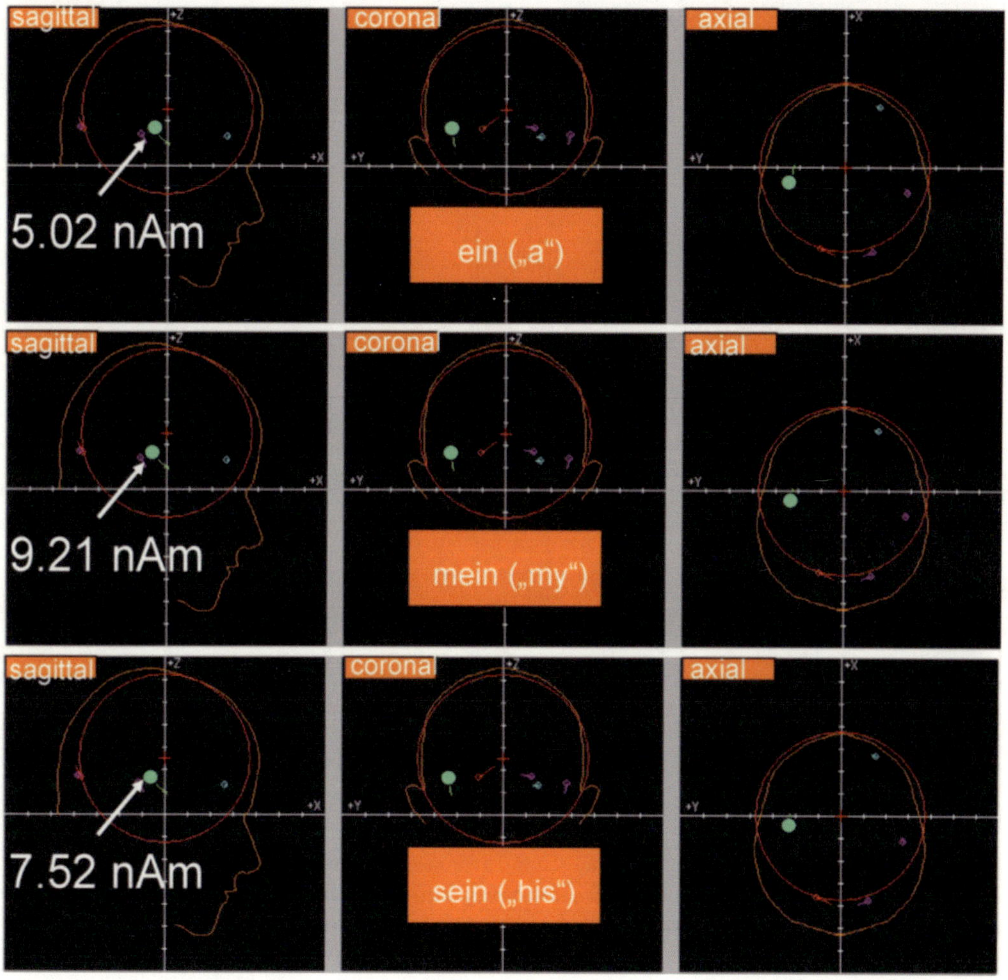

Figure 4. MEG source localisation results. Source localization for the later time range (500–800 ms): for the averaged data set (across 22 participants) the magnetic field distributions related to all three kinds of pronoun are displayed for a particular time point within the time window from 500 to 800 ms, which was found to include significant differences over left temporal and left fronto-temporal sensors depending on the kind of pronoun. The localized dipole in this respective region shows stronger brain activity as reflected by dipole strength (nA m) related to both personal pronouns compared to the

neutral pronoun (strongest activity in the "mein"("my") condition). The location of this dipole is interpreted as left temporal. Most likely it is the left insular cortex that is able to discriminate between self and other (adapted from Walla et al., 2007 with permission).

The above-mentioned EEG study by Walla et al. (2008) revealed very supportive similar findings. Together with the MEG findings the "multiple aspect theory" of self-awareness was created and the insular cortex was suggested to be critical for self-reference processing. In an independent EEG study by Herbert et al. (2011a), confirmative date were collected with respect to a self-other distinction (Figure 5), and these self-reference findings were even extended to the emotion domain. From 350 ms onwards, processing of self-related unpleasant words (e.g. my fear) elicited larger frontal negativity compared to unpleasant words that were related to the other (e.g. his fear) or that had no reference at all (e.g. the fear).

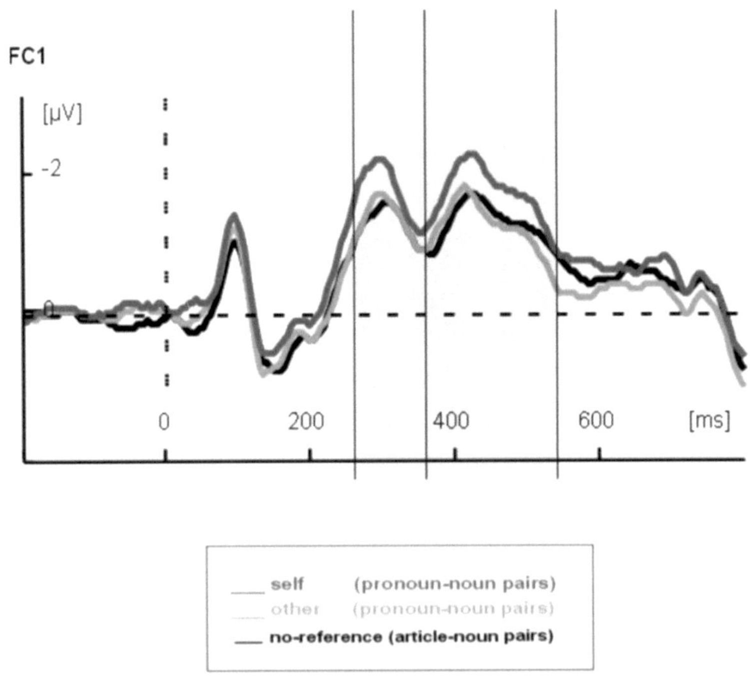

Figure 5. Main effects of self–other reference. Grand average ERP waveforms at posterior and anterior electrodes during reading of self- and other-related pronoun–noun pairs and non-referential article–noun pairs (adapted from Herbert et al., 2011a with author permission).

The results of a recent fMRI study by Herbert et al. (2011b) revealed the neural structures that mediate self-reference in emotional conditions. The study demonstrates that the activity level of the amygdalae and the insular cortex depends on stimulus reference (as described below). The authors further conclude that brain structures implicated in affective and self-related processing might be crucial prerequisites for a subjective experience of emotions.

Reading unpleasant words increased activity in the amygdala and the insular cortex regardless of self, other or no reference (Figure 6 and 7). This confirms the role of these two structures in processing negatively valenced stimuli (negative affective information processing). Interestingly, positively valenced nouns preferentially increased amygdala and insular cortex activity in case of self-reference compared to other or no reference (Figure 6 and 7). In addition, pleasant nouns were rated more pleasant in case of self-reference, which mirrors underlying neurophysiology on the behavioural level.

Taken together, the above-mentioned studies highlight that "emotion"-related brain activity begins at the subcortical level (section 3.), and that self-reference seems to play a specific role for at least some of emotion-related information (section 4.).

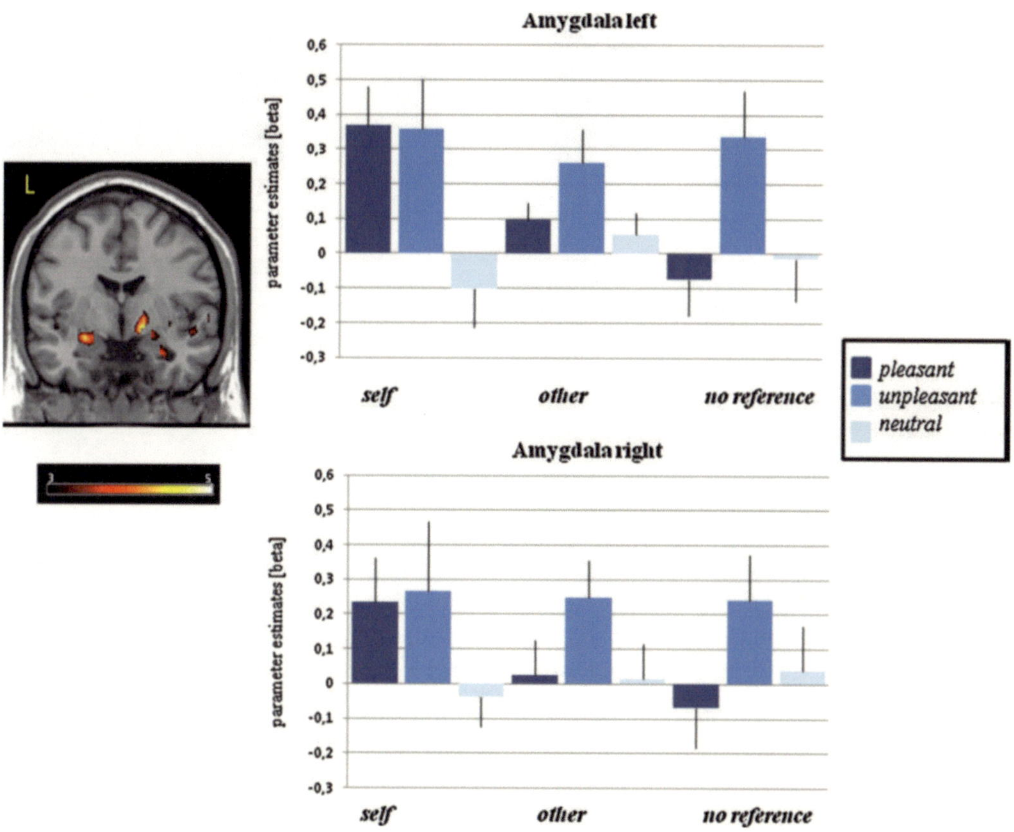

Figure 6. Right panel: Mean signal changes (mean and standard errors) in the left and right amygdala during processing of emotional and neutral self-related, other-related and unreferenced nouns. The picture on the left (left panel) displays significant changes in the amygdala during processing of self-related emotional nouns, $p < 0.005$. Color bars represent T-values. (adapted from Herbert et al., 2011b with permission).

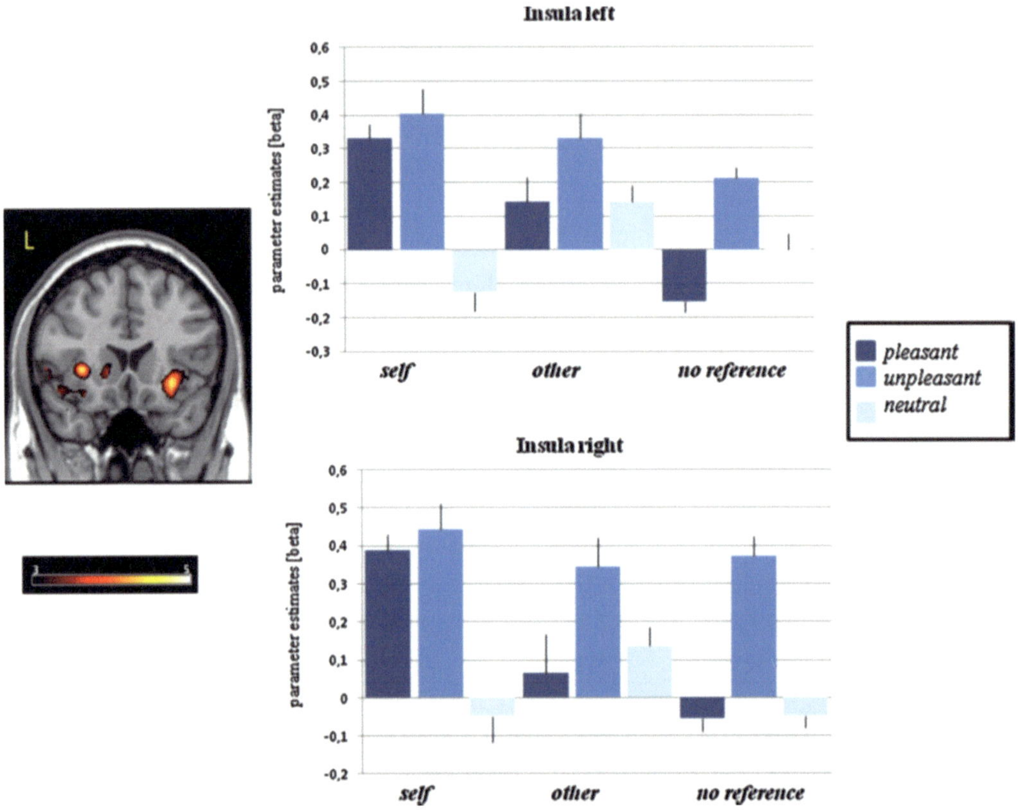

Figure 7. Right panel: Mean signal changes (mean and standard errors) in the left and right insula during processing of emotional and neutral self-related, other-related and unreferenced nouns. The picture on the left (left panel) displays significant changes in the insula during processing of self-related emotional nouns, $p < 0.005$. Color bars represent T-values. (adapted from Herbert et al. (2011b) with permission).

6. Problems and inconsistencies

Because of the many levels of control of all emotion-related processes within the neuroaxis, scholars from different disciplines discussing emotion issues easily misinterpret what others say. Some feel that emotions arise from higher brain regions where cognitions and affects intermingle; some think that discussions of emotions in animals must be constrained to the behavioral level only (LeDoux, 1996, 2012); yet others think that emotions are epiphenomena and can have no causal influence on the control of behavior. The view of too many behavioral neuroscientists - that there is no possibility of a sound science of experienced affective processing (feeling) - avoid the most robust evidence against their beliefs: Almost everywhere in the brain emotional behavior can be induced with DBS and can serve as "rewards" and "punishments" in the control of behavior. If behaviorist skeptics wish to have it their way, their responsibility is to list the diverse "rewards" and "punishments" which control human behavior that are not experienced in our species. In our experience, none have yet to be put forward. And from this vantage, experienced affective processing (feeling) has to be defined as much in neural terms as in psychological/verbal ones—for the confusion exists primarily at the later level.

If one is after a definition of emotion it turns out that almost as many definitions exist as textbooks are available. Just as some scholars would call the engine of a car "car", while others would call driving a hunk of sculpted metal a "car" without realizing that the engine is essential for driving, but it actually is a separate thing deserving its own label. Additionally, many original articles in emotion research report about emotions elicited in observers after presentations of facial expressions. Does a facial expression really elicit the same emotion-related activity in the observer's brain as the one that caused the facial expression in the person the face belongs to? It seems that the answer is, no it doesn't (see Sabatinelli et al., 2011; Britton et al., 2005, 2006). Looking at 157 neuroimaging studies, Sabatinelli found that only the amygdala demonstrated consistent activity independent from stimulus category (face or scene). Ideally, the science community needs a more specific definition of emotion in order to make consistent progress and to promote research communication within and across disciplines.

In the frame of this chapter we tried to consistently use the terms "affective information" and "emotion". In the original articles these terms were used interchangeably and even mixed with further terms including cognitive aspects. As mentioned in the introduction, we want to generate awareness about the inconsistent and broad use in particular of the term emotion. Feeling the urge to do something about this is not new. We are not the first to address this issue and we are certainly not alone. In 1981, Kleinginna and Kleinginna created awareness about the wide variety of approaches to labeling emotion by providing a list of no less than 92 emotion definitions. They classified these definitions into 11 categories depending on their theoretical basis. Some of these categories are based on subjective aspects of emotion (affective and cognitive), others on external stimuli, or on physiological mechanisms. Some are based on expressive behavior, on functional consequences or on disruptive or adaptive effects. Others are based on the multi-aspect nature of emotional phenomena and some distinguish emotion from other processes or emphasize the overlap between emotion and motivation. Finally, the authors found some statements that question the usefulness of the entire "emotion" concept. No doubt, the variety is big. Kleinginna and Kleinginna also stated that more recent definitions are as inconsistent as the earlier ones. This reflects the state of research up to the year 1981.

In 1995, LeDoux emphasized in the abstract of a paper entitled "Emotion: Clues from the Brain" that scientists at that time have not been able to reach a consensus about what emotion is and what place emotion should have in a theory of mind and behavior. Some emotions were considered more basic than others. To what extent do emotional responses contribute to emotional experiences? What can we say about interactions between cognition and emotion and finally how important are conscious versus unconscious processes in emotion research. A few years later, Cabanac (2002) mentioned that there is still no consensus in the literature on a definition of emotion and even today, a decade later, not much progress has been made. Perhaps, due to the appealing possibilities of neuroimaging methods researchers were spoiled by eye-catching colored brain images that looked nice and were easy to sell, but after all they neglected to make progress in terms of identifying a better concept of emotion and providing a more specific evidence-based definition. Fed by multi-used terms for brain functions that occur from sensory input to actual behavior, ongoing research is obviously not focused on clarifying terminological issues around "emotion", so semantic confusions prevail. To date, we still lack a useful definition and a distinct and common terminology of related functions.

However, we would suggest that a nested hierarchical view of both brain and mind may go a long way toward clarity, in that discourse in the area, especially as related to human emotions, has been primarily at what we call the tertiary process level. If we consider that primary-process analysis, best pursued in animal models (Panksepp, 1998, 2011a,b), provides the most robust evidence for cross-mammalian genetically-ingrained infrastructures for emotionality, not only in terms of behavior but raw phenomenally significant affective experiences, we may need to cultivate new ways to discuss the full complexity of the brain and mind (Solms & Panksepp, 2012). The single fact that highlights the affective phenomenology that arises from these ancient circuits is the simple fact that wherever in the brain investigators have evoked, with deep brain stimulation, coherent instinctual expressions of emotional behaviors, those central states always serve as rewards and punishments in the control of simple learned approach and escape behaviors (even in the absence of neocortex). Since all major "rewards" and "punishments" that control human behavior are also experienced affectively, we have no good reasons to conclude, other than pervasive biases promoted by long-standing beliefs, that the primitive subcortical foundations of emotional integrations that are experienced as affects cannot be cognitively interpreted by our brains. We think they can, but this requires a new marriage between animal and human research, where one recognizes how powerfully cognitive aspects of mind can influence affective functions and vice versa. How those findings relate to the abundant correlative data from human brain imaging is an open issue (Lindquist et al., 2012), but one needs to conceptualize and evaluate the cognitive and affective issues independently for the reciprocal interactions can be huge (Liotti and Panksepp, 2004; Northoff, et al., 2009).

An informative review paper by Phan et al. (2002) summarizing 55 Neuroimaging studies (Positron Emission Tomography (PET) and functional Magnet Resonance Imaging (fMRI)) nicely demonstrates that authors label "emotion" almost anything that happens in the brain without discriminating between affective processing, actual subjective experiences and other aspects (Figure 8). Phan et al. stated as one of the inclusion criteria that only studies about "higher-order mental processes of emotion" were entered in their analysis, while excluding lower-order processes including "sensory or motor processes, such as gustatory/olfactory or pain induction". This distinction together with the wide distribution of relevant brain areas highlights that emotion-related brain processing does have many aspects, but many traditional distinctions do not really help to better understand them nor do they help to better define emotion. In fact, many facets of the current debate about the nature of emotions continue to contribute to the many confusions that have long characterized this field (for a many examples, and suggested solutions, see Lindquist, et al., 2012).

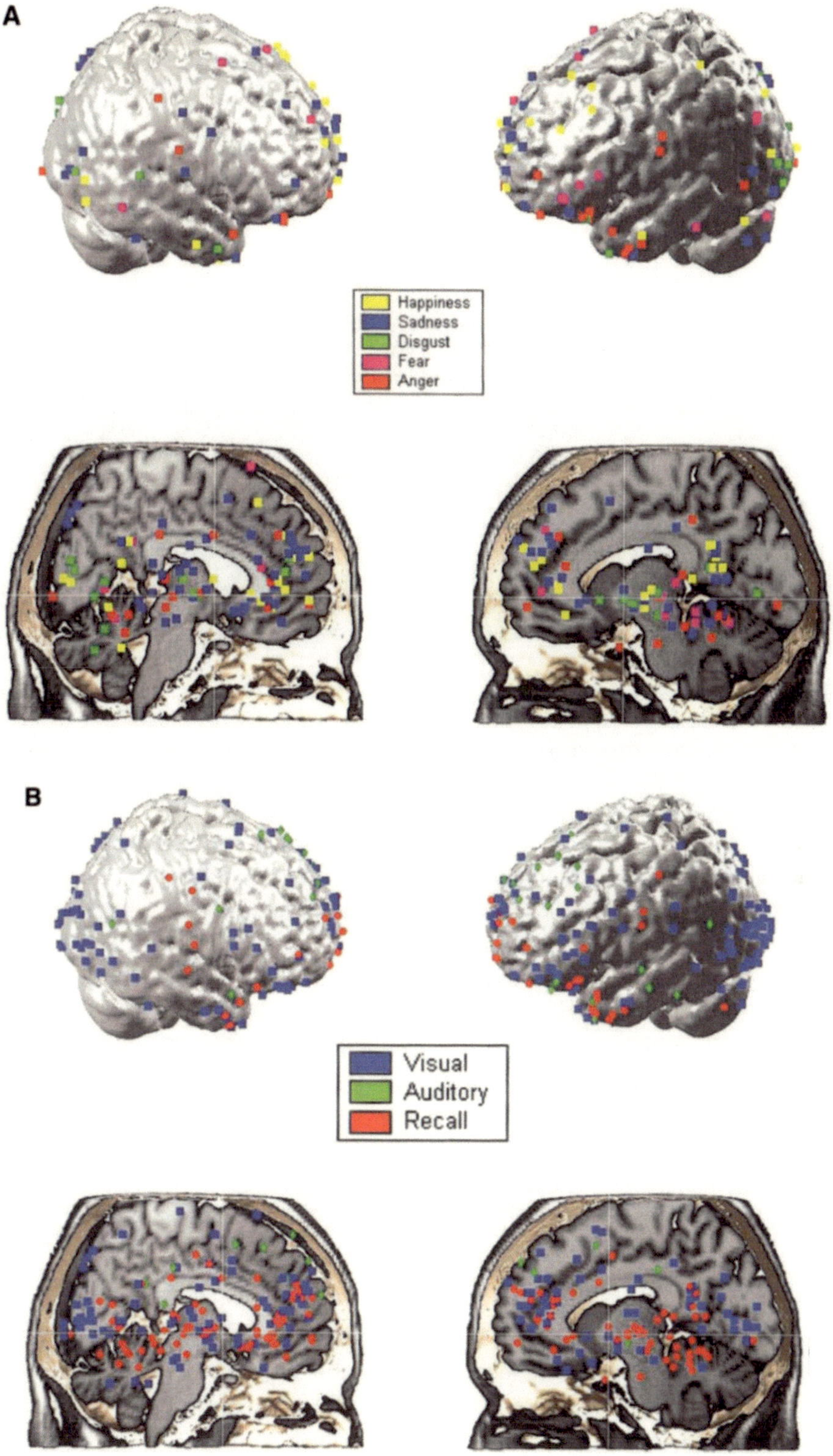
A
Happiness
Sadness
Disgust
Fear
Anger
B
Visual
Auditory
Recall

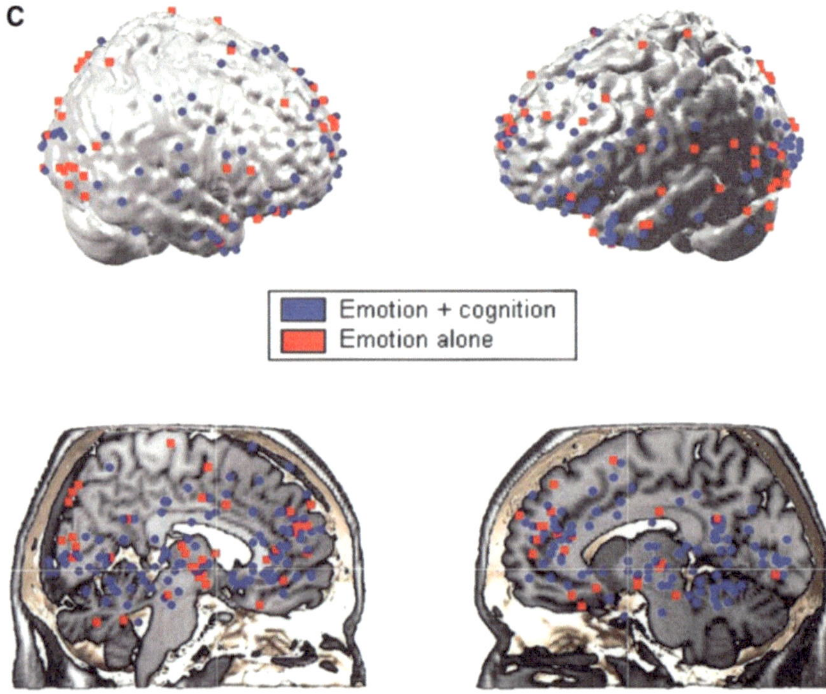

Figure 8. Phan et al. (2002) study: Overlay of neuroimaging findings from emotion studies showing emotion-relevant brain areas. (A) Activation foci: Individual emotion. (B) Activation foci: Induction method. (C) Activation foci: Cognitive demand. Adapted from Phan et al. (2002) with permission.

Too many chefs spoil the soup and too many scholars from different disciplines spoil the definition of emotion. For cognition, the sibling of affective information processing (both system are meant to support behaviour adaptation), you can say that it basically means "thinking", but breaking emotion down to a single term seems to be a rather difficult challenge. The reason for that is because emotion is the output and not the processing. If you place affective information processing on the level of cognitive information processing you could say that affective processing means "evaluating". In this chapter, it is suggested that the term emotion be reserved for only the behavioral aspects of it. After all, the Latin word emotion means to *move out*. It is about movement and movement equals behavior (in terms of neurobiology). The alternative is that emotion be simply seen as a class-identifier—an umbrella concept—that includes all the major aspects that are traditionally subsumed by this concept, namely the behavioral, autonomic-physiological, neural, cognitive and affective attributes. The reason we suggest the more minimalist solution is that the broader concept has led to so much trouble already, and at this stage of history we find many people talking past each other (as is well summarized in Lindquist, et al., 2012).

This would allow the experiential issues to be discussed more cogently without the excess historical baggage that now clutters the field and continually impedes clear discourse. If we were to reserve the term "emotion" to the visually evident behavioral displays, and discussed affective states independently at several distinct levels—e.g., the primal affective-experiential level, the secondary-process learning level, and the tertiary-process thoughtful cognitive level, we may be able to disentangle the conceptual Gordian Knot that is the major current historical dilemma of the field. If we do this, we can envision the study of affect related cognitive information-processing to highlight many of the unique properties of the affective life in humans, and the many ancestral affective value schemata apparently shared homologously in all mammals (maybe even all vertebrates) to provide a level of fundamental psychological analysis that is best pursued constitutionally and causally in animal models of emotionality. This would still leave the many important autonomic-visceral arousals that accompany emotions as a field that can be equally illuminated by human and animal research. Such an approach would also allow for several different affects and perhaps emotions to occur simultaneously as a result of one set of external stimuli, affective stimuli.

7. The proposed Emotion-Model

The proposed Emotion-Model (figure 9) follows the idea that simpler schemes are better than complex ones, especially in the early phases of investigation, where we still are despite thousands of published papers. Our model gives the ambiguous term "emotion" a distinct place (and meaning) rather than using it interchangeably for various different processes that should all have their own separate labels. We were inspired by numerous neuroimaging studies (e.g. especially Damasio et al., 2000), which mainly demonstrated the engagement of subcortical structures in processing of affectively experienced states. We follow Panksepp's idea that "emotions" have their behavioural-action roots deep in the brain, and they also generate raw feelings, and label the roots "affective processing". We also accept that the lower levels of processing are strongly influenced by higher brain functions which are most effectively studied in humans (e.g, Liotti & Panksepp, 2004; Northoff, et al., 2006; Lindquist, et al., 2012). Because the foundational structures for emotionality are old in evolutionary terms and because it is often claimed that conscious experiences rely on cortical structures, we believe that "emotions", as behaviors, all have an unconscious origin, while at the same time, through some kind of poorly understood emergent "field dynamics" those emotion-related systems provide a foundation for the origin of raw affective feelings. Their origin is ultimately rooted in primal affective action routines as well as higher affective information processing. Still, the first level of affective information processing, as reflected in basic mechanisms of learning and memory is unconscious by nature. It does not always promote emotional displays, while still processing stimulus-related life supportive or detrimental aspects. In other words, the intermediate secondary-process level that lies between our lower and higher psychological functions may help parse action patterns in space and time, and thereby provide more discrete pieces of information for higher brain processing. Many human emotions are possible consequences of such unconscious processing of affective states into more discrete components that are discrete motor expressions in one way or another. They occur in humans and certainly in various other nonhuman mammals. It may even be that such affective processing without creating any new emotional reactions occurs in some if not all lower vertebrates. In humans, such intermediate levels of affective processing provide enormous amounts of new information that is grist for thought, as well as the generation of enormous affective and emotional nuances.

The behavioural aspects of emotions (or expressive aspects) were highlighted by several authors. Even Darwin focussed on the expressive nature of an emotion rather than anything else, although he never denied the affective power of emotions. We now know more about the underlying processes that lead to an emotion, and what we can derive from the evidence is that not all affective processes (especially sensory and homeostatic ones) necessarily lead to emotion responses, although they guide our behaviour on the basis of evaluating life supportive or detrimental aspects of information representing the outer world. If these processes do not lead to emotions and also not to feelings, which are experienced affective processes they remain non-conscious and are thus a type of incidental encoding, which we call here incidental affective encoding.

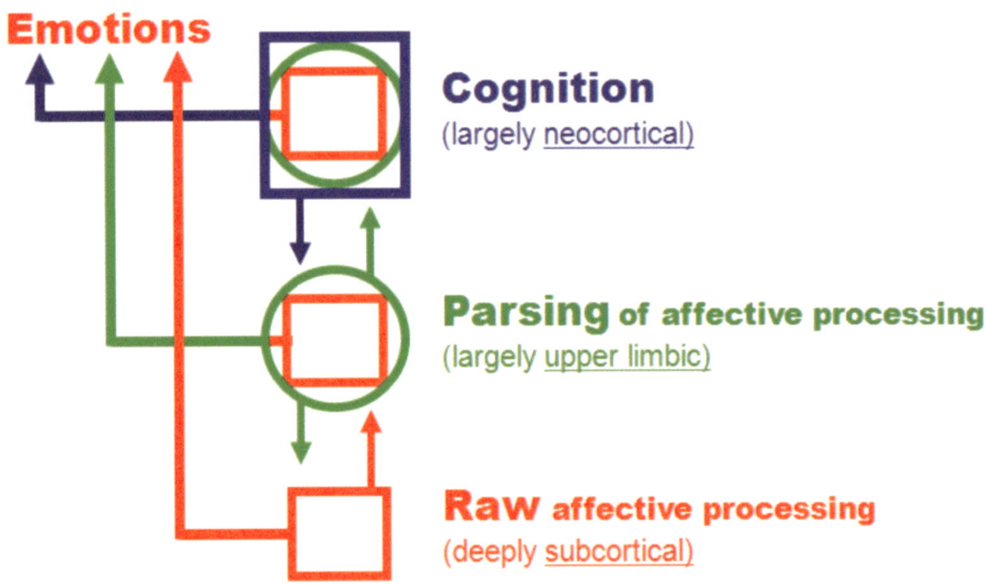

Figure 9. The proposed emotion model. Emotions are consequences of raw affective processing. They can be modified by information of higher order processes. Thus, raw affective information is able to elicit more than just one emotion, while these multiple emotions can even be differently valenced. However, affective processing also occurs in the absence of emotion generation. Finally, emotions are principally independent from cognition. Adapted from Solms and Panksepp (2012).

To summarise the proposed Emotion-Model, an emotion is always caused by implicit affective information processing. Even emotional displays in humans are thus the result of affective information processing. Affective information processing in humans typically evaluates the world outside and only sometimes, when certain intrinsic types of within-brain action readiness schema are aroused, create both emotional responses and emotional feelings. It may well be that the crucial factor for creating an emotion and/or a feeling as a result of affective processing is deep "self reference" as it may occur in brain regions as deep as the PAG (Panksepp, 1998) as well as higher order "self reference" as it may occur in the insular cortex (Walla et al., 2007; Herbert et al., 2011b) and various medial cortical zones (Northoff, et al., 2006).

"Emotion" research is a field with wide implications. Basic researchers, clinicians, product developers and also advertisers and marketers – they all deal with emotion, yet they don't seem to bother too much about the fact that one term – emotion – is in use to explain a whole complex chain of brain processes and perhaps different functions and/or sub-functions. The present multi-tiered evolutionary model that we propose here may help to guide scientific inquiries and explain scientific findings in more coherent, and hopefully understandable ways. It must be noted that most other animals do not have such massive higher reflections of cognitively experienced affective processing, so in them instinctual emotional behaviours may veridically reflect corresponding affective states (Panksepp, 1998, 2011a,b). Thus, animal research may help illuminate the subcortical emotional and affective infrastructures of human minds that are comparatively inaccessible through human research. An example of how this may promote understanding of human emotional responses is currently well-represented in the emerging field of neuroeconomics (Knutson & Greer, 2008) as well as consumer neuroscience, where intuition, or in other words the well known "gut-feelings", are in discussion as implicit affective processes, perhaps merged with non-conscious cognitions. For instance, startle reflex modulation is considered to be a methodological approach that allows to quantify affective information processing in the human brain (e.g. Walla et al., 2010; Walla et al., 2011; Geiser et al., 2011; Grahl et al., 2012).

Our final statement relates to the idea that affective information processing is adaptive and supports the fitness of an organism as usually seen from an evolutionary perspective (see Gross, J.J., 1999). We believe that at least in humans this is not always the case, since the primary-process subcortical networks for affective processing emerged long before the human neocortex, which permits self-reflective thoughtfulness about ones affective feelings. It may well be that affective information processing and emotions do play an adaptive role, but obviously they can be life threatening as in cases of severe depression. Depressions are assumed to have affective origins, closely related to various primary-process affective systems (Coenen, et al., 2011; Panksepp & Watt, 2011). They can cause enormous life problems if not adequately dealt with. Perhaps, this issue often does not relate to affective processing alone, but often occurs as a result of affective processing associated with "internal information" such as information stored in episodic memory, which can lead to ruminative dwelling on one's emotional problems.

If so, psychotherapy without concurrent use of optimal medications may not be as effective as with the use of affectively appropriate medications, which can now be developed through the use of animal models that respect and study the emotion related feelings of other animals (e.g., Burgdorf, et al., 2011; Panksepp, 2012). Indeed, if the "primary affective processing" substrates have been sensitized (e.g., elevated responsivity of the FEAR system in chronic anxiety and PTSD), then pharmacological somatic approaches may need to be implemented promptly to alleviate distress. Since such circuit changes are not easily monitored in individual clients, it may be judicious to assume such changes may have transpired in the underlying primal emotional substrates, and evaluate whether modest doses of appropriate medications can facilitate psychotherapeutic interventions. The Emotion-Model as proposed here does not yet include a full discussion of optimal psychotherapeutic aspects. However, the stratified emotion model we have been working with (Figure 9) highlights how higher and lower aspects of affective information processing may need to be envisioned for the generation of a comprehensive model (for further development of this nested-hierarchical model, see Northoff, et al., 2011; Panksepp, 2011). We simply offer this chapter as an introductory start. The model will be further developed and future investigations will show whether the suggested hierarchical structure can accommodate the fuller complexity of human affective information processing, its accompanying affective states and accompanying emotional responses.

Author details

Peter Walla
School of Psychology, University of Newcastle,
Center for Translational Neuroscience and Mental Health, Australia

Jaak Panksepp
Department of VCAPP, College of Veterinary Medicine, Washington State University, USA

8. References

Alcaro, A., Huber, R., & Panksepp, J. (2007). Behavioral functions of the mesolimbic dopaminergic system: An affective neuroethological perspective. *Brain Research Reviews, 56*, 283–321.

Alcaro, A. & Panksepp, J. (2011). The SEEKING mind: primal neuro-affectie substrates for appetitive incentive states and their pathological dynamics in addictions and depression. Neuroscience & Biobehavioral reviews, 35(9): 1805-20.

Adolphs, R., Tranel, D., Damasio, H., and Damasio, A. R. 1995. Fear and the human amygdala. J. Neurosci. 15: 5879–5891.

Barrett, Mesquita, et al. (2011). "Context in Emotion Perception." Current Directions in Psychological Science 20(5): 286-290.

Bechara, A., Tranel, D., Damasio, H., Adolphs, R., Rockland, C., and Damasio, A. R. (1995). Double dissociation of conditioning and declarative knowledge relative to the amygdala and hippocampus in humans. Science 269: 1115–1118

Berlin, H.A. (2011). The neural basis of the dynamic unconscious (with commentaries). *Neuropsychoanalysis, 13*, in press.

Berridge, K.C., Winkielman, P. (2003). What is an unconscious emotion? (The case for unconscious "liking"). Cognition and Emotion, 17(2): 181-211.

Britton, J.C., Phan, K.L., Taylor, S.F., Welsh, R.C., Berridge, K.C., and Liberzon, I. (2005). Neural correlates of social and non-social emotions: an fMRI study. Neuroimage, 31(1):397-409.

Britton, J.C., Taylor, S.F., Berridge, K.C., Mikels, J.A., Liberzon, I. (2006). Differential subjective and psychophysiological responses to socially and nonsocially generated emotional stimuli. Emotion 6(1):150-155.

Burgdorf, J., Panksepp, J., & Moskal, J. R. (2011). Frequency-modulated 50kHz ultrasonic vocalizations: a tool for uncovering the molecular substrates of positive affect. Neurosci Biobehav Rev, 35(9): 1831-1836.

Cabanac, M. (2002). What is emotion? Behavioural Processes 60: 69-83.

Calder, A. J., Young, A. W., Rowland, D., Perrett, D. I., Hodges, J. R., and Etcoff, N. L. (1996). Facial emotion recognition after bilateral amygdala damage: Differentially severe impairment of fear. Cogn. Neuropsychol. 13: 699–745.

Coenen, V.A., Schlaepfer, T.E., Maedler, B., Panksepp, J. (2011). Cross-species affective functions of the medial forebrain bundle-implications for the treatment of affective pain and depression in humans. *Neuroscience & Biobehavioral Reviews*, 35(9): 1971-81.

Craig, A.D., How do you feel--now? The anterior insula and human awareness. *Nat. Rev. Neurosci.* 2009, *10*, 59-70.

Damasio, A.R., Grabowski, T.j., Bechara, A., Damasio, H., Ponto, L.L., Parvizi, J., et al. (2000). Subcortical and cortical brain activity during the feeling of self-generated emotions. Nature Neuroscience, 3: 1049–1056.

Damasio, A., Damasio, H. & Tranel, D. (2012). Persistence of feelings and sentience after bilateral damage of the insula. Cerebral Cortex, in press. doi:10.1093/cercor/bhs077

Darwin, C. R. 1859. On the origin of species by means of natural selection, or the reservation of favoured races in the struggle for life. London: John Murray. [1st edition].

Ekman, P., Friesen, W. V., O'Sullivan, M., Chan, A., Diacoyanni-Tarlatzis, I., Heider, K., Krause, R., LeCompte, W.A., Pitcairn, T., Ricci-Bitti, P. E., Scherer, K.R., Tomita, M., & Tzavaras, A. (1987). Universals and cultural differences in the judgments of facial expressions of emotion. Journal of Personality and Social Psychology, 53(4), 712-717.

Garrett, A.S., Maddoc, R.J. (2006). Separating subjective emotion from the perception of emotion-inducing stimuli: an fMRI study. Neuroimage, 33: 263-274.

Geiser, M., Walla, P. (2011). Objective measures of emotion during virtual walks through urban environments. Applied Sciences, 1: 1-11.

Grahl, A., Greiner, U., & Walla, P. (2012). Bottle shape elicits gender-specific emotion: a startle reflex modulation study. Psychology, 3(7): 548-554.

Gross, J.J. (1999). Emotion regulation: Past, Present, Future. Cognition and Emotion, 13(5): 551-573.

Halgren, E., Walter, R. D., Cherlow, D. G., and Crandall, P. H. (1978). Mental phenomena evoked by electrical stimulation of the human hippocampal formation and amygdala. Brain 101: 83–117.

Hamm, A.O., Weike, A.I., Schupp, H.T., Treig, T., Dressel, A., and Kessler, C. (2003). Affective blindsight: intact fear conditioning to a visual cue in a cortically blind patient. Brain, 126: 267-275.

Herbert, C., Herbert, B.M., & Pauli, P. (2011b). Emotional self-reference: Brain structures involved in the processing of words describing one´s own emotions. Neuropsychologia, 49, 2947-2956.

Herbert, C., Herbert, B.M., Ethofer, T., & Pauli, P. (2011a) His or mine? The time course of self-other discrimination in emotion processing. Social Neuroscience, 6, 277-288.

Izard, C. E. (1971). The face of emotion (Vol. 23): Appleton-Century-Crofts New York.

Kaplan-Solms, K. and Solms, M. (2000). Clinical Studies in Neuro-Psychoanalysis: introduction to a depth neuropsychology. London: Karnac Books.

Kleinginna, P.R.Jr., and Kleinginna, A.M. (1981). A Categorized List of Emotion Definitions, with Suggestions for a Consensual Definition. Motivation and Emotion, 5(4: 345-379.

Knutson, B., & Greer SM. (2008). Anticipatory affect: neural correlates and consequences for choice. *Philosophical Transactions of the Royal Society*, London B Biological Sciences. 363: 3771-3786.

Ikemoto, S. & Panksepp, J. (1999). The role of the nucleus accumbens dopamine in motivated behavior: a unifying interpretation with special reference to reward-seeking. Brain Research. Brain Research Review, 31(1): 6-41.

LeDoux, J.E. (1993). Emotional memory systems in the brain. Behavi. Brain Res. 58: 69–79.

LeDoux, J.E. (1995). Emotion: Clues from the Brain. Annu. Rev. Psycho, 46:209-235.

LeDoux, J. (1996). *The emotional brain*. New York: Simon & Schuster.

LeDoux, J. (2012). Rethinking the emotional brain. Neuron, 73: 653-676.

Lindquist, K.A., Wager, T.D., Kober, H., Bliss-Moreau, E., and Barrett, L.F. (2012). The brain basis of emotion: A meta-analytic review. Behavioral and Brain Sciences, 35: 121-202.

Lindquist, K. A., Wager, T. D., Bliss-Moreau, E., Kober, H., & Barrett, L. F. (2012). What are emotions and how are they created in the brain? Behavioral and Brain Sciences, 35: 175-184. response to comments.

Liotti, M., & Panksepp, J. (2004). On the neural nature of human emotions and implications for biological psychiatry. In Panksepp J (ed) *Textbook of Biological Psychiatry*, pp. 33-74. Wiley, New York.

Mauss, I.B., and Robinson, M.D. (2009). Measures of emotion: a review. Cognition and Emotion, 23(2): 209-237.

Morris, J.S., Öhman, A., and Dolan, R.J. (1999). A subcortical pathway to the right amygdala mediating "unseen" fear. Proc. Natl. Acad. Sci., 96(4): 1680-1685.

Narumoto, J., Okada, T., Sadato, Fukui, K., Yonekura, Y. (2001). Attention to emotion modulates fMRI activity in human right superior temporal sulcus. Cognitive Brain Research, 12: 225–231.

Northoff, G., Henzel, A., de Greck, M., Bermpohl, F., Dobrowolny, H., & Panksepp, J. (2006). Self-referential processing in our brain—A meta-analysis of imaging studies of the self. *Neuroimage,* 31, 440-457.

Northoff, G., Schneider, F., Rotte, M., Matthiae, C. Tempelmann, C., Wiebking, C., Bermpohl, F., Heinzel, A., Danos, P., Heinze, H.J., Bogerts, B., Walter, M., & Panksepp,

J. (2009). Differential parametric modulation of self-relatedness and emotions in different brain regions. *Human Brain Mapping,* 30, 369-382.

Northoff, G., Wiebking, C., Feinberg, T, and Panksepp, J. (2011). The'resting-state hypothesis' of major depressive disorder – a translational subcortical–cortical framework for a system disorder. Neurosci. Biobehav. Rev. DOI: 10.1016/j.neubiorev.2010.12.007

Öhman A. 2002. Automaticity and the amygdala: nonconscious responses to emotional faces. Curr.Dir. Psychol. Sci. 11:62–66

Panksepp, J. (1992). A critical role for affective neuroscience in resolving what is basic about basic emotions. Psychological Review, 99, 554-60.

Panksepp J. (1998). Affective Neuroscience: The Foundations of Human and Animal Emotions (Series in Affective Science). Oxford University Press, New York, New York.

Panksepp, J. (2005). On the embodied neural nature of core emotional affects. *Journal of Consciousness Studies,* 12, 158-184.

Panksepp, J. (2011a). Cross-species affective neuroscience decoding of the primal affective experiences of humans and related animals. PloSOne, 6(9).e21236.

Panksepp, J. (2011b). The basic emotional circuits of mammalian brains: do animals have affective lives?. Neurosci Biobehav Rev, 35(9): 1791-804.

Panksepp, J. (2012). The vicissitudes of preclinical psychiatric research: justified abandonment by big pharma? *Future Neurology,* 7: 1-3.

Panksepp, J. & Biven, L. (2012). *Archaeology of Mind: The Neuroevolutionary Origins of Human Emotions.* New York: Norton.

Panksepp, J. & Moskal, J. (2008). Dopamine and SEEKING: subcortical "reward" systems and appetitive urges. In: Elliot, A. (Ed.), Handbook of Approach and Avoidance Motivation. Mahwah, NJ: Lawrence Erlbaum Associates, pp. 67-87.

Panksepp, J., & Watt, D. (2011). What is basic about basic emotions? Lasting lessons from affective neuroscience. Emotion Review, 3, 387–396.

Phan, K.L., Wager, T., Taylor, S.F., and Liberzon, I. (2002). Functional Neuroanatomy of Emotion: A meta-Analysis of emotion activation studies in PET ans fMRI. Neuroimage, 16: 331-348.

Sabatinelli, D., Fortune, E.E., Li, O., Siddiqui, A., Krafft, C., Oliver, W.T.,Beck, S., Jeffries, J. (2011). Emotional perception: Meta-analyses of face and natural scene processing. NeuroImage, 54(3): 2524–2533.

Solms, M. & Panksepp, J. (2012). The 'Id' Knows More than the 'Ego' Admits: Neuropsychoanalytic and Primal Consciousness Perspectives on the Interface between Affective and Cognitive Neuroscience. *Brain Science,* 2, 147-175. doi:10.3390/brainsci2020147

Tracy, J.L. and Randles, D. (2011). Four models of basic emotions: a review of Ekman and Cordaro, Izard, Levenson, and Panksepp and Watt. Emotion Review, 3(4): 397-405.

Tracy, J. L., & Robins, R. W. (2008). The automaticity of emotion recognition. Emotion, 8(1), 81-95.

Walla, P. (2011). Non-Conscious Brain Processes Revealed by Magnetoencephalography (MEG), Magnetoencephalography, Elizabeth W. Pang (Ed.), ISBN: 978-953-307-255-5, InTech, Available from:
http://www.intechopen.com/books/magnetoencephalography/non-conscious-brain-processes-revealed-by-magnetoencephalography-meg-

Walla, P., Brenner, G., and Koller, M. (2011). Objective measures of emotion related to brand attitude: A new way to quantify emotion-related aspects relevant to marketing. PlosOne, 6(11): e26782. doi:10.1371/journal.pone.0026782.

Walla, P., and Deecke, L. (2010). Odours Influence Visually Induced Emotion: Behavior and Neuroimaging. Sensors, 10(9):8185-8197.

Walla, P., Richter, M., Färber, S., Leodolter, U., and Bauer, H. (2010). Food evoked changes in humans: Startle response modulation and event-related potentials (ERPs). Journal of Psychophysiology, 24(1): 25-32.

Walla, P. (2008). Olfaction and its dynamic influence on word and face processing. Progress in Neurobiology: Cross-modal integration. Progress in Neurobiology, 84: 192-209.

Walla, P., Duregger, C., Greiner, K., Thurner, S., and Ehrenberger, K. (2008). Multiple aspects related to self awareness and the awareness of others: an Electroencephalography (EEG) study. Journal of Neural Transmission, 115(7):983-92.

Walla, P., Greiner, K., Duregger, C., Deecke, L., and Thurner, S. (2007). Self awareness and the subconscious effect of personal pronouns on word encoding: a magnetoencephalographic (MEG) study. Neuropsychologia, 45: 796-809.

Zachar, P., & Ellis, R. (Eds.). (2012). *Emotional theories of Jaak Panksepp and Jim Russell.* Amsterdam: John Benjamins.

Zajonc, R. B. (2000). Feeling and thinking: Closing the debate over the independence of affect. In J. P. Forgas (Ed.), Feeling and thinking: The role of affect in social cognition (pp. 31–58). New York: Cambridge University Press.

Chapter 7

Neuroimaging for the Affective Brain Sciences, and Its Role in Advancing Consumer Neuroscience

Peter Walla, Aimee Mavratzakis and Shannon Bosshard

Additional information is available at the end of the chapter

http://dx.doi.org/10.5772/51042

1. Introduction

To fully understand the driving behaviour of a car it is absolutely inevitable to investigate all its hidden parts underneath the surface and to find out what their functions are. To fully understand human behaviour we need to complete traditional behavioural measures with neuroimaging data that allow us to look inside the brain. Only via neuroimaging methodology do we have access to underlying brain processes that guide our behaviour without leading to any conscious reportable traces that show up in questionnaires. On top of that, especially when emotion-related explicit responses are required questionnaires provide us with biased responses due to cognitive influences. These responses can be far away from true underlying emotion-related information. The discrepancy between biased and unbiased emotion-related information processing is of utmost interest for both basic affective neuroscience and consumer neuroscience.

2. Emotion specificity in the brain revealed by functional Magnet Resonance Imaging (fMRI)

This section will begin by reviewing major milestones in emotion research achieved by way of fMRI. It focuses on advances in our understanding of the structures involved in the visual perception of emotion and how this has changed the way researchers look at the role of the amygdala, particularly its role in the coordination of emotion responses beyond the fear response. New leads in perception research using functional MRI methods are then reviewed including the possible primacy of cognition in emotion perception, as well as the often neglected role of the endocrine system in modulating perceptual ability.

2.1. Structural and functional organisation of emotion perception

The discrimination of affective signals in visual sensory input is thought to begin in the early stages of visual perception (LeDoux, 1996). The structures facilitating this are intertwined with visual processing to consistently produce rapid and sometimes unconscious emotional responses to the surrounding environment before the individual consciously recognises exactly what they are seeing (Whalen et al., 1998). The efficiency of visual-emotion discrimination despite its complexity has caught the attention of visual, perceptual and emotion researchers. The role of the amygdala in visual emotion discrimination is a primary focus in emotion perception research. The amygdala is a small almond size subcortical structure found bilaterally in the medial temporal lobe of mammalian brains. Neuroimaging studies show that neural pathways projecting from nuclei of the amygdala innervate multiple cortical and subcortical regions (Sah, Faber, De Armentia, & Power, 2003). All of these findings have obviously made the amygdala a primary region of interest for understanding the nature and organisation of emotion activity in the brain.

2.1.1. The direct subcortical pathway model

Modern theory suggests that the amygdala evolved early in the evolution of species as a mechanism specialised for rapidly detecting and responding to perceived threat (LeDoux, 1996), which has been described as an 'alarm signal' (e.g. Liddell et al., 2005; Tamietto & de Gelder, 2010). According to this theory, the neural communication of 'raw' or consciously unprocessed emotional information bypasses comprehensive visual processing stages, allowing the rapid transmission of threat signals to the amygdala via a pathway that crosses only the superior colliculus and pulvinar nucleus of the thalamus (see figure 1a). This adaptive function of this structural organisation is in line with the discovery of direct efferent connections from the amygdala to the hypothalamus, which coordinates autonomic and reflexive bodily responses to motivationally salient stimuli (Risold, Thompson, & Swanson, 1997) and which has long been recognised for its direct involvement in emotional behaviour (Swanson, 2000). This fear detection system is also found in less cortically developed mammals (LeDoux, 1996), suggesting that the direct subcortical processing pathway was an evolutionary achievement, and one that has been left unaltered across time and species due to its efficient design and salient purpose. This theory is also in line with findings from human studies focusing on emotion processing below the level of consciousness, where the subcortical alarm system was shown to operate independent of conscious awareness, presumably allowing for the preparation of motivational responses to threat even before such cues are consciously seen (Morris, Öhman, & Dolan, 1999; Whalen, et al., 1998). Despite the perseverance of the subcortical threat-detection pathway model, several phenomena challenge its comprehensiveness (A comprehensive discussion of these issues is provided by Pessoa & Adolphs, 2010). A central problem unaccounted for by this model of emotion processing is the modulation of early visual emotion processes by higher cognitive influences, which this section now turns to.

2.1.2. Multiple pathways in early visual perception

The functional capacity of the direct subcortical pathway model fails to adequately address possible mechanisms of this early cognitive interaction given that a main proposition of the model is that rapid subcortical processing involves the exclusive processing of affective signals, bypassing any higher cortical involvement. Pessoa and Adolphs (2011) in fact point out that there is no empirical evidence to suggest that affective information 'bypasses' cortically-bound circuits, but rather that multiple pathways are involved in the construction of visual emotion perception, and that each pathways likely specialises in selective attributes of information processing, but that none of these pathways involves the exclusive use of emotional information relative to other pathways.

There is general widespread agreement regarding the existence of an interaction between bottom-up and top-down factors in emotion processing (Gros, 2010; Ochsner et al., 2009). The New Look framework (Bruner, 1957) in particular states that the construction of perception is influenced by top down factors such as individual needs and expectations. While it is not yet known exactly what stage/s of visual perception are influenced by cognition it has been traditionally assumed that cognitive input influenced later categorisation stages of visual processing, and that earlier stages involved the pure bottom up extraction of basic features from sensory signals. Several recent experiments suggest, however, that top-down modulation by cognition may reach much deeper into the early visual stages of perception than current theory anticipates. Gilchrist and Nesberg (1952) showed that hungry individuals overestimated the brightness of pictures of food compared to other pictures, while more recently Radel and Clement-Guillotin (2012) extended this work by directly attributing the perceptual effect to an early perceptual processing stage. They examined differences in reaction times when hungry and satiated individuals were asked to identify food from non-food pictures as fast as possible and found that hungry individuals did recognise pictures of food fastest, directly pointing to an early unconscious level of semantic encoding that precedes the processing of motivationally relevant information.

In another recent study investigating the relationship between emotion word concepts and facial expression recognition, a direct interaction was found between higher semantic centres and early emotion perception. In this study, the authors temporarily inhibited accessibility of an emotion word via a technique called semantic satiation, whereby repeatedly saying the word (in this case 30 times) causes the temporary exhaustion of action potential generation along this region, thereby briefly inhibiting conscious access to the word. Using this technique, the researchers investigated whether semantically satiating an emotion word label such as 'anger' affected participants ability to recognise an angry face. Indeed they found that after 30 repetitions of the emotion word participants were slower to recognise an angry facial expression compared to when the word had not been satiated by repetition beforehand (Gendron, Lindquist, Barsalou, & Barrett, 2012), demonstrating the widespread and dynamic involvement of cortical areas in modulating emotion perception.

While these studies do not provide direct evidence for the involvement of the amygdala as an interception point of higher cognitive processes, there are many empirical examples demonstrating a correlational relationship between amygdala activity and cognitively based emotion tasks (For a review see Phelps, 2006). In addition, it is known that there are extensive connections between the amygdala and multiple cortical regions (see figure 1). However, possibly one of the strongest cases supporting a primitive role for cognition in visual processing comes from recent imaging data of the visual cortex and amygdala, which this chapter now turns to.

2.1.3. The serial re-entry model of emotion discrimination in visual perception

An emerging theory of the discrimination of emotion content during visual perception is the idea that sequential stages of communication occur between the amygdala and the visual pathway via a 'serial re-entry' style of emotion processing. This concept is based on the idea that affective signals received early in the discrimination process travel through 'predictive pathways' that initiate and modulate the preparation of an appropriate bodily response via efferent amygdala projections. Serial modification of the affective response is thought to occur as the affective signal cascades along the visual pathway and the emotional nature of the inputted information becomes clearer.

Current empirical anatomical research provides support for the notion that the amygdala plays a key role in gauging emotional value of visual affective information, however it is still unclear which visual structures participate in this process and what their function may be. Accumulated analysis of previous research suggests that visual emotion discrimination is likely to occur hierarchically, with affective signals originating through rostral inferior temporal-amygdala interactions, an area that has been implicated in basic unconscious identity and semantic processing (See Storbeck, Robinson, & McCourt, 2006 for an indepth discussion) and response initiation originating later through amygdala-extra striatal interactions. Testing this kind of theory requires access to both temporal and spatial properties of processing events. However, the limitations imposed by scalp recorded electroencephalography have challenged researchers to develop novel ways to empirically demonstrate evidence of a re-entrant style of visual-emotion processing. Sabatinelli and colleagues (Sabatinelli, Lang, Bradley, Costa, & Keil, 2009) attempted to answer this question using rapid-sampling event-related-fMRI, a technique that, although not feasible for whole brain analysis, can be useful for examining a specific set of proximally located regions of interest. In this study, relative onset of activation of specifically defined regions along one plane were examined including the inferior temporal cortex, amygdala, medial occipital gyrus and calcarine fissure. They found relative differences in BOLD signal onset related to emotional valence at successive stages of visual processing including the inferior temporal cortex and the amygdala (See Figure 2). The data suggests that re-entrant input begins with connections between the inferior temporal cortex and the amygdala. Discrimination of emotional from non-emotional signals is evident by increases in BOLD activations to emotional stimuli located in the amygdala and the inferior temporal cortex (V2; Secondary occipital cortex) approximately ~1 second before emotional discriminatory activation is seen in the extra striatial cortex. Despite its anatomical placement early in the visual processing pathway, the primary visual cortex does not, however, respond to emotional stimuli, and is instead consistently activated by both emotional and non-emotional stimuli suggesting its non-involvement in emotion detection. Further to this, the amygdala has been shown to have direct feed-forward and feed-back connections with not just subcortical structures but also multiple cortical structures located in the parietal cortex, the frontal cortex, cingulate cortex, orbito-frontal cortex (OFC) and the Insula. Therefore it is possible that at many stages of visual processing regions directly connected to the amygdala can influence emotional responses to visually perceived emotional stimuli.

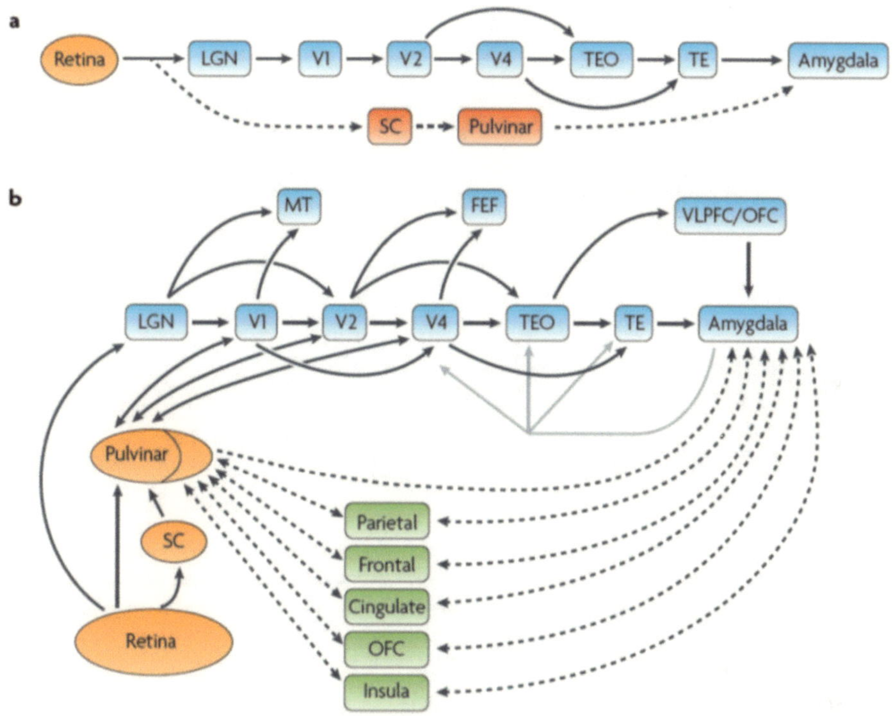

Figure 1. | **Visual pathways. a** | A traditional flowchart of visual processing typically emphasizes the LGN –v1–v2–v4–teO–te pathway, although the scheme is not strictly hierarchical. The amygdala, in particular, is a recipient of visual signals from the anterior visual cortex. According to the 'standard hypothesis', a subcortical pathway involving the superior colliculus and the pulvinar nucleus of the thalamus provides fast and automatic access to the amygdala. **b** | An alternative view of the flow of visual signals includes multiple pathways, including both alternative routes (for example, LGN to Mt) and shortcuts (for example, v2 to teO). Only some of these are shown. The flow of visual information may be more appropriately viewed in terms of 'multiple waves' of activation that initiate and refine cell responses at a given processing 'stage'. For simplicity, feedback pathways, which are known to be quite extensive, have been omitted. The existence of such feedback pathways dictates, however, that a complex ebb-and-flow of activation sculpts the neuronal profile of activation throughout the visual cortex, and likewise the amygdala responses. Some of the connections between the pulvinar and visual cortex, and between the pulvinar and 'associational' areas, are also indicated. The line in the pulvinar is intended to schematically separate the medial pulvinar (to the right of the line) from the rest of the structure. FeF, frontal eye field; LGN, lateral geniculate nucleus; Mt, medial temporal area (also known as v5); OFc, orbitofrontal cortex; sc, superior colliculus; te, inferior temporal area te; teO, inferior temporal area teO; v, visual cortex; vLPFc, ventrolateral prefrontal cortex. Figure and caption adapted with permission from Pessoa, L. and Adolphs, R. (2010). Emotion processing and the amygdala: from a 'low road' to 'many roads' of evaluating biological significance. Nature Reviews Neuroscience, 11(11), 773-783.

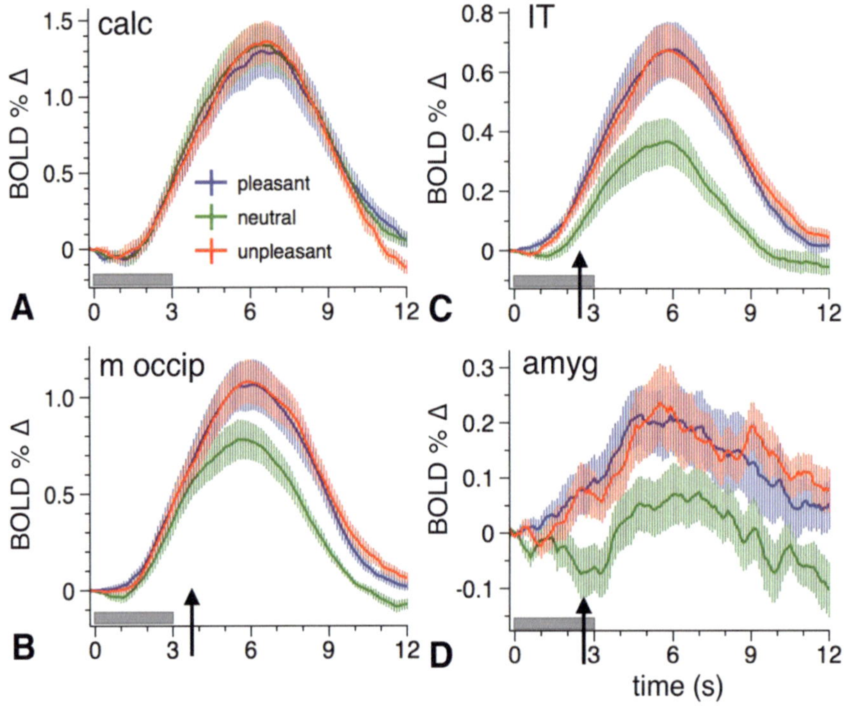

Figure 2. Average time courses (n17) of picture-driven BOLD signal in amygdala, inferotemporal cortex, middle occipital gyrus, and calcarine fissure. Blue and red lines represent pleasant and unpleasant pictures, and green represents neutral pictures. The gray bar on the abscissa signifies the picture presentation period. Arrows indicate the point at which BOLD signal during an arousing picture presentation is significantly greater activity than BOLD signal during neutral pictures. Figure and caption adapted with permission from Sabatinelli, D., Lang, P. J., Bradley, M. M., Costa, V. D. and Keil, A. (2009). The timing of emotional discrimination in human amygdala and ventral visual cortex. The Journal of Neuroscience, 29(47), 14864-14868.

2.2. Mediation of emotion perception by the endocrine system

Many homeostatic mechanisms function as feedback cycles. The hypothalamus is the principle structure that maintains homeostasis through its influence on the endocrine and autonomic nervous system. This dynamic system is only recently being investigated via brain imaging methods in terms of its influence on emotion-related information processing, and there is still much to learn regarding how the endocrine system interacts with and modifies the perception and expression of emotion. Nevertheless, this area of investigation presents a unique opportunity for understanding organisational and functional principles underlying emotion and motivated behaviour.

2.2.1. Hormones influence non-verbal emotional behaviour

Reproductive hormone levels have traditionally been associated with emotional behaviour. Researchers are now beginning to understand how this relationship unfolds in the brain. It is already known that reproductive hormone receptors exist in amygdaloidal regions (Österlund & Hurd, 2001) and that hormones act on physiological processes, altering morphology, which in turn modifies behavioural expressions (See Becker et al., 2005 for an extended discussion). Several behavioural experiments have demonstrated a correlation between fluctuations in specific hormone levels and a perceptual bias towards recognition of threatening stimuli. For example, Pearson and Lewis (2005) reported highest accuracy for fear during the late preovulatory phase when estrogen levels are highest, and lowest accuracy for fear during the menstrual phase when estrogen levels are lowest. Raised progesterone levels have also been associated with a bias towards the recognition of threatening stimuli (Conway et al., 2007; Derntl et al., 2008a) suggesting that elevated progesterone levels are associated with increased sensitivity to facial cues carrying sources of threat or negative contagion. Derntl and colleagues also found a general ovulatory phase effect in females, further suggesting an evolutionary consistent relationship between pregnancy and increased behaviour consistent with protection and caution.

Recent examinations of the neural activity underlying hormonally-modulated perceptual biases have been performed during natural fluctuations in hormone levels and during controlled administration conditions, with the accumulated evidence to date suggesting an important role for reproductive hormones in modulating neural plasticity related to threat vigilance. For example, using BOLD fMRI, Van Wingen and colleagues (2007a; 2007b) found that the administration of a single dose of progesterone was associated with increased amygdala activity during an emotion matching task, but in an emotion memory task, administered progesterone was associated with decreased amygdala activity. Derntl and colleagues (2008b) found somewhat different effects when they separated female participants into two groups based on cycle phase: The early follicular phase (lower estradiol and lower progesterone levels) and the late Luteal phase (higher estradiol and higher progesterone levels). They reported a correlation between amygdala activation, recognition accuracy and female hormone levels such that amygdala activation was stronger during the follicular stage (low progesterone levels), coinciding with improved emotion recognition performance across five discrete emotion categories, including negative and positive emotions (Figure 3; Figure 4). According to the authors of the study, increased amygdala activity during the luteal phase is likely to be related to perceptual sensitivity biases towards threatening emotional stimuli, facilitating cautious behaviour associated with lower risk-taking. While during the follicular phase increased amygdala activity may be associated with heightened social awareness. At the behavioural level this may enable an underlying social advantage for fertile females in that the higher accuracy displayed during the fertile phase mediates more successful social interactions, a skill vital for selecting the best mate.

3. Section summary

This section has described some of the major advances in our understanding of what factors modulate emotion processing during visual perception as well as current leads in hormone and gender based emotion research. Current evidence holds that the amygdala acts not only as a hub for facilitating the rapid signalling of threatening stimuli to initiate hypothalamic

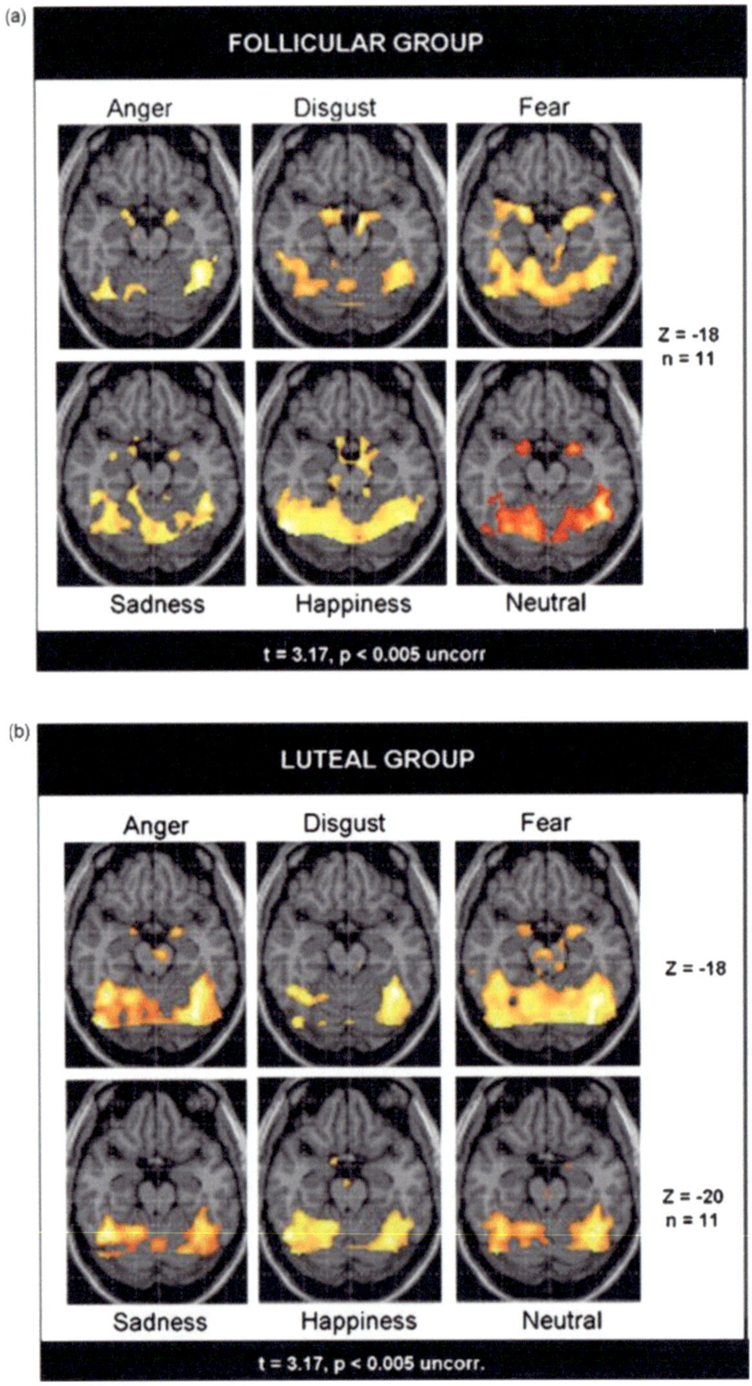

Figure 3. Results of whole-slab analysis showing activation maps of random effects analysis on one coronal slice (Y = 0) comprising the amygdala for FPG (a) and for LPG (b) (threshold: $t = 3.17$ and $p < 0.005$ uncorrected).

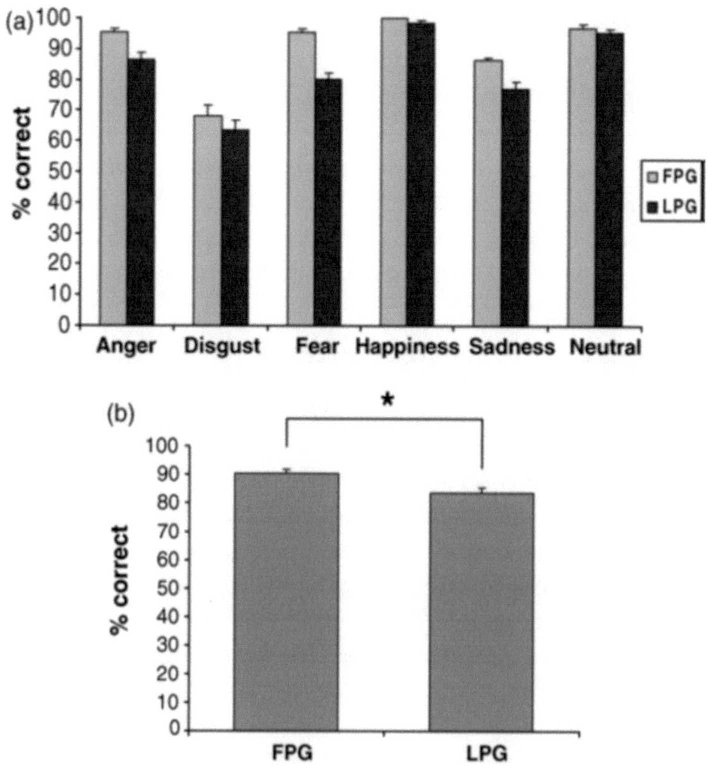

Figure 4. Recognition accuracy with standard error of mean for all emotions across females in the follicular phase (FPG) and females in the luteal phase (LPG) is presented in (a). Mean percent correct across all stimuli for FPG and LPG females are illustrated in (b). Results of the repeated measures ANOVA revealed a significant phase effect ($p = 0.011$) with a better performance of the FPG group–—illustrated with an asterisk in (b) without any significant emotion-by-phase interaction ($p = 0.373$). Figures 3 and 4 and captions adapted with permission from Derntl, B., Windischberger, C., Robinson, S., Lamplmayr, E., Kryspin-Exner, I., Gur, R. C. and Habel, U. (2008). Facial emotion recognition and amygdala activation are associated with menstrual cycle phase. Psychoneuroendocrinology, 33(8), 1031-1040.

mediated autonomic responses, but also as a central relay station for the widespread communication of emotional information to areas throughout subcortical and cortical regions. Affective signals are now thought to originate from IT-amygdala interactions, with modulation and response formation occurring shortly thereafter via complex interconnections between the amygdala and successive stages of the visual system.

Modelling of the BOLD signal in ER-fMRI may be a valuable technique for better understanding the functional basis of emotion discrimination in visual perception based on the time course of BOLD related activity. It is also important to remember, however, that in evolutionary terms the most important objective of all affective neuroscience and perception is not the speed at which the first neural activation occurs, but the speed at which the first behavioural response occurs. De Gelder, Van Honk and Tamietto (2011) point out that these two events are not necessarily linked. In other words, it cannot be assumed that adaptive behavioural responses will be explainable in terms of functions involving the first neural pathway to respond to the emotional stimuli. Rather, adaptive responses are more likely to be the result of the fastest pathway to initiate a biologically relevant motivational response, which may or may not be independent of initial activations. Better understanding the effect of hormones on the modulation of emotion perception is one avenue for increasing our understanding of the functional organisation underlying emotion perception, particularly given that this method is highly related to understanding principles of evolution, as well as understanding many underlying factors influencing social behaviours.

4. Neuromarketing/Consumer Neuroscience

Over the last few decades the merging of marketing with neuroscience has captured the attention of both the academic and corporate world. Neuromarketing enables marketers and researchers to better understand what consumers react to and how intense their reaction is. What makes it more interesting is that these questions can be answered without the need to explicitly ask the consumer for their opinion. Neuromarketing is able to tap into one's non-conscious and collect answers to questions such as: Is the colour, shape or smell of a particular product a good selling point? Although in its infancy, this new field has already had a major impact on the way many businesses market their products. With the formation of over 150 neuromarketing firms in the last 10 years, and almost 5000 times the number of Google searches between 2002 and 2004 (Figure 5; Plassmann, Zoëga Ramsøy & Milosavljevic, 2012) there is no surprise that this field has had such an impact across a vast number of disciplines.

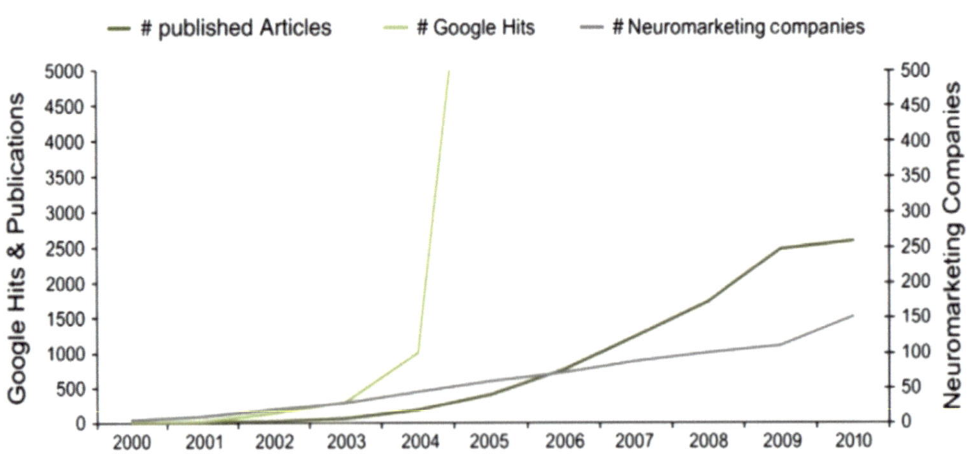

Figure 5. Graphical depiction of the increase in Google searches and published articles relating to neuromarketing as well as the increase in neuromarketing companies (plassmann et al., 2012; with permission).

Although it is undeniable that neuromarketing is a useful field of study, along with its success, has come a major dilemma pertaining to the way that it perceived by consumers and the media. Throughout this section, I will no longer refer to neuromarketing as such, but instead as consumer neuroscience. Since the formation of neuromarketing, consumers and those alike have held the opinion that the aim of this field was force consumers to buy things that they do not want nor need. It is a common misconception that neuromarkeitng aims to find the 'buy button' in the brain (provided one actually exists). This is neither the current aim of neuromarketing/consumer neuroscience nor should it ever be. Instead, the term consumer neuroscience emphasises that this field aims to study the interactions between products, the market and consumers rather than an attempt to coerce consumers into buying products.

Before we can appreciate the field of consumer neuroscience, we must have an understanding of what neuroscience is and what it can bring to the field of marketing. Neuroscience, through studying the nervous system, seeks to better understand the biological basis of behaviour. However, according to Plassmann et al. (2012), due to the complex nature of consumer behaviour, it is essential that we focus specifically on systems neuroscience rather than cellular neuroscience. Systems neuroscience is a sub-discipline of neuroscience which focuses on how different neural circuits function, either together or separately. Rather than focusing on behaviour at a neuronal level, systems neuroscience focuses on both the cognitive and affective (emotional) aspects of consumer behaviour. It is common knowledge that much of our behaviour is driven by our unconsciousness (Chartrand, 2005). For this reason, it is justified that neuroimaging be used to better understand consumer behaviour.

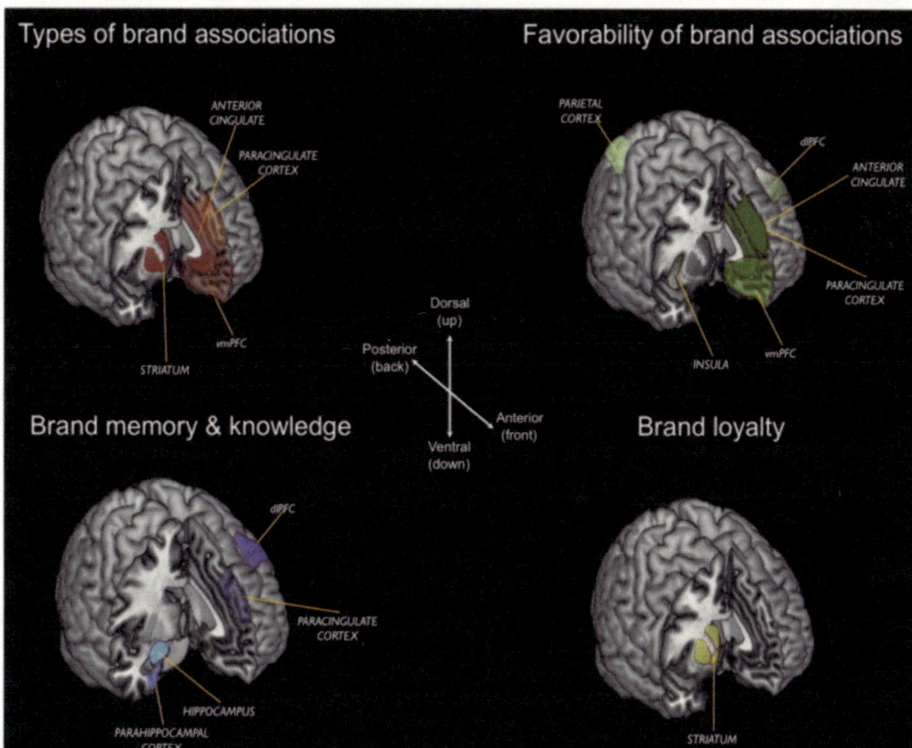

Figure 6. An excerpt taken from Plassmann et al. (2012) (with permission) depicting the many regions involved in the processing of brand information.

This section of the chapter will focus on how neuroimaging studies have identified specific neural circuits that are involved in the different aspects of the decision-making process. The figure above (Figure 6.) illustrates that the areas activated within the brain depending on the interaction that the consumer has with abrand. In many cases, several regions are responsible for the processing of a single cue. More specifically, the image gives a summary of the location of some of the processes that are involved in the psychology of brands (Plassmann et al., 2012).

In the following, we will focus on several current neuroimaging techniques and how their introduction into the field of marketing has influenced our understanding of consumer neuroscience. Branding, package design and labelling will be discussed because they are a major focus of a large number of studies. In addition, they are of particular interest to the marketing community because the results can be applied to the marketing of products and services.

4.1. Branding

When looking to purchase a product, brand name is an important factor, but plays only a partial role in the final decision made by the consumer. According to Keller and Lehmann (2006), consumers rely on well-known brands because they know that these brands are either of a higher quality or that the performance of the product is superior to that of the competition. Studies have shown that more often than not, it is only when a lesser-known brand is offered at a lower price, that they are chosen over well-known brands (Sethuraman & Cole, 1999).

In one of the most famous consumer neuroscience studies, McClure et al. (2004) revealed that in some cases, brand name is everything. In this study, a comparison between Coca Cola and Pepsi was made. Prior to the commencement of the study, it was established that there was roughly an equal preference for both Coca Cola and Pepsi. During the second phase of the experiment participants were shown either a picture of a Coke can prior to receiving Coke or a Pepsi can prior to receiving Pepsi. Participants that received Coke showed significant levels of activation in the dorsolateral prefrontal cortex (DLPFC), the hippocampus and midbrain. No such finding was reported when Pepsi was delivered after participants viewed a Pepsi can. Furthermore, when the delivery was preceded with a light instead of a Coke can, significant differences in activation were seen between the two forms of cues (Figure 7). According to Mclure et al. (2004) suggest that the activation seen in the DLPFC, hippocampus and midbrain provides evidence that Coke possesses a greater wealth of cultural meaning than that associated with Pepsi.

As seen in the above study, functional magnetic resonance imaging (fMRI) is a useful means of measuring the significant levels of activation in the brain. As an area of the brain becomes more active, it requires more oxygen. It is these changes in oxygen levels that fMRI aims to measure. However, fMRI is not the only method utilised by researchers to understand how the brain reacts to stimuli. Another tool used to investigate brain activity within a consumer setting is the less prominent magnetoencephalography (MEG). In contrast to fMRI, MEG measures brain activity by recording the magnetic fields produced by the naturally occurring electrical currents in the brain. In a study conducted by Junghofer, Kissler, Schupp, Putsche, Elling and Dobel (2010), investigated which brain regions were responsible for the early processing (>120ms) of man made stimuli. During the study, two separate measures of consumer behaviour were collected. Self-report data was collected from participants via a survey in which they expressed activities related to their consumer behaviour toward specific brands of shoes or motorcycles. Moreover, a brain-based measure was also collected in which participants were exposed to images of different brands of motorcycles and shoes. The most interesting finding presented by Junghofer et al., was the discrepancy between the self-report data and the data collected from the brain responses. Explicitly, self-report data showed a clear difference in consumer behaviour and brand expertise between each gender, however this was less evident from the results of the brain measures. Figure 8 shows that although activity in the occipito-temporal regions differed between males and females, many participants showed rather similar activation to both shoes and cars.

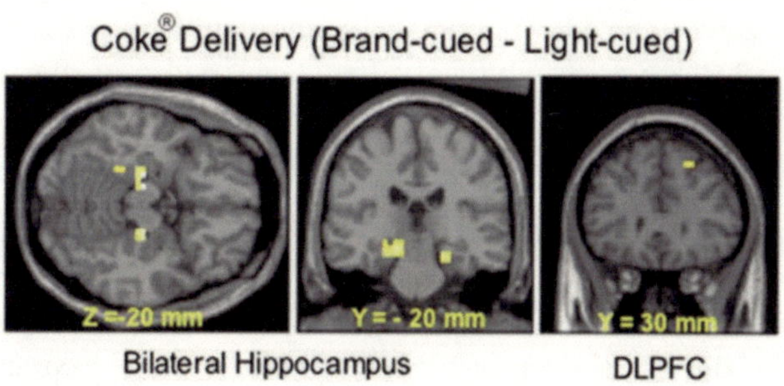

Figure 7. Significant activations between Coke delivered following an image of a Coke can and Coke delivered following the presentation of a light cue. Significant activations were found bilaterally in the hippocampus, the left parahippocampal cortex, midbrain and dorsolateral prefrontal cortex. These findings were exclusively found with Coke (McClure et al., 2004) (with permission).

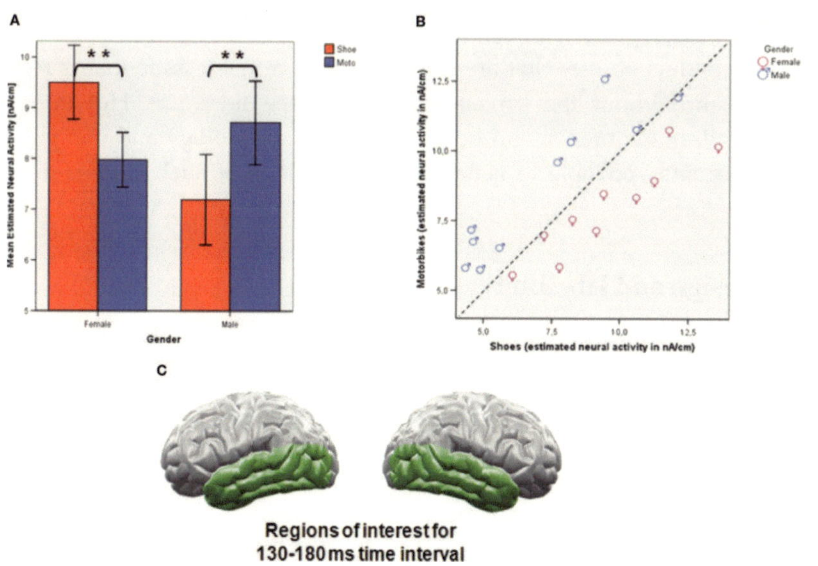

Figure 8. Image taken from Junghöfer et al. (2010) (with permission) indicating the difference in activation of the occipito-temproal cortex (except for the primary visual areas) in males and females when viewing motorcycles and shoes.

The study conducted by Junhöfer et al. (2010) present findings similar to those expressed in a number of pieces of research. It is repeatedly reported that a discrepancy exists between subjective and objective measures of consumer behaviour. From a marketing perspective, these findings illustrate the continuing problems that arise when consumers are asked questions in relation to their willingness to buy, rather than obtaining a response via subconscious processes.

In sum, the study conducted by McClure et al. (2004) presented findings that explain the success that Coca Cola has had over its rival, Pepsi. However, the only conclusions we can draw from this study is that there are strong neurocorrelates related to Coke, but not to Pepsi. Although we know that Coke has a greater wealth of knowledge associated with it in comparison to Pepsi, there is little we can do with these findings in terms of marketing. More specifically, we are unable to generalise the findings to that of other products, we are unable to draw conclusions as to why Coke has developed a greater amount of cultural meaning and Pepsi has not, and most importantly, we can not use these findings to improve Pepsi as a product to help it better compete with Coke.

In a similar manner, the study conducted by Junhöfer et al. (2010) have no immediate translational value, however, there is the possibility that these findings can help companies to better understand trends in consumer behaviour. Furthermore, these trends can then be used to assist in the development in activities related to their products. Again, the only conclusion that we are able to draw from this study is that a product liked by consumers may initiate activation in the occipito-temporal cortex. However, although this study may be seen as useless for companies that have already released their products onto the market, companies that are looking to release their product and wish to investigate how well it will compete with existing products may find this study more relevant.

The inability to conduct studies that are translational is a major issue that is repeated time and time again throughout the consumer neuroscience literature. However, consumer neuroscience is still in its infancy and hopefully, as the technology and methods are better understood, it becomes possible to generalise the findings of such studies to the field of marketing.

4.2. Package design and labelling

It should come as no shock that a more appealing product is capable of initiating a much more positive emotion. Previous studies have shown that individuals have been seen to express heightened levels of emotion toward attractive product packaging in comparison to unattractive product packaging (see Honea & Horsky, 2011). Have you ever wondered why when you buy something as expensive as a piece of jewellery, the packaging is usually made to look rather plain. Some products that are assumed to be of high value, highly experiential and have a positive influence on sensory systems, have been known to be presented in rather plain boxes as this neutralises the expectations of the individual, thus results in intensified subsequent emotions (Honea & Horsky, 2011). In addition to modifying the emotional responses of consumers, product aesthetics are able to alter the expectations of consumers. In many cases, the effect that product aesthetics has on consumer behaviour can be seen without the use of any neuroimaging techniques. Simply, the modification of product packaging can be used to mislead consumers into believing that products are larger or hold more than they actually do. There are many reasons that companies modify the packaging of their products, however the focus of this section is not to report how product packaging is used to mislead consumers (European Parliament, 2012), but rather identify the areas involved in processing packaging using neuroimaging techniques.

So what happens at a non-conscious level that affects which products we find appealing and which of those we do not? When shopping, it is usually the case that the decisions we make are made non-consciously and in a matter of seconds (Milosavljevic, Koch & Rangel, 2011), so it is imperative that the product being marketed stands out from its competitors. So how do companies decide what their new product packaging should look like and whether or not the public will find them enticing? Well the answer lies with neuroscience. A new branch of neuroscience termed "neuroaesthetics" has been used to address the questions surrounding the way the brain is activated in the presence of product packaging. Given that much of consumer behaviour is driven by processes at a non-conscious level (Chartrand, 2005), it would be inappropriate to simply ask for a verbal response as to which product or packaging they would be more likely to purchase. Moreover, previous research has shown us time and time again that there are discrepancies between self-report measures (subjective measures) and neuroimaging measures (objective measures; Walla, Brenner & Koller, 2011).

Several studies conducted by Reimann, Zaichkowsky, Neuhaus, Bender & Weber (2010) investigated the effect that good aesthetic properties had on brain activity. Interestingly, the first two of their studies revealed that participants chose products with aesthetic properties more often than products with standard packaging, even when a well-known brand was used (Figure 9). It was also reported that participants took longer to make the choice that resulted in the product with the aesthetic packaging being chosen.

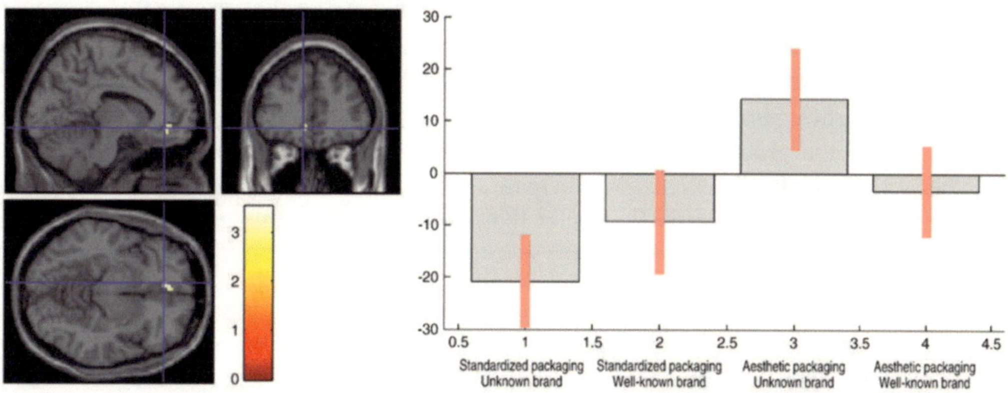

Figure 9. Left: Significant levels of activation in the vmPFC regarding brand and type of packaging (standardised vs. not standardised). Right: Percentage of activation change in the vmPFC (Reimann et al. 2010) (with permission).

To assess which regions of the brain were responsible for the increase in affective processes, Reimann et al. (2010) conducted an fMRI study and found that participants engage specific brain areas when assessing aesthetic package design. More specifically, significant increases in activation were seen in the ventromedial prefrontal cortex (vmPFC), the striatum (especially in the right nucleus accumbens) and also in the cingulate cortex (Figure 10). In addition, the heightened levels of activation in the vmPFC due to aesthetic packaging were witnessed for both well-known and unfamiliar brand names.

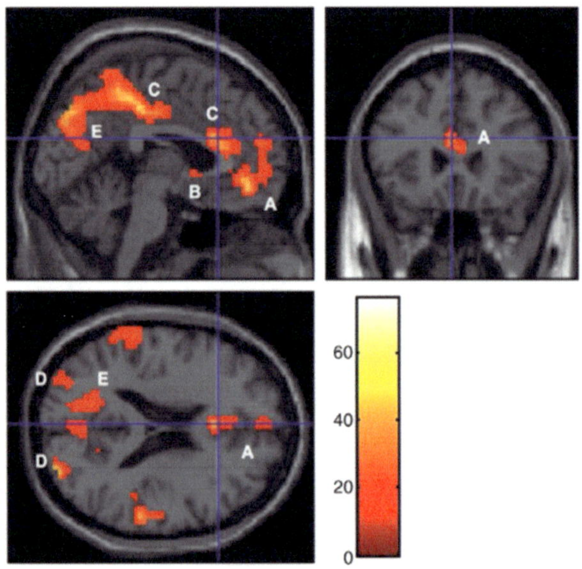

Figure 10. Significantly larger levels of activation in the vmPFC (A), striatum, particularly nucleus accumbens (B), cingulate cortex (C), primary visual cortices (D), and precuneus (E) during aesthetic product presentations (Reimann et al. 2010) (with permission).

Each of the abovementioned regions of the brain plays an important role in the processing of aesthetic features of products. The literature repeatedly shows that the vmPFC becomes activated when an individual is rewarded (McClure et al. 2004; Plassmann et al., 2012). In this case, the reward was considered to be when participants saw a product that possessed aesthetic properties. Similarly, the striatum (in this case the right nucleus accumbens) also plays a role in the processing of aesthetic properties. However, in contrast, the striatum becomes activated when participants anticipate a reward. According to Reimann et al. (2010) these regions of the brain work in sync at the point when the consumer views a product with aesthetics.

In another study that focused on the way that products are labeled rather than the way that the products are packaged, it was reported that in obese individuals, several regions of the brain are more highly activated when an item of food is perceived to be of a higher calorie content (Ng, Stice, Yokum & Bohon, 2011). During this study, an identical milkshake was delivered to obese and lean participants (based on their body mass index), however one was labeled as low fat and the other as regular. Obese participants were seen to show higher levels of activation in the somatosensory, gustatory, and reward evaluation regions when presented with a regular milkshake versus an identical milkshake labeled 'low-fat'.

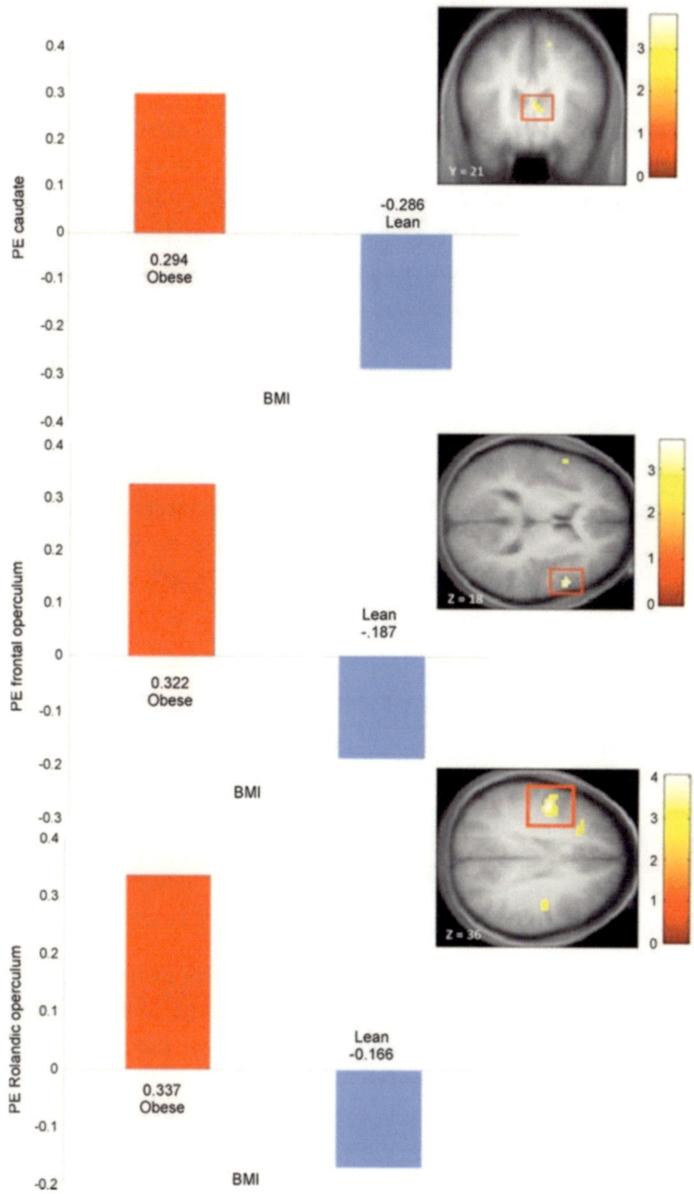

Figure 11. Difference in activation between lean and obese women. Activation of the caudate was due to anticipated intake of high-fat versus water. Activation of the frontal operculum was due to anticipated intake of high fat versus low fat milkshakes. Activation of the Rolandic operculum was due to the receipt of high fat versus low fat milkshake (Ng et al. (2011)) (with permission).

With regard to the obese individuals in their study, Ng et al. (2011) found significantly higher activation of the Rolandic operculum (gustatory cortex) and caudate. These areas were reported as becoming activated when participants anticipated the intake of food. In addition, obese women were also seen to have a more active posterior cingulate gyrus and hippocampus, parrahippocampal gyrus and vmPFC. Ng et al. stated that these areas may have been responsible for the encoding of the reward value. Figure 11 shows the difference in the activation of the caudate, operculum and Rolandic operculum between lean and obese women.

According to Ng et al. (2011), the findings from their study offer an explanation as to why obese people remain obese even when they focus on eating low-fat foods. When an individual eats a food that is high in calories, the reward experience during consumption increases the expectation of reward, thus eating continues and may result in overeating. In contrast, when eating low calorie foods, people may overeat in order to compensate for the relative reduction of pleasantness and reward.

This study provides an excellent example of the translational value of consumer neuroscience. Although it does not allow businesses to increase the monetary value of its products, it identifies why consumers behave differently depending on the labeling of the product. There is no doubt that the findings presented by Ng et al. (2011) may be beneficial to not only the health industry, but the way that supermarkets interact with consumers. Many supermarkets promote products that are 'low fat' with the expectation that consumers will be buy these products and consume less calories, however it may be having the opposite effects.

Moreover, the study conducted by Ng et al. (2011) shows that obese people show more activation in several brain regions when they are not only expecting to receive food, but when eating something that is labeled as low fat rather than regular. Although the findings of Reimann et al. cannot be generalized to specific marketing contexts at present, the ability to generalize these findings to specific products and consumer scenarios will become better understood as this field continues to grow.

4.3. Final statement

It is undeniable that consumer neuroscience is of benefit to both the research and marketing world. However, it is possible that the technology reported within this chapter is not well enough understood to be able to generalise the findings to the field of marketing and have it result in benefits to a company. The studies presented above show a correlation between neuroimaging and buyer behaviour, however the ability to generalise these findings to specific consumer contexts is difficult. In the early development of consumer neuroscience, simply stating that neuroscientific methods were being used resulted in an increase in sales. From the studies provided throughout this summary, it can be speculated that the technology being used in consumer neuroscience studies may be far ahead of our comprehension. However there are more basic forms of neurophysiological technologies available which appear to be much more promising.

In addition to the use of fMRI or MEG within a consumer neuroscience setting, another recent development within this field is the use of startle reflex modulation (Walla, Brenner &

Koller, 2011). This method involves the presentation of several stimuli, some of which are associated with a loud startle probe designed to initiate a startle response in the participant. In humans, it is found that for pleasant or positive stimuli, the startle response is reduced in comparison to that witnessed when unpleasant or negative stimuli are presented. The startle reflex has been used within a marketing context (Walla et al., 2011; Grahl et al., 2012) and provides a direct measure of emotion that can be directly linked to a participant's like or dislike. In Walla et al.'s study (2011), it acknowledges that a discrepancy exists between participants' stated preference for a brand and what their startle reflex shows. In addition, it shows a significant difference in eye blink response between liked and disliked brands (Figure 12).

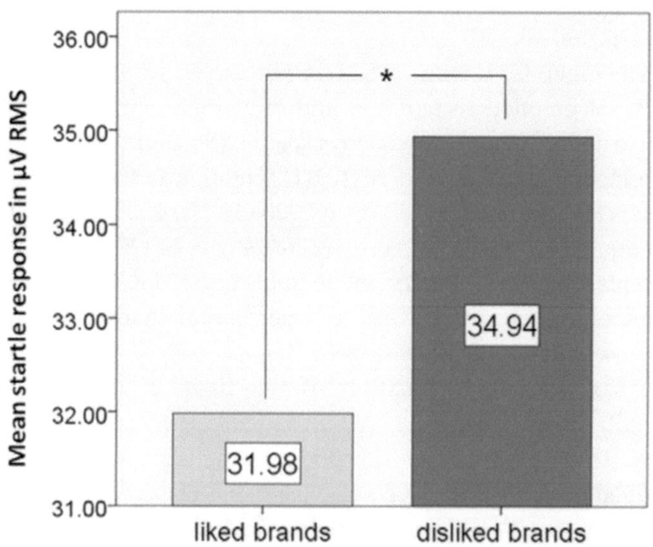

Figure 12. Mean eye blink response to liked versus disliked brands. (with permission)

It is plausible that the findings presented by Walla et al. (2011) indicate that physiological techniques may be more beneficial in the earlier stages of product development. Through the use of startle reflex modulation; it may be possible to determine whether or not consumers are likely to react positively to a product before it reaches markets. This process may also allow businesses to determine how to make their products more appealing before they are marketed. It is clear that the potential of neuroscience to benefit the marketing world is present, however it may be a few more years away.

Author details

Peter Walla, Aimee Mavratzakis and Shannon Bosshard
University of Newcastle, School of Psychology, Centre for Translational Neuroscience and Mental Health Research, Australia

5. References

Becker, J. B., Arnold, A. P., Berkley, K. J., Blaustein, J. D., Eckel, L. A., Hampson, E., et al. (2005). Strategies and methods for research on sex differences in brain and behavior. *Endocrinology, 146*(4), 1650-1673.

Bruner, J. S. (1957). On perceptual readiness. *Psychological review, 64*(2), 123.

Conway, C., Jones, B., DeBruine, L., Welling, L., Law Smith, M., Perrett, D., et al. (2007). Salience of emotional displays of danger and contagion in faces is enhanced when progesterone levels are raised. *Hormones and Behavior, 51*(2), 202-206.

Chartrand, T. L., (2005). The role of conscious awareness in consumer behaviour. *Journal of Consumer Psychology, 15*(3), 203–210.

Derntl, B., Kryspin-Exner, I., Fernbach, E., Moser, E., & Habel, U. (2008a). Emotion recognition accuracy in healthy young females is associated with cycle phase. *Hormones and Behavior, 53*(1), 90-95.

Derntl, B., Windischberger, C., Robinson, S., Lamplmayr, E., Kryspin-Exner, I., Gur, R. C., et al. (2008b). Facial emotion recognition and amygdala activation are associated with menstrual cycle phase. *Psychoneuroendocrinology, 33*(8), 1031-1040.

de Gelder, B., van Honk, J., & Tamietto, M. (2011). Emotion in the brain: of low roads, high roads and roads less travelled. [10.1038/nrn2920-c1]. *Nat Rev Neurosci, 12*(7), 425-425.

Gendron, M., Lindquist, K. A., Barsalou, L., & Barrett, L. F. (2012). Emotion words shape emotion percepts. *Emotion.*(Advance online publication. doi: 10.1037/a0026007).

Gilchrist, J., & Nesberg, L. S. (1952). Need and perceptual change in need-related objects. *Journal of experimental psychology, 44*(6), 369.

Gros, C. (2010). Cognition and Emotion: Perspectives of a Closing Gap. *Cognitive Computation, 2*(2), 78-85.

Grahl, A., Greiner, U., & Walla, P. (2012). Bottle shape elicits gender-specific emotion: a startle reflex modulation study. Psychology, 3(7): in press.

Honea, H., and Horsky, S. (2011). The power of plain: Intensifying product experience with neutral aesthetic context. Springer Science and Business Media.

Junghöfer, M., Kissler, J., Schupp, H. T., Putsche, C., Elling, L., & Dobel, C. (2010). A fast neural signature of motivated attention to consumer goods separates the sexes. *Frontiers in Human Neuroscience, 4*, 179.

Keller, K. L., & Lehmann, D. R. (2006). Brands and branding: Research findings and future priorities. *Marketing Science, 25*(6), 740.

LeDoux, J. (Ed.). (1996). *The emotional brain*. New York: Simon & Schuster.

Liddell, B., Brown, K., Kemp, A., Barton, M., Das, P., Peduto, A., et al. (2005). A direct brainstem-amygdala-cortical [] alarm'system for subliminal signals of fear. *Neuroimage, 24*(1), 235-243.

McClure, S.M., Li, J., Tomlin, D., Cypert, K.S., Montague, L.M., and Montague, P.R. (2004). Neural Correlates of Behavioral Preference for Culturally Familiar Drinks. Neuron, Vol. 44, 379–387.

Morris, J., Öhman, A., & Dolan, R. (1999). A subcortical pathway to the right amygdala mediating "unseen" fear. *Proceedings of the National Academy of Sciences, 96*(4), 1680.

Ng, J., Stice, E., Yokum, S., & Bohon, C. (2011). An fMRI study of obesity, food reward, and perceived caloric density. Does a low-fat label make food less appealing? *Apetite*, 65-72.

Ochsner, K., Ray, R., Hughes, B., McRae, K., Cooper, J., Weber, J., et al. (2009). Bottom-up and top-down processes in emotion generation. *Psychological science, 20*(11), 1322.

Österlund, M. K., & Hurd, Y. L. (2001). Estrogen receptors in the human forebrain and the relation to neuropsychiatric disorders. *Progress in Neurobiology, 64*(3), 251-267.

Pearson, R., & Lewis, M. B. (2005). Fear recognition across the menstrual cycle. *Hormones and Behavior, 47*(3), 267-271.

Pessoa, L., & Adolphs, R. (2010). Emotion processing and the amygdala: from a 'low road' to 'many roads' of evaluating biological significance. [10.1038/nrn2920]. *Nat Rev Neurosci, 11*(11), 773-783.

Pessoa, L., & Adolphs, R. (2011). Emotion and the brain: multiple roads are better than one. [10.1038/nrn2920-c2]. *Nat Rev Neurosci, 12*(7), 425-425.

Phelps, E. (2006). Emotion and cognition: Insights from studies of the human amygdala. *Annual review of psychology, 57*, 27-53.

Plassmann, H., Ramsøy, T. Z., & Milosavljevic, M. (2012). Branding the brain: A critical review and outlook. *Journal of Consumer Psychology*, 18-36.

Radel, R., & Clément-Guillotin, C. (2012). Evidence of Motivational Influences in Early Visual Perception Hunger Modulates Conscious Access. *Psychological science*.

Reimann, M., Zaichkowsky, J., Neuhaus, C., Bender, T., & Weber, B. (2010). Aesthetic package design: A behavioral, neural, and psychological investigation. Journal of Consumer Psychology, 20, 431-441.

Risold, P., Thompson, R., & Swanson, L. (1997). The structural organization of connections between hypothalamus and cerebral cortex. *Brain Research Reviews, 24*(2), 197-254.

Sabatinelli, D., Lang, P. J., Bradley, M. M., Costa, V. D., & Keil, A. (2009). The timing of emotional discrimination in human amygdala and ventral visual cortex. *The Journal of Neuroscience, 29*(47), 14864.

Sah, P., Faber, E., De Armentia, M. L., & Power, J. (2003). The amygdaloid complex: anatomy and physiology. *Physiological reviews, 83*(3), 803-834.

Schupp, H. T., Junghöfer, M., Weike, A. I., & Hamm, A. O. (2003). Attention and emotion: an ERP analysis of facilitated emotional stimulus processing. *Neuroreport 14*, 1107–1110

Sethuraman, R., & Cole, C. (1999). Factors influencing the price premiums that consumers pay for national brands over store brands. Journal of Product and Brand Management, 8(4), 340–351.

Storbeck, J., Robinson, M., & McCourt, M. (2006). Semantic processing precedes affect retrieval: The neurological case for cognitive primacy in visual processing. *Review of General Psychology, 10*(1), 41.

Swanson, L. (2000). Cerebral hemisphere regulation of motivated behavior. *Brain research, 886*(1-2), 113-164.

Tamietto, M., & de Gelder, B. (2010). Neural bases of the non-conscious perception of emotional signals. *Nature Reviews Neuroscience, 11*(10), 697-709.

Walla, P., Brenner, G., & Koller, M. (2011). Objective measures of emotion related to brand attitude: A new way to quantify emotion-related aspects relevant to marketing. *Plos one, 6*(11).

Whalen, P., Rauch, S., Etcoff, N., McInerney, S., Lee, M., & Jenike, M. (1998). Masked presentations of emotional facial expressions modulate amygdala activity without explicit knowledge. *Journal of Neuroscience, 18*(1), 411.

Van Wingen, G., van Broekhoven, F., Verkes, R., Petersson, K., Bäckström, T., Buitelaar, J., et al. (2007a). Progesterone selectively increases amygdala reactivity in women. *Molecular Psychiatry, 13*(3), 325-333.

van Wingen, G., van Broekhoven, F., Verkes, R. J., Petersson, K. M., Bäckström, T., Buitelaar, J., et al. (2007b). How progesterone impairs memory for biologically salient stimuli in healthy young women. *The journal of Neuroscience, 27*(42), 11416-11423.

Chapter 8

Transcranial Magnetic Stimulation and Neuroimaging Coregistration

Elias P. Casula, Vincenza Tarantino, Demis Basso and Patrizia S. Bisiacchi

Additional information is available at the end of the chapter

http://dx.doi.org/10.5772/50076

1. Introduction

The development of neuroimaging techniques is one of the most impressive advancements in neuroscience. The main reason for the widespread use of these instruments lies in their capacity to provide an accurate description of neural activity during a cognitive process or during rest. This important advancement is related to the possibility to selectively detect changes of neuronal activity in space and time by means of different biological markers. Specifically, functional magnetic resonance imaging (fMRI), positron emission tomography (PET), single-photon emission computed tomography (SPECT), and near-infrared spectroscopy (NIRS) use metabolic markers of ongoing neuronal activity to provide an accurate description of the activation of specific brain areas with high spatial resolution. Similarly, electroencephalography (EEG) is able to detect electric markers of neuronal activity, providing an accurate description of brain activation with high temporal resolution. The application of these techniques during a cognitive task allows important inferences regarding the relation between the detected neural activity, the cognitive process involved in an ongoing task, and behaviour: this is known as a *"correlational approach"*.

Besides the fascinating perspective that neuroimaging techniques offer, their correlational nature also represents one of the main limitations since it does not permit to establish causal inferences on brain-cognition-behaviour relations. The development of tools such as transcranial magnetic stimulation (TMS) and transcranial direct current stimulation (tDCS)[1] have compensated for this limit. These instruments, in fact, are able to actively interfere with the ongoing brain activation, permitting to establish a directional (i.e., causal) link between a

[1] The tDCS technique will not be covered in this chapter. Its use with concurrent neuroimaging is very recent since only a few studies so far have investigated this possibility (see [10], for a review).

brain area and a cognitive process. Transcranial magnetic stimulation generates a brief and strong current through a stimulation coil which, in turn, induces a perpendicular, high time-varying magnetic field that penetrates the cranium unimpeded and painlessly [1]. The changing magnetic field induces a transitory electric current that causes depolarisation of a focal population of neurons. Traditionally, this feature has been used to provide a non-invasive measure for neurophysiologic investigation of the central and peripheral nervous systems. Only in the last twenty years the TMS capacity of inducing a transient and focal depolarisation has been utilised in cognitive neuroscience research to allow inferences regarding the role of cerebral areas during the execution of cognitive tasks [2].

However, despite the widespread use of TMS, its exact mechanism of action and interaction with ongoing neural activity is still unclear. In fact, some studies have reported contrasting effects of the same TMS protocol both in cognitive performance, whose execution can be facilitated or inhibited (e.g., [3,4]) and in therapeutic protocols of repetitive TMS (see section 1.2), which can generate the opposite effect in cortical excitability modulation though keeping the same parameters of stimulation [5]. Recent studies have stressed the importance of clarifying the physiological mechanism of TMS [6] and the need to disambiguate its effects on the physiological and behavioural domains [7]. A univocal explanation of the contrasting outcomes after TMS application has not been provided yet, probably because of its complex and variable interaction with brain activity, which can result in the aforementioned unpredictable outcomes. Depolarisation induced by TMS might in turn activate both local neurons under the coil and neurons that project axons far away from the site of stimulation [8]. Moreover, the TMS pulse might activate a mix of neurons, both excitatory and inhibitory. This could be another factor that can lead to contrasting effects [9]. To this end, neuroimaging techniques potentially offer a promising contribution through the description of brain activity evoked by TMS. Recently, many studies have combined TMS with neuroimaging techniques in a coregistration approach and currently this methodology represents a promising answer to some of the unsolved questions regarding the brain-cognition-behaviour relationship.

In this chapter the combined use of TMS and neuroimaging will be widely discussed with particular regard to its advantages as well as its methodological and technical aspects. In the first section the novelty value of TMS-neuroimaging coregistration will be covered with a discussion of how TMS can compensate for the limits of neuroimaging techniques and, vice versa, how neuroimaging could extend the results provided by TMS. In the second section common methodological aspects among the different TMS-neuroimaging coregistrations will be discussed. The third section will focus on TMS-EEG coregistration with regard to the advantages, clinical and research applications, and technical issues that greatly concern the simultaneous use of these two instruments. Finally, the last section of the chapter provides a review of coregistration studies with the other techniques (fMRI, PET, SPECT and NIRS) that will be carried out. The use of such techniques in combination with TMS is more recent than TMS-EEG coregistration. Thus, the review of these methodologies will be relatively shorter in comparison to the discussion on the more popular TMS-EEG methodology.

2. From correlation to coregistration

2.1. What can neuroimaging add to TMS?

One of the most controversial aspects of TMS lies in its complex physiological mechanism. In fact, despite the widespread use of TMS in current research, its mechanism of action is still poorly understood. The ability of TMS to interfere with brain activity is based on the principle of the electromagnetic induction of an electric field, namely Faraday's Law. According to this law the exposition of a material to a time-changing magnetic field causes the induction of an electric field. When TMS is applied to the brain, these electric currents cause a transient and non-invasive depolarisation of cell membranes and thereby neuronal activation in the stimulated area [1]. The application of TMS to the hand representation in the primary motor cortex, for example, induces a depolarisation of the neurons of the corticospinal tract, which evokes a muscle twitch in the contralateral hand. The size of the motor-evoked potential (MEP) reflects the excitability of the corticospinal system. This is one of the few "visible effects" that TMS induces when it is applied to the brain and currently most of the knowledge on the physiological mechanisms of TMS is based on the analysis of such peripheral markers. At the end of the 1980s, the TMS capacity of inducing a non-invasive, transient, and relatively focal depolarisation was used for the first time as a "disruptive" technique, whose effects were interpreted in terms of "virtual brain lesions" [11]. This term was proposed considering the TMS effect as inducing a temporary, reversible lesion in the stimulated area. The "virtual lesion" interpretation of the TMS mechanism was widespread for two main reasons: first, it was supported by early studies on cognitive processes (e.g., [12]); second, it was the most parsimonious and simple explanation of the TMS effect. With the development of neuronavigation systems (see section 4.1), the idea of TMS as a "point and shoot" methodology grew further, until several experiments showed that TMS could also result in the facilitation of cognitive performance (e.g., [4,13]). These "paradoxical" facilitation effects revealed the inadequacy of a "virtual lesion" hypothesis in explaining TMS effects, leading to a reconceptualisation of its mechanisms. Recently, new evidence from biophysical and neuroimaging studies (e.g., [14,15]) offered new insights into basic properties of TMS, leading to an interpretation of its effect in terms of a random-induced neuronal activity ([16]). This activity can be thought of as "neural noise" since is not directly associated with the activity of the stimulated area. For these reasons, its effect can result in interference or facilitation of a cognitive performance depending on the relationship between the noise (i.e., TMS-evoked activity) and the signal (i.e., target activity) [16]. Nevertheless, besides the credible contribution of these kinds of studies clear evidence of the TMS physiologic mechanisms has not yet been provided.

Neuroimaging techniques offer an important contribution to TMS mechanism comprehension through the description of the neural activation evoked by the electromagnetic pulse. For instance, electroencephalography (EEG) can detect the response of a cortical area to the TMS pulse (i.e., cerebral reactivity) based on the related electric markers of its activity, namely TMS-evoked potentials (TEPs). The analysis of TEP characteristics such as latency, amplitude, polarity, and waveform can offer an insight into the physiological state of the stimulated brain area, allowing researchers to tackle inference with TMS mechanisms. On the other hand, techniques such as fMRI, PET, SPECT, and NIRS, which provide better spatial resolution than EEG, offer a detailed picture of responses to TMS throughout the brain. One of the most direct exemplifications of a neuroimaging contribution is the demonstration of the spread dynamics of TMS-evoked activity from the stimulated area to the connected regions. Ilmoniemi and colleagues ([17] – discussed below in section 2.2) were the first to provide direct evidence of this phenomenon. The authors mapped the ongoing activity evoked by the stimulation of the primary motor cortex and primary visual cortex in the ipsilateral and contralateral homologous regions. This evidence had a high novelty value in the field of TMS research, considering that traditionally its effects were evaluated only in regard to the stimulated area. Besides the elucidations on the general TMS mechanism, neuroimaging techniques can also provide direct evidence on the effect of a single TMS parameter. An example was provided by Käkhönen and colleagues [18]. The authors investigated reactivity variations of the prefrontal cortex and primary motor cortex across different stimulation intensity conditions. All the different contributions that each neuroimaging technique provides to TMS will be further discussed in the following sections of this chapter.

2.2. What can TMS add to neuroimaging?

The correlational nature of neuroimaging techniques does not allow any conclusion about the causal role of an activated brain region in task performance. Basing on fMRI data for example it can be demonstrated that an *X* cerebral area is activated while a *Y* cognitive process is performed. However, from a logical point of view this evidence is not sufficient to establish that if the *X* area is activated, the *Y* process is being performed [19]. This argument, which has not been legitimated by scientific logic, is known as "reverse inference" [20]. Furthermore, besides the accurate spatio-temporal information, neuroimaging instruments cannot account for most of the complex variability in neurobiological mechanism modulation. One of the main limitations of these techniques in fact is the poor information about the nature of the brain activation. Basing on PET or fMRI data for example it cannot be established whether the observed activity is excitatory or inhibitory [21]. This is a crucial aspect since the activity detected in a certain area might also reflect inhibitory activation aimed to stop or inhibit processes competing with the function of the area. Moreover, a brain area could merely be accidentally activated by a cognitive process [21]. Finally, in the presence of diffuse brain activation during a multi-componential cognitive task, functional neuroimaging cannot discriminate between the different contributions of the activated brain areas within the ongoing cognitive process [22]. These factors pose several problems in demonstrating the role of a certain area within a cognitive process. In summary, since a brain region can be considered crucial in an "*X*" cognitive process only if the modulation of its activity affects cognitive performance (i.e., facilitation/disruption of the performance), the manipulation of brain activation as a variable is a critical factor in establishing its particular causal role. This feature is provided by transcranial magnetic stimulation technique.

The active interference provided by TMS is used frequently in current neuroscience research to make causal inferences regarding the functional contribution of a stimulated brain area.

There are three main TMS protocols, and their use generally depends on the goal of the application: "single-pulse" (spTMS), "paired-pulse" (ppTMS), and "repetitive" (rTMS). Single-pulse stimulation is mostly used to transiently "interfere" with instantaneous cerebral process, providing an accurate description of the cerebral processing timing. This stimulation is commonly used in the investigation of motor and cognitive process functioning. Regarding the first, spTMS provides precise measures of corticospinal excitability, such as motor threshold (MT) and cortical silent period[2], which are common indices in TMS studies. Regarding cognitive processes, spTMS allows the study of cognitive processing in a causal way through the measurement of reaction times and the accuracy of a performance while delivering a pulse at different time intervals from the stimulus onset (e.g., [23]). The high time resolution provided by spTMS can be used to identify critical periods during which the stimulated area and its connections cover a crucial role within the ongoing process (i.e., mental chronometry – [2]).

Paired-pulse stimulation consists of two pulses and is mostly used in the study of inhibitory processes of motor and premotor cortices. This stimulation can be delivered by one or two coils located in two different areas; in the latter case, we refer to it as "twin-coil" stimulation [24]. This procedure permits the investigation of motor-associated area interactions by analysing variations in MEP amplitude evoked by a test coil placed over the primary motor cortex [24,25]. The other coil, referred to as conditioning coil, is placed over another scalp site. If the conditioning stimulus, which is given prior to the test stimulus over M1, induces a variation in the amplitude of the test MEP (i.e., facilitation or inhibition), a functional connectivity between the two sites with regard to its timing and nature (i.e., facilitatory or inhibitory) might be inferred. Pulse intensities and inter-stimulus-intervals (ISIs) also provide different effects. An ISI of a few milliseconds is generally used in the investigation of short-interval cortical inhibition processes (SICI – [26]), whereas a longer ISI (e.g., 50-200 ms) is generally used in the study of long-interval cortical inhibition processes (LICI – [27]). Different effects can be observed also by varying the intensities of the two stimuli: lower intensities and short ISI generally deliver facilitatory effects [28], whereas inhibitory effects are often observed with higher intensities [24].

Repetitive stimulation consists of a "train of pulses" delivered in a certain time frequency. In the literature, stimulation with a frequency higher than 1Hz is referred to as "high-frequency rTMS", whereas stimulation with a frequency of less than 1Hz is referred to as "low-frequency rTMS" [29]. Repetitive TMS, unlike spTMS and ppTMS, can produce an effect on the excitability of a stimulated area for a period that lasts beyond the duration of the TMS application, depending on the stimulation parameters. For this reason, it has been used frequently both in cognitive studies (e.g., [30] – discussed in section 1.3) and in clinical applications, especially regarding major depression (e.g., [31]), Parkinson's disease (e.g., [32]), and epilepsy (e.g.,[33]) it has been generally established that a low-frequency rTMS protocol produces an inhibitory effect on cortical excitability, while a facilitatory effect is

[2] The motor threshold is the lowest TMS intensity necessary to evoke MEP in a target muscle in 50% of trials [35]. The cortical silent period is referred to as the suppression of electromyographic activity (EMG) in the voluntarily contracted target muscle after the induction of a MEP [36].

often observed after a high-frequency rTMS protocol. Unfortunately, in these cases, the literature also often reports different and equivocal outcomes generated by the same rTMS protocol [5]. In general, now TMS is likely to be classified as a "brain-interference method" rather than a brain imaging method.

2.3. Methodological aspects of TMS-neuroimaging coregistration

Because of the electrical and magnetic principles TMS and neuroimaging are based upon, their simultaneous use (i.e., coregistration) poses several technical problems. The TMS pulse, in fact, induces an electromagnetic artefact that can affect data acquisition when it is performed during neuroimaging (i.e., "on-line" approach), especially when TMS is combined with electroencephalography (EEG) or functional magnetic resonance imaging (fMRI). Such technical problems can mostly be avoided by applying rTMS before or after neuroimaging (i.e., "off-line" approach). Currently, with the exception of MEG, all the other neuroimaging techniques have been successfully used in combination with TMS, both in on-line and off-line approaches.

On-line and off-line approaches provide different information and pose different technical and methodological issues. The choice of one approach instead of the other is generally established based on the target of the study, as well as on the setting and the instruments available. The on-line approach allows direct evaluation of the instantaneous effect of magnetic stimulation on brain tissue. More specifically, TMS is used to interfere with ongoing neuronal activation whose variations in brain activity are detected by neuroimaging. Besides the information provided on the reactivity of the stimulated area and its connectivity to other areas, this approach also has potential value from a technical point of view since it permits researchers to clarify the interaction of TMS effect on the brain. One of the first examples of this kind of study was performed by Bohning and coworkers ([34] – discussed in section 3), who aimed to directly measure the exact magnetic field produced by TMS in human subjects. The authors used two TMS coils suitable for concurrent fMRI (i.e., constructed with non-magnetic materials) to map the magnetic fields generated by TMS in the human brain. This study was the first one that combined TMS and MRI in an on-line approach.

Off-line coregistration can be performed using neuroimaging before or after TMS. In the first case, neuroimaging can be used to guide the exact coil positioning in a localised brain area. This procedure is used particularly in cognitive neuroscience studies since neuroimaging techniques can reliably identify one or more brain areas that are activated during a cognitive task. Subsequent TMS can be applied over the identified area to interfere with ongoing neuronal processing while participants are performing a task that is supposed to involve the stimulated area. This procedure potentially provides important elucidation regarding the possible contribution to a cognitive process of a certain brain region or its interconnected areas. A famous study by Cohen and colleagues [30] provides a direct example of this approach. The authors based their work on previous neuroimaging studies on people who were blind from an early age, which showed prominent activation of the occipital visual areas during Braille reading [37]. Starting with this evidence, they applied short trains of 10-Hz rTMS to different cortical areas in subjects who were blind from an early age while they were involved in the identification of Braille or embossed Roman letters. When TMS was delivered over the occipital visual cortex tactile perception was distorted, resulting in a large number of errors in both tasks. In contrast, the same stimulation in healthy volunteers affected their visual performance, but not their tactile performance. These data confirmed that blindness from an early age generates a cross-modal reorganisation that causes the recruitment of the visual cortex in somatosensory processing. Neuroimaging techniques such as MRI can also be used to define specific anatomical targets based on individual brain images for subsequent TMS. With MRI-guided frameless stereotactic neuronavigation, precise coil placement can be obtained with a high degree of reproducibility across different sessions (e.g., [38] – discussed in section 2.1). This application will be further discussed in the section related to TMS-MRI coregistration.

A different application of the off-line approach consists of using neuroimaging after rTMS to investigate and map the long-term effects of the stimulation. This application offers important insights into functional cortical plasticity as well as elucidation of the TMS mechanism's after-effects. Since the spTMS and ppTMS effects are instantaneous, the only protocol suitable for this approach is rTMS, whose after-effects may last for a variable time. For this reason, neuroimaging should start quickly after the rTMS protocol to ensure that even short-duration after-effects were detected [39]. An example of this application is provided by Lee and colleagues [40]. The authors explored the effects on regional excitability caused by low-frequency rTMS over the primary motor cortex. The authors applied 1 Hz rTMS for 30 minutes, and then activation was mapped through PET at rest and during freely selected finger movements. The results showed an effect of rTMS both locally, with a major activation in the stimulated motor area, and throughout the brain regions engaged in the task. In summary, on-line and off-line approaches provide different insights into the TMS effects on brain activity and imply different methodological and technical precautions. However, the use of one approach does not exclude the other one; conversely, the utilisation of neuroimaging both before and after TMS is an optimal method to detect the effects of the stimulation on neuronal activity.

3. TMS-EEG coregistration

Neural activity generates electric as well as chemical signals. The electric signals generated from the simultaneous activity of large neuron populations can be detected and measured by electrodes applied on the scalp (usually placed according to the 10-20 system). Such signals can be recorded from the scalp since brain, skull, and scalp tissues passively conduct the electric (as well as magnetic) currents generated by the neurons' activity. The recording of tension variations between different electrodes is referred to as electroencephalography (EEG). One of the main EEG applications in clinical and in research settings is the detection of electric responses evoked by cognitive, motor, or sensorial processes. These responses are referred to as event-related potentials (ERPs). The time-varying magnetic field generated by the TMS pulse produces currents in the cortical layers of the brain and a subsequent depolarisation of cell membranes so that action potentials are initiated after the ion channels are opened [17]. The subsequent post-synaptic activation can be recorded in the EEG. The analysis of EEG signals can be used to localise and measure the synaptic activations, thus allowing direct inferences about the reactivity of cerebral areas and their functional connectivity. The first published attempt to measure TMS-evoked brain responses was performed by Cracco and coworkers [41]. The authors recorded responses to TMS from the homologous area contralateral to the stimulation site with an onset latency of 9-12 ms. This study was the first attempt to examine cerebral connectivity by combining TMS and EEG. Three years later, the same research group used a cerebellar stimulation and recorded responses from the interaural line [12]. However, these early attempts were not replicated immediately, probably because of the various technical limitations. Indeed, voltage changes induced by the TMS pulse between scalp electrodes are six orders of magnitude larger than microvolt-level EEG signals [42]. Such high voltage levels can lead to the saturation of a standard EEG amplifier, which can last for hundreds of milliseconds. The subsequent development of TMS-compatible multi-channel EEG recording systems allowed the measurement of instant and direct neuronal effects of TMS from multiple scalp locations, which was impossible with previous technologies. The first study that used these systems was conducted by Ilmoniemi's group. Technical and methodological aspects relative to these systems will be discussed in section 2.3.

The main capacity of TMS lies in its ability to non-invasively interfere with brain activity by modulating the voltage over the membranes of the cortical neurons. In a complementary way, the main potential of concurrent EEG lies in its ability to measure the instantaneous cortical activation induced by TMS with a millisecond time scale, which is currently not possible with any other brain imaging method. Techniques such as PET, SPECT, and fMRI, in fact, are unable to detect the temporal sequence of increased cerebral activity with a sampling frequency similar to that of neural signal transmission because changes in blood flow and oxygenation take several seconds after changes in neuronal activity. On the other hand, EEG does not provide as accurate a spatial resolution as the other techniques do. The next section will address the nuts and the bolts of TMS-EEG coregistration, providing a detailed view of its characteristics and methodology.

3.1. Advantages of TMS-EEG coregistration

This section discusses how the combined use of TMS and EEG can provide precise details on both the initial activation of the stimulated area (i.e., cortical reactivity) and the subsequent spread to connected regions (i.e., cortical connectivity). Cerebral reactivity is defined by the response of a certain brain area to stimulation. Traditionally, TMS was used to assess the reactivity of areas that offer a peripheral marker of central excitability, namely the primary motor cortex and the primary visual cortex. When TMS is applied to the primary motor cortex, a muscle twitch is elicited, measurable with EMG. Similarly, when the V1 area is stimulated, the subject may perceive a moving/flashing phosphene. Excluding these two regions other areas of the cortex are behaviourally silent and their reactivity can be investigated only through the combined use of TMS and EEG. In TMS-EEG studies, cortical reactivity is examined through an analysis of the characteristics of TMS-evoked potentials, such as latency, amplitude, scalp distribution, and waveform (e.g., [18]). These indices represent quantifiable markers of the cerebral neurophysiological state of the stimulated area [43]. In particular, the study of how cortical response varies across different physiological states and/or cognitive conditions is a topic of central interest in the literature. For example, different modulation of reactivity can be generated in comparing responses during a cognitive task and at rest (e.g., [44] – discussed in section 2.3) or in comparing different physiological states after a pharmacological treatment or a TMS protocol. A recent example of the latter application has been provided by Lioumis and coworkers [45]. In this study, the authors aimed to study the responses to TMS of the left primary motor cortex and the prefrontal cortex in a test-retest design. TMS was applied at three intensities in two sessions with a 1-week interval between them. Accurate repositioning of the coil was guaranteed by a neuronavigation system. The results showed high reproducibility in cortical responses after the two TMS sessions, providing evidence of the reliability of TMS-EEG investigation of cortical excitability changes in test-retest designs.

From a technical point of view, the study of how an area reacts to a TMS pulse might be useful in clarifying the effect of a single TMS parameter on brain activity. An example of this application is provided by Kommsi and colleagues [46]. The authors aimed to directly evaluate the effect of the stimulus intensity on TMS-evoked cortical responses. TMS was applied over the primary motor cortices of seven healthy volunteers at four intensities (60%, 80%, 100%, and 120% of MT). The results showed a similar distribution of the potentials for the four intensities, whereas an increment in response amplitude was observed with higher intensities. The evidence provided by the study offered interesting elucidations on the effects of stimulus intensity on TEPs. First, TMS can evoke measurable brain activity even at subthreshold intensities (60% of motor threshold); second, the analysis of the relationship between the stimulus and response potentially offered insights into the state of activation of the brain.

Connectivity studies with traditional TMS-EMG setup were limited to the investigation of motor-associated area interaction (i.e., with "twin-coil" stimulation – discussed in section 1.2). With the development of TMS-compatible multi-channel EEG, the study of connectivity in non-motor areas has become possible. In TMS-EEG coregistration studies, cerebral connectivity is evaluated by tracing the spread of TMS-evoked activity by reconstructing the activity-sources and/or based on the latency of EEG deflections. The first procedure is realised through the application of the minimum-norm estimate, which localises the source of the electric signals [47]. The first study that successfully applied this procedure was performed by Ilmoniemi group [17]. These authors applied TMS at a 0.8 Hz frequency over the primary motor and visual cortices of healthy volunteers. The spread of the TMS-evoked activity was traced using inversion algorithms that localised an immediate response locally to the stimulation. They observed that 5-10 ms after the magnetic pulse, the activation spread to the adjacent ipsilateral motor areas; furthermore, after 20 ms, activation reached the homologous regions in the opposite hemisphere. This activation pattern was observed stimulating both areas. The study by Ilmoniemi and colleagues was the first that provided direct information about cortico-cortical connections through the use of TMS-EEG coregistration. In recent years, many other research studies have confirmed the results obtained by these authors, also providing important insights into the study of the spread dynamics of TMS-induced activity (e.g., [48,49] – discussed in section 2.2).

The analysis of the latencies of scalp-recorded EEG deflections offered a different approach in the investigation of cortico-cortical connectivity. The high temporal resolution of EEG allows the reliable identification of the temporal progress of TMS-evoked activity spread. This permits researchers to infer the causal relations of the TMS-evoked activation. An example of this procedure was provided by Iramina and colleagues [50]. The authors applied TMS at three different intensities (90%, 100%, and 110% of MT) over the cerebellum (20 mm above the inion) and recorded frontal positive potential deflections at Cz with a latency of 9 ms and at Fz with a latency of 10 ms. The results obtained by the authors offered a possible demonstration of occipito-frontal connectivity and, on the other hand, provided evidence of the reliability of TMS-EEG coregistration as a precise methodology in connectivity studies. To this end, a further demonstration of TMS-EEG feasibility has been obtained by examining changes in the spread of TMS-evoked activity while placing the coil over different sites. Kommsi and coworkers stimulated five sites in the left sensorimotor cortex of six healthy volunteers while they monitored responses throughout the brain [38]. To ensure the precise localisation of the anatomic locus of stimulation the authors used a frameless stereotactic method (see section 3). A consistent pattern of response both ipsilaterally and contralaterally was recorded with a latency of 17-28 ms. More important, contralateral responses showed consistent changes when different loci were stimulated. Two conclusions may be drawn from these data. First, the importance of coil positioning is critical since even a small shift in its position caused a different response. Second, the precise recording of ipsi- and contralateral responses revealed a corresponding high spatiotemporal resolution of TMS-EEG methodology in detecting the spread dynamics of TMS-evoked activity.

3.2. Methodological approaches

As suggested by Miniussi and Thut [43], TMS-EEG applications can be grouped into three approaches: inductive, interactive, and rhythmic. Within the "inductive approach" TMS-EEG coregistration is used to provide insights into the neurophysiological state of the brain through TEP analysis across different conditions. The "interactive approach" aimed to investigate the temporal course and the spatial spread of TMS-induced activity during cognitive performance. Finally, in the "rhythmic approach", TMS is used as a technique to interact with oscillatory brain activity.

From an inductive approach perspective, TEPs are considered an index of the cerebral neurophysiological state in areas that does not produce a peripheral marker in response to a TMS pulse. TEP analysis has useful application in clinical and research studies as well as in technical studies. As discussed above, cortical responses evoked by TMS potentially offer important insights into brain activity both locally in the stimulated area and in connected regions. More specifically, the inductive approach aims to infer brain activity dynamics focusing on TEP characteristics and distribution (e.g., [17,38]) without considering behavioural outcomes (which are more relevant in interactive approach studies). Rather, inductive studies are more interested in comparing conditions generated from different neurophysiological states of the brain (e.g., [48,49]). An interesting example of this approach has been provided by Massimini and colleagues, who aimed to investigate connectivity changes across different states of consciousness [49]. The authors applied TMS at a subthreshold intensity (90% of MT) over the rostral portion of the right premotor cortex of six healthy volunteers. The results revealed a critical difference in the spread of TMS-evoked activity between the state of wakefulness and non-REM sleep. A prominent spread of the activity from the stimulation site to ipsi- and contralateral areas was observed during quiet wakefulness. In contrast, during non-REM sleep, the authors observed a rapid decrease in the initial response that did not spread beyond the stimulation site. Thus, the authors concluded that states of consciousness are strictly related to cerebral connectivity efficiency (Massimini et al., 2005). The data provided by this study are a direct exemplification of TEP's potential to reveal important information on the local and distant spread dynamics of cerebral activity.

Regarding technical applications, TEP analysis in combination with a systematic and methodical manipulation of TMS parameters can potentially provide important information on which parameters (e.g., stimulation intensity, coil orientation) are the most effective in producing a certain neuronal modulation. As seen previously in this chapter, the studies by Kommsi group [38,46] provided direct evaluation of the effects of stimulation intensity and coil positioning. Another example of this approach was provided by Bonato and colleagues. The authors applied TMS over the left primary motor cortex of six healthy volunteers, varying the coil orientation. Two orientations were compared: one at 45 degrees with respect to the sagittal plane (which was found to be optimal by previous studies – [52,53]) and one at 135 degrees with respect to the sagittal plane. The authors found that the two orientations evoked a similar pattern of electric potentials but with different amplitudes. From a technical point of view, TMS-EEG can thus provide useful insights into the comprehension of the unclear neurophysiological correlates of the TMS parameters. Future research studies investigating the effects of other TMS parameters might provide important contributions regarding the real outcomes of TMS on brain tissue.

The TMS-EEG interactive approach aims to investigate "where, when and how TMS interacts with task performance" ([43] p. 252). Therefore, interactive approach studies are particularly relevant in cognitive neuroscience research since they aim to study how the effects of TMS correlate with behaviour. More specifically, this approach focuses on the precise determination of which areas are affected by the pulse (i.e., "where") during cognitive performance; the definition of the cognitive process timing course, which is the critical temporal interval in which TMS affects cognition (i.e., "when"); and, finally, the clarification of the TMS effect in terms of the facilitation or inhibition of task performance (i.e., "how"). One example of this approach was offered by a study from Taylor and coworkers [54]. The authors aimed to investigate a frontal-parietal network interaction during a spatial attention task. TMS was applied in short trains of 5 pulses at a frequency of 10 Hz over the right frontal eye field (FEF). When rTMS was delivered during the cueing period, the authors found that the neural activity evoked by visual stimuli was significantly affected. In another study, the same group of research [55], applied a similar rTMS protocol (3 pulses at 10Hz) over the dorso-medial frontal cortex (dMFC) to test its role in conflict resolution through an Eriksen flanker task [56]. The results were interesting: when contralateral (right-hand) incongruent trials occurred, TMS disrupted performance by increasing error rates. Both the results of these studies offered clear anatomo-functional contributions to FEF [54] and to dMFC [55]. Moreover, they provided interesting data on TMS focality since in both studies no effects were observed after the stimulation of a control site that was physically closer to the target areas. In summary, this evidence offers a demonstration of the value of TMS-EEG coregistration as a reliable technique in the study of TMS effects during cognitive tasks with high temporal and spatial resolution.

The TMS technique has different applications in the study of cerebral oscillatory activity [9]. Currently, the rhythmic approach represents one of the most promising avenues for clarifying the TMS mechanisms of interaction with brain activity [57]. The rhythmic approach uses the capacity of TMS to interact with brain rhythms, allowing the opportunity both to investigate the meaning of rhythmical activity and to induce a synchronisation of cerebral oscillations. A study by Sauseng and colleagues offered an exemplification of the first aspect [58]. The authors of the study aimed to investigate the relation between 10 Hz oscillatory activity and cortical excitability. To address this question they applied TMS to the primary motor cortex of six healthy volunteers. Their results showed that when the pre-stimulation level of alpha power was low, an MEP was evoked more easily, and vice versa. Moreover, this effect occurred only at the stimulation site. The results of the study offered insight into the relation between motor cortex excitability and local alpha oscillations. In contrast, other studies have focused on the capacity of rTMS to induce a pattern of oscillatory activity. Brignani and colleagues, for example, investigated the effects of low-frequency rTMS on the EEG oscillatory activity [59]. The authors applied rTMS at a 1 Hz frequency over the primary motor cortex of six healthy volunteers. The results showed an increment in the alpha band related to the period of the stimulation. These data confirm the TMS capacity to induce a synchronisation of the background oscillatory activity locally to the stimulation site. The induction of a certain rhythm of brain oscillation might also have potential value in the cognitive domain. More specifically, brain oscillations at a certain frequency are induced, and then their effect can be tested during the performance of a cognitive task. If a systematic effect on performance is observed, an inference regarding the causal relation between brain rhythm and cognitive processes could be established [7]. Some studies have explored this possibility. In a study by Klimesch and coworkers [60], for example, the authors applied rTMS at individual alpha frequency (IAF) to influence the dynamics of alpha desynchronisation leading to an improvement of cognitive performance [61]. Repetitive TMS was delivered over the mesial frontal cortex (Fz) and the right parietal cortex (P6) while subjects performed a mental rotation task. The results confirmed the authors' hypothesis: rTMS improved task performance by enhancing the extent of alpha desynchronisation. This study, besides providing evidence of the rTMS capacity to interact with cerebral rhythms, also demonstrated the functional relevance of oscillatory neuronal activity in the alpha band during cognitive processing. Recently, more studies have investigated a possible relation between alpha oscillations and cognition. In particular, recent research studies that used visual tasks identified a relation between the occipito-parietal alpha amplitude and the perception of visual stimuli (e.g., [62]). Therefore, the use of the rhythmic approach in TMS-EEG studies also appears promising in cognitive domain research, and in the future more cognitive processes needed to be investigated in relation to brain rhythms.

3.3. Technical issues

The simultaneous use of TMS and EEG, like the other TMS-neuroimaging combinations, poses several technical issues due to artefacts of different nature. In this part of the chapter, technical problems concerning the combined use of TMS and EEG will be discussed. The aim is to review the strategies developed so far to obtain a reliable EEG recording during TMS. As mentioned above, the main problem of this methodology is caused by the high TMS-induced electrical field, which can saturate recording EEG amplifiers.

A great portion of the studies that have analysed the EEG response to TMS have focused on the cortical response (TEP) evoked by a single pulse on the primary motor cortex at rest (e.g., [38,45,49,51,63-65]). The TEP components detected in most of these studies are: N15, P30, N45, N100, P180, and N280. The large number of studies that observed this pattern of TEPs demonstrated the high reproducibility of TMS-evoked deflections, contrary to motor-evoked potentials, whose amplitude is highly variable [66]. In spite of the high consistency of TMS-evoked EEG potentials, only the N100 is considered a "universal" response since it is the most evident, pronounced, and reproducible component evoked by TMS over the motor cortex (e.g., [45,49,63,64,67]). On the other hand, the occurrence of the other components can vary depending on TMS-related factors (e.g., coil positioning or orientation – [38,51]) as well as subjective-related factors (e.g., state of the cortex and state of consciousness – [67,49]). Different TMS parameters, for example, can determine a temporal shift in the potentials, even of a few milliseconds (e.g., [51,65]). Currently, the origin of TEPs is still unknown with the exception of the N45 component, which has been localised in the central sulcus (ipsilateral to the stimulation) and whose amplitude is directly related to the stimulus intensity [63].

Interestingly, most of the studies mentioned above were unable to detect cortical responses before 10-15 ms from the TMS pulse onset or even later. This latency period that precedes TEP recording is due to the high voltages induced by the TMS pulse between scalp electrodes. These currents can cause saturation of the amplifier, which might last hundreds of milliseconds before the system resumes working appropriately. Thus, all attempts to apply TMS during an EEG recording have faced these technical issues. In recent years, the development of new technologies and solutions has gradually led to an improvement of the temporal resolution of EEG recording during TMS. Such strategies can be divided in two types: on-line strategies, which consists of the creation of technologies that are able to avoid saturating the EEG amplifiers during TMS (e.g., [42]) and off-line strategies, which aim to remove artefacts once the coregistration is completed (e.g., [44,68]).

In 1997, TMS-compatible multi-channel EEG systems were introduced, allowing the instantaneous measurement of TMS effect on brain activity from multiple scalp locations. The 60-channel EEG system developed by Virtanen group [42], guaranteed its TMS-compatibility through the use of gain-control and sample-and-hold circuits, which permit the locking of EEG signals for several milliseconds (i.e., "gating period") immediately post-TMS. This technology avoids the saturation of the recording by preventing the passage of the artefact along the amplifier circuits. Such a blocking system is controlled by an external trigger, which is activated about 50 μs before the TMS pulse and is released 2.5 ms after the pulse. In the study performed by Virtanen group in 1999, the authors successfully recorded EEG responses while TMS was applied over FCz with an intensity of 100% and 120% of MT and a frequency of 1 Hz. In spite of the novelty value of this system, some problems remained unsolved. For instance, the gating period lasts much longer than the TMS pulse itself, which lasts only about 300 μs. This did not allow the recording of the signal immediately after the stimulation. Other TMS-compatible EEG amplifiers have been developed recently. In 2003, Iramina and colleagues ([50] - discussed in section 2.1) developed a 64-channel system based on a sample-and-hold circuit and were able to measure EEG activities 5 ms after the TMS pulse onset. Another system developed by Thut and coworkers [44] was based on a slew-rate limiter: this technology allowed continuous recording and prevented saturation during TMS. Today, new TMS-compatible EEG systems are able to avoid saturation due to TMS pulse, which results in a very short-duration artefact. This feature permits continuous EEG recording during TMS, allowing researchers to see what happens in the EEG signal around the TMS pulse. Bonato and colleagues ([51] – discussed in section 2.2), for example, used TMS-compatible DC amplifiers that were able to tolerate the high time-varying magnetic field induced by TMS. This characteristic allowed the recording of cortical response to TMS with high temporal and spatial resolution. In spite of the high temporal resolution recording provided by these new systems, some technical questions remain unsolved. For instance, it is still difficult to distinguish between the cortical and non-cortical (i.e., magnetic) currents that characterise at least the early part of the response after TMS [69]. All these considerations reflect the relevance that artefact investigation still has in the literature and its characterisation as a crucial factor to differentiate artefactual activity from cortical activity.

Off-line strategies, unlike on-line ones, aim at removing the artefact only after the complete acquisition of the TMS-EEG coregistration. This aim is achieved through the use of software strategies (i.e., algorithms, off-line filters) or experimental procedures. Off-line strategies have been developed recently: the first work that used a similar approach was performed by Thut group (see below). Two main approaches can be distinguished: a subtractive approach and a correctional approach. Both procedures although based on different logics aim to correct, reduce, or remove the TMS-induced electromagnetic artefact. In the subtractive approach, a template artefact is generated by delivering stimulation in a control condition (e.g., [44]) or applying TMS over a phantom (e.g., [64]). The subtraction of the template artefact from experimental data permits the isolation of the target response. The studies of Thut group [44,70], as mentioned above, were the first to use a subtractive approach that aimed to isolate cortical responses related to a visual task (VEPs). To this end, they created a control condition in which TMS pulses were delivered at rest. This procedure permits the isolation of only the artefact without task-related responses. This condition was then subtracted from the visual task condition to isolate only the task-related TEPs. A similar procedure was followed by Bender and coworkers [64], who aimed to investigate the influences of cerebral maturation on TMS-evoked N100. The authors used a glass head dummy covered by a cloth soaked with water (simulating the impedances of skull and scalp, respectively) to generate a template artefact. The study of only the N100 component was permitted by subtracting phantom artefacts from human-evoked potentials.

The correctional approach comprises all procedures aimed at reducing or removing artefacts through the use of algorithms and off-line filters. These procedures are more common in technical studies, often performed by biomedical and computer engineering equipment (e.g., [68,71]). Morbidi and colleagues, for example, proposed an off-line Kalman filter as a new effective and low-cost strategy for artefact reduction [71]. The solution proposed by the author allowed the modelling of the dynamic components of TMS-EEG signal through the use of time-varying covariance matrices. The authors compared the dynamic Kalman filter with stationary filters such as the Wiener filter, concluding that the first one guarantees a more efficient deletion of TMS-induced artefacts while preserving the integrity of EEG signals around TMS pulses. Another example of artefact correction via software was performed by Litvak group [68]. The authors used a method developed by Berg and Scherg [73], originally applied for ocular artefact correction, based on a multiple-source approach. Using a set of artefact topographies, the authors constructed a source model and a set of brain topographies that consisted of multiple dipoles that model brain activity. From this source model a linear inverse operator was computed that decomposed the data into a linear combination of brain and artefact activities, which were subtracted from the data. The results showed that the modelled brain activity was not altered after the correction process. In summary, off-line procedures also potentially offer a wide range of possible solutions to clean EEG recordings from TMS artefacts. Nevertheless, since this approach is still in an early stage, other research studies are needed to develop and improve new ad hoc strategies that provide an optimal dissociation between cortical and artefactual TMS-related activity.

Besides the relevance of the aspects just discussed, many other factors play an important role in providing a reliable signal-to-noise EEG with concurrent TMS. These aspects are mainly referable to TMS (e.g., parameters of stimulation, stimulator devices[3]) and to EEG setup (e.g., electrodes, wires, cap). Recently, several research studies have investigated the effect of specific TMS parameters, such as TMS frequency, intensity, waveform (e.g., [69]), ISI (e.g., [65]), or coil orientation (e.g., [51]) on artefact characterisation. In their study, Veniero and colleagues manipulated several TMS parameters to observe their effect in the electromagnetic artefact amplitude and latency [69]. The authors compared three TMS devices (two biphasic and one monophasic), four types of figure-of-eight coils, ten intensities (from 10% to 100% of the maximum output), three frequencies (spTMS; rTMS at 5 Hz; rTMS at 20 Hz), and two sham conditions (i.e., performed with a placebo coil and with a

[3] TMS stimulators can be categorized into two types based on the waveform generated: monophasic and biphasic. Recent studies have underlined their different effects on neural tissue (e.g., [78,79]).

real coil turned over). Furthermore, EEG artefact generated by TMS delivered over the scalp was compared to the EEG artefact generated by TMS over two phantoms (i.e., a melon and a human knee). The authors found that the artefact produced by the magnetic pulse lasted approximately 5 ms after TMS onset in all conditions. Its duration, therefore, was not affected by different parameters of stimulation. In contrast, the artefact amplitude was higher when evoked by a monophasic pulse compared to a biphasic one. Other studies that manipulated the TMS ISI and coil orientation did not find a prominent effect of these parameters on cortical response except for minor variations in the latency of some components [65,51].

Regarding EEG-related factors, the type of electrode is one of the most influential variables in performing an efficient TMS-EEG coregistration. Because of the strong electric field generated by TMS, an electrode suitable for TMS-EEG coregistration should satisfy numerous physical requirements to work appropriately. Small dimensions are necessary, first to prevent the forces caused by the induced currents from affecting the electrode too much, and second to avoid overheating. Moreover, to provide the best interface with the skin, it should be coated with a suitable surface material [73]. For these reasons, traditional electrodes (made of silver or tin and with a diameter of ~1 cm) are not suitable for concurrent TMS since they are more affected by the induced currents. This can result in both a larger artefact and a higher risk of skin burns [74-76]. Additional problems can result from electrode polarisation, caused by electric currents between the electrolyte and the electrode. When an electrode is polarised, the artefact might cause an EEG baseline shift that can last for hundreds of milliseconds. Currently, the most frequently used electrodes in TMS-EEG systems are small Ag/AgCl pellet electrodes. These characteristics, other than reducing temperature by more than 50% [73,77], permit excellent recording during TMS [77]. Another technical aspect that influences the artefact amplitude is electrode impedance which has to be kept at low values (generally below 5 kΩ). High values of impedance in fact can lead to greater artefacts [73]. Generally, low values of electrode impedance are reached with skin scrubbing and cleaning with alcohol or ad-hoc products, and several strategies may be implemented to achieve this result. A study conducted by Julkunen and colleagues, for example, found a significant reduction of TMS-induced artefacts after puncturing the epithelium under the electrode contacts with custom-made needles [80]. Finally, recent studies have observed that the electrode wire arrangement can also play an important role in reducing TMS-evoked artefacts (e.g., [69,81]). Sekiguchi and coworkers, in particular, tested the effect of coil direction relative to the orientation of the stimulated electrode wire [81]. The authors observed a great reduction in the artefact amplitude when the coil was placed perpendicularly to the wire direction of the stimulated electrode. Their results suggested that the rearrangement of the lead wires relative to the fixed coil orientation can significantly reduce TMS artefacts from EEG recordings.

Besides the electric effect on the brain, TMS application can affect EEG recording also as a result of multimodal sensory stimulation. A TMS pulse, in fact, has multiple "indirect" effects; for instance, it produces a "click" of 100-120 dB [82] that elicits an auditory response which, in turn, might produce a startle reflex that can affect behavioural data, especially in reaction time detection [83]. Furthermore, there is evidence of auditory and sensorial-evoked potentials related to the TMS click that should be considered and controlled for, especially in the electrophysiological analysis of TMS evoked-potentials [84,85]. A solution to avoid this problem is using earplugs or masking the coil click with white noise (e.g., [63,86]) or a sound with a similar spectral content (e.g., [49]). Alternatively, if the experimental design does not allow the use of earplugs, some authors have created a control condition to isolate and exclude the auditory artefacts (e.g., [64]). Finally, TMS-elicited muscle activity (e.g., involuntary stimulation of a facial nerve) or electrode movement can also be source of artefacts during EEG recording. In these cases only slight modifications of the setting can improve the record, for instance by reorienting the coil, reducing the intensity, or trying to avoid direct contact of the coil with the recording electrodes.

3.4. Clinical applications

Electromiographic activity alterations induced by TMS, such as the prolongation of the silent period, have been used as an index in several neurological and psychiatric conditions and reported in patients with Parkinson's disease, dystonia, and Alzheimer's dementia [87,89]. The evaluation of cortical oscillatory activity extended and fostered the relevance of TMS-EEG coregistration, particularly focusing on the non-motor regions of the cortex (e.g., the prefrontal cortex – [59,90]). Moreover, differences between healthy and pathological patterns were reported in patients with schizophrenia [91,92]. The combined use of the TMS-EEG method by Manganotti group, interestingly, proved to be effective during sleep state and has inspired many works devoted to studying clinical samples [93]. Another example is provided by the group of Massimini and Tononi, who investigated cortical effective connectivity during loss-of-consciousness states [49,94]. These research studies are relevant in that they could be used for both diagnostic aims and treatment in pathologies related to minimally conscious states as well as in communication disorders such as aphasia, akinetic mutism, and catatonic depression.

A remarkable application of combined TMS-EEG involved pathologies (e.g., epilepsy, migraine) that are commonly excluded from TMS application. Manganotti group [95,96] evaluated the effects of sleep deprivation on cortical reactivity to TMS in patients suffering from juvenile myoclonic epilepsy (JME). They administered single-pulse TMS over the left motor area during continuous EEG recording, assessing TMS-evoked responses during waking, sleep deprivation, and different sleep stages. In these patients, sleep deprivation produced increased short-latency intracortical facilitation and decreased inhibition of motor areas, as well as, *de facto,* an overall increase in corticospinal excitability. In JME patients, the frontal excitability is a distinctive trait since it behaves in the opposite way with respect to the response to sleep deprivation in healthy controls, which is reduced. However, most studies have evaluated EEG states before and after a TMS treatment (e.g., epilepsy or migraine – [97,98]).

4. TMS-MRI coregistration

Magnetic resonance imaging (MRI) is an imaging technique based on the properties of the atomic nuclei of biological tissues. This technique measures their spin precession within a strong magnetic field induced by the MRI scanner. More specifically, the MRI-induced magnetic field causes an alignment of some atomic nuclei in the body parallel to the magnetic field itself. The radio frequency fields subsequently applied systematically perturb the alignment of the magnetised nuclei in a predictable direction. The rotating magnetic field produced by the nuclei is detectable by the MRI scanner, which records this information to construct an image of the scanned area. The images generated by an MRI scanner have a high spatial resolution of a few millimetres and provide detailed structural information on brain anatomy. However, since this method provides only static information, only a few research studies have focused on the simultaneous use of TMS and MRI. Most of the studies acquired TMS and structural data separately in time (i.e., by the off-line approach), avoiding most of the technical problems that characterise on-line coregistration.

The main technical problem in performing simultaneous TMS-MRI coregistration lies in the presence of the coil within the MRI scanner since it is made of ferromagnetic material. New MRI-compatible coils are suitable for concurrent MRI and fMRI since they are not made of magnetic material. The first study that used this kind of coil was performed by Bohning and colleagues [34]. The authors could measure and characterise the magnetic field generated by TMS in healthy human brains using a standard 1.5 T MRI scanner. Specifically, they obtained 3D maps of the magnetic field created by two TMS coils.

The combined use of TMS and MRI can have useful applications for both research and clinical purposes. Since TMS, as stated above, provides precious insights into the physiological state of brain regions, such information, if appropriately combined with detailed images provided by an MRI scanner, might reveal important correlations between physiological indices (e.g., cortical reactivity and connectivity) and structural measures. An example of this kind of study was provided by Boorman and coworkers [99]. The authors investigated the relationship between a physiological measure of functional connectivity and a measure of structural connectivity during the execution of a decision-making test. Functional connectivity was investigated (i.e., through a twin-coil approach – see section 1.2) by applying TMS over the dorsal premotor cortex and the primary motor cortex. The structural anatomic network, linking the brain regions involved in the task, was reconstructed using diffusion-weighted imaging (DWI). The results of the study revealed a relationship between individual differences in functional and structural connectivity in action choice-related brain networks. The potential contribution of TMS-MRI combined use in revealing possible correlations between physiological data (i.e., provided by TMS) and structural data (i.e., provided by MRI) is also evident in clinical studies. A study by Sach and colleagues, for example, used TMS capacity to non-invasively investigate the central-motor conduction in relation to changes in tissue structure due to the degeneration of corticospinal fibres, detected by MRI [100]. The authors applied single-pulse TMS over the primary motor cortex of fifteen patients with amyotrophic lateral sclerosis (ASL), six of whom had no clinical signs. The results showed a negative correlation between central-motor conduction time and fractional anisotropy. This evidence offered insights into the diagnosis of motor neuron disease before clinical symptoms become apparent.

Regarding off-line TMS-MRI combined applications, these might not be strictly considered as coregistration approaches. However, the use of MRI imaging before TMS is highly popular especially in cognitive neuroscience research to perform neuronavigated TMS (for a recent review, see [101]). This procedure consists, first, of the acquisition of high-resolution structural images. Then, the subject's head outside the scanner is co-registered to MR images based on anatomical landmarks that are easily identifiable such as nasion, inion, and auricular deflexions. This permits precise guidance for the placement of the TMS coil over a particular brain region based on the subject's anatomy. Moreover, such a system allows on-line control of the TMS position, which can be monitored and fixed during a session of stimulation. Therefore, the highly reproducibility of TMS positioning and orientation across different sessions is guaranteed. In current cognitive neuroscience studies that use TMS, as stated before, the use of neuronavigation systems is now very common, even with the use of an MRI template, in case subjects do not have personal MRI scans.

5. TMS-fMRI coregistration

Functional magnetic resonance imaging (fMRI) is a functional imaging technique that uses magnetic resonance imaging to detect and measure the activation of a brain area. This procedure consists of the image of variations in regional blood flow, measured by changes in endogenous oxy- and deoxyhemoglobin concentration, which reflect the energy use of brain cells. The detection of such variations is based on the magnetic properties of deoxyhemoglobin and oxyhemoglobin, which are paramagnetic and diamagnetic, respectively. The local magnetic field variations caused by the quantity of oxygen in haemoglobin are detected by fMRI, offering a measure of the activation of a certain brain area. As mentioned above, fMRI is able to detect the activation of certain brain regions with high spatial resolution (i.e., with millimetre precision) and poor temporal resolution since changes in blood flow last longer than the underlying neural responses (i.e., a few seconds).

The combined use of TMS and fMRI is a promising methodology in determining the limitations of both techniques, as stated in section 1 of this chapter. However, the simultaneous use of the two techniques is technically challenging because of the high magnetic field strength of MRI scanners, which can vary from 1.5 to 7 T. The mere presence of TMS coils within the scanner can affect the homogeneity of the fMRI static magnetic field. This problem can lead to a signal loss in echo-planar images as well as spatial distortions. A recent study by Bungert and coworkers used some shims made of thin patches of austenitic stainless steel to reduce the effect of the TMS coil on the magnetic field [102]. The results showed a reduction of about 80% of the effect of the coil, which permitted the elimination of the associated artefact. Many technical problems arise from the simultaneous functioning of TMS and fMRI. A TMS stimulator, for example, may generate radiofrequency noise that can affect the MRI signal. This problem is generally managed through the use of radiofrequency filters [39]. Recently, another type of image artefact generated by leakage currents in a TMS system was investigated by Weiskopf and his group [103]. The authors characterised the image artefacts through the use of numerical simulations and the application of different coil geometries in phantom studies. The problem was solved by devising a relay-diode combination that was inserted in the TMS circuit, reducing the leakage current. Furthermore, as in TMS-EEG coregistration, the TMS pulse itself can be a source of different artefacts during fMRI. Distortions caused by the TMS pulse were investigated at 2.0 T by Bestmann and colleagues [104]. The authors found that both the echo-planar imaging section orientation (EPI) relative to the plane of TMS coil and the temporal gaps between TMS and image acquisition play a crucial role in artefact generation. Based on the results of the study, the authors concluded that TMS should be applied at least 100 ms before EPI to avoid stimulation during imaging. To our knowledge, the first study that demonstrated the feasibility of TMS application during fMRI acquisition was performed by Bohning group. The authors used non-ferromagnetic TMS coil to stimulate the primary motor cortex of three healthy volunteers inside a 1.5 T MR scanner. They observed significant responses in the motor cortex during the TMS condition compared to a rest condition, proving that the combined use of the two techniques is possible.

Besides the technical issues posed by the simultaneous use of TMS and fMRI, this methodology has potential value for different purposes. The on-line coregistration of the two techniques might reveal the effect of TMS in neural circuits with respect to its spatial resolution, which is provided by MRI with high precision. This procedure can be performed at rest with the aim of investigating the basic mechanism of TMS-brain interaction and measuring the reactivity and connectivity of stimulated areas for neurophysiological applications. One example of these applications was provided by Bestmann and collaborators [107]. The authors applied high-frequency rTMS (3.12 Hz) over the left sensorimotor cortex of healthy volunteers. They compared stimulations with intensities above and below the active motor threshold of the subjects. The two intensities produced different results: suprathreshold rTMS produced high activation in the stimulated area (sensorimotor cortex) and in its connected regions, both cortical (supplementary motor area, dorsal premotor cortex, cingulate motor area) and subcortical (putamen, thalamus), whereas subthreshold rTMS elicited a similar pattern of activation but no MRI-detectable activity in the stimulated sensorimotor cortex. These results, on one hand, offered insight into the cerebral motor system's connectivity and reactivity; on the other hand, they showed interesting evidence regarding the TMS mechanisms of action regarding its different dynamics depending on the stimulation. Interestingly, its effects spread not only in cortical areas but also in subcortical structures.

Concurrent TMS-fMRI studies also potentially provide contributions to cognitive neuroscience research. TMS applied during a task permits establishment of the causal role of an area within a cognitive process. This inference can be reinforced by mapping with high spatial resolution the TMS-induced activity through concurrent fMRI. Sack and coworkers, for example, investigated the role of the parietal cortex in visuospatial judgements [107]. The authors applied TMS to the left and right parietal cortices during fMRI while the participants performed a visuospatial task. The behavioural results revealed impaired performance when TMS was applied over the right parietal cortex, whereas left stimulation produced no effect. Furthermore, fMRI detected a change in the activity of a specific fronto-parietal network in the right hemisphere, which had a significant correlation with the impaired cognitive performance. This result revealed a specific right fronto-parietal activation during the task, corroborating the previous hypothesis of a distributed fronto-parietal network underlying visuospatial processes.

Useful applications can also be obtained using rTMS and fMRI separately in time (i.e., off-line approach). In a study performed by Tegenthoff and colleagues, for example, the authors aimed to investigate the effects of high-frequency rTMS in tactile perception as well as in cortical plasticity [108]. rTMS was applied at a frequency of 5 Hz over the cortical representation of the right index finger of the primary somatosensory cortex. Stimulation of this area caused a lowering of the discrimination threshold of the right index finger. This data was corroborated by subsequent fMRI, which detected an enlargement of the right index finger's somatotopic representation. The results obtained by the authors provided evidence of the effects of rTMS on perceptual as well as on cortical plasticity. Concurrent TMS-fMRI can, thus, have potential in establishing causal links between cognition, perception, motor processes and their cortical correlates.

Clinical applications of TMS-fMRI coregistration have mainly focused on the long-term effects of either a cerebral dysfunction or a rehabilitation program. The residual cortical activity was considered to be a variable indicating cerebral plasticity. Several studies conducted by Li's group were devoted to evaluating the cortico-cortical network in depressant patients and the influence of medications on this network. In their first study, Li and colleagues administered cycles of 1 Hz rTMS on the prefrontal cortex, interleaving fMRI measurements of the regional changes in BOLD response [109]. Through principal component analysis (PCA), they were able to describe the network of brain areas that increased activity, which included the stimulated area as well as deep limbic regions, critical in the treatment of depression. Later, these authors applied the stimulation in a temporal window after administering lamotrigine and valproic acids and demonstrated the reliability of TMS-fMRI coregistration in the assessment of the effect of medications both locally and in cortical networks [110]. Hamzei and coworkers assessed the effects of rehabilitative therapy after a stroke (of either the middle cerebral artery or internal capsule) that involved the motor functions of the hand area [111]. Paired pulse was applied to investigate intracortical inhibition and intracortical facilitation; BOLD response was measured following passive and active movements of either the affected or the non-affected hand. Their study was important since it was the first one to investigate the efficacy of a treatment using a multiple-view perspective obtained from several techniques. Although appealing, this kind of study is really rare, perhaps because of the several challenges posed by the combination of these methods.

6. TMS-PET and TMS-SPECT coregistration

The functioning of PET is based on the detection of pairs of gamma rays generated by the collision of positrons (emitted by an isotope that is introduced into the body as a tracer) with electrons. Through the detection of the exact points where gamma rays are generated, PET allows the reconstruction of three-dimensional images of tracer concentration within the body. Different radioactive tracers (e.g., carbon-11, oxygen-15) provide different indices, such as the regional cerebral blood flow (rCBF), which are strictly related to neuronal activity. Thus, PET images are able to detect selective activations of the brain both at rest and during a task with a spatial resolution of about 5 mm. Like PET, SPECT is a nuclear medicine tomographic imaging technique whose functioning is based on gamma ray detection. Since the two techniques are very similar, their combined use will be discussed together.

As far as we know, the first study that applied TMS during PET was performed by Paus' group [112]. In this study, the authors tested previous evidence of anatomical fronto-occipital connectivity provided by studies on monkeys [113]. Transcranial magnetic stimulation was delivered over the left frontal eye fields (FEF) in different trains of pulses (5, 10, 15, 20, 25, and 30 trains) at a frequency of 10 Hz with an intensity at 70% of the maximum output of the stimulator. The authors found a significant positive correlation between the number of TMS pulses and cerebral blood flow. More specifically, prominent activation was found in the stimulation site in the left medial parieto-occipital cortex and in the left and right superior parietal cortices. The results corroborated previous studies that investigated FEF connectivity on macaque monkeys [113] and provided clear evidence of the reliability of the combined TMS-PET technique in the study of cerebral connectivity. As demonstrated by the above mentioned study, the use of TMS during PET poses fewer technical problems compared to other neuroimaging coregistrations. Moreover, TMS-PET combined use guarantees distinctive advantages. First, during PET acquisition, it is possible to monitor the coil positioning since it is clearly visible; this is not possible during fMRI acquisition. Furthermore, during PET, even long rTMS sessions can be delivered without temporal limits, allowing researchers to see the effect of the stimulation both in the stimulated area and in the connected regions. On the other hand, this also represents a limitation since PET is unable to detect the effects of a single-pulse TMS or even of a short sequence of pulses. Therefore, because of its poor temporal resolution, only cumulative rTMS effects on brain activity can be detected by a PET scan [39].

Simultaneous TMS-PET coregistration has also been used in the study of cognitive processes. Motthaghy and colleagues, for example, tested the effect of rTMS on a working memory task and on regional blood flow changes [114]. Repetitive TMS was applied in 30 s trains at a frequency of 4 Hz over the dorsolateral prefrontal cortices (DLPFC) and over the midline frontal cortex as a control site. In the same time, subjects were required to perform a verbal working memory task. The results showed worse performance on the task when the stimulation was applied over the left and right DLPFC. Concurrently, significant reductions in regional blood flow changes were detected both locally and in connected regions. The results obtained by the authors represent one of the first direct evidence showing the disruptive effects of rTMS in a cerebral region within a network involved in a cognitive task. Other studies have focused on rTMS effects on motor cortical excitability, offering interesting elucidation regarding its neurophysiological mechanisms; an example of this approach was provided by Lee's group [40], whose study was discussed in section 1.3.

Regarding therapeutic applications, few studies have used TMS-PET coregistration for clinical purposes. The PET and SPECT techniques are suitable for detecting changes in plasticity due to the TMS therapy, especially given that rTMS has mostly been used with patients resistant to pharmacological treatments. As a consequence, a relatively large body of literature on mood disorders, such as depression, has allowed the mapping of long-lasting activity changes and cortical reorganisation [115-117]. Frontal-lobe rTMS was also proposed as a treatment for Parkinson's dementia: studies conducted by Straffella's group tried to determine the modification caused by rTMS in the cortical functioning and in the neurotransmitters tied to the development of this kind of dementia [118]. Apart from these examples, the situation clearly suggests that TMS combined with these techniques for clinical purposes is limited to the study of the long-lasting effects of the TMS technique itself. Therefore, in the future, there will probably be no attempts to apply the simultaneous recording of PET/SPECT with TMS.

7. TMS-NIRS coregistration

Near-infrared spectroscopy (NIRS) is a spectroscopic method of detecting changes in haemoglobin concentrations through the measurement of the absorption of near-infrared light by neural tissue. This permits the detection of changes in brain activity with good spatial resolution, limited to the cortical regions. Since this method does not make use of magnetic fields, it is suitable to be combined with TMS without particular technical precautions. However, compared to other TMS-neuroimaging coregistrations, a smaller number of studies have used NIRS during TMS; therefore, technical details regarding this coregistration are still lacking.

One of the first studies that successfully applied TMS during NIRS was performed by Oliviero and colleagues [119]. The authors compared cerebral variations in oxyhemoglobin, deoxyhemoglobin, and cytochrome oxidase-induced magnetic and electrical stimulation. Stimulation was delivered at a frequency of 0.25 Hz over the NIRS probe on the anterior right frontal region. Repetitive TMS immediately induced a significant increase in oxyhemoglobin and a decrease in cytochrome oxidase, whereas this effect was not observed after electrical stimulation. The results of the study underlined the different effects provided by magnetic and electric stimulation, suggesting that rTMS induced higher regional cerebral blood flow rate and, consequently, an increase in the activation of the stimulated area. Interestingly, some studies have also evaluated the effect on metabolic activity after single-pulse TMS (e.g., [120,121]), which is otherwise impossible with other neuroimaging techniques such as PET and SPECT (see section 5). In a study by Mochizuki and coworkers, for example, the authors applied single-pulse TMS over the left primary motor cortex at different intensities (100%, 120%, or 140% of the active motor threshold) both at rest and during contraction of the right first dorsal interosseous muscle [121]. The results showed an increase in oxyhemoglobin in the active condition when TMS was delivered at 100% intensity. In contrast, significant decreases in deoxyhemoglobin and total haemoglobin were observed under the resting condition with TMS at 120% and 140% intensity. The authors interpreted the decrease as a lasting inhibition induced by higher-intensity TMS that results in a reduction in the baseline firing of corticospinal tract neurons. Moreover, combined TMS-NIRS studies have also evaluated the effect of rTMS at higher frequencies such as 1 Hz (e.g., [122]) and theta-burst stimulation[4] (e.g. [123]), on the regional cerebral haemoglobin rate.

However, compared to the other techniques NIRS is a very new methodology. Therefore, more studies are needed in this field. Clinical research, for example, is lacking at the moment, but all indications suggest that this combination would be a worthwhile field of application for several pathological conditions (e.g., learning disabilities).

8. Conclusions

The combined use of different neuroimaging techniques is currently one of the most promising methodological approaches to the study of human brain functioning. Neuroimaging and TMS represent two complementary methodologies whose combined use is likely to be more widespread in the future. In this chapter, we have stressed the high potential of this integrative trend, as shown by the large number of studies discussed. Nevertheless, besides the fascinating perspective opened by the coregistration approach, several technical problems have limited advancement in some application fields. Therefore, many of the studies mentioned aimed to solve such technical problems. Once a reliable technical basis is established, many of the unsolved questions will be answered and future perspectives deepened. Specifically, more studies are needed to explore the clinical potential of a coregistration approach concerning both diagnostic and rehabilitation applications. Furthermore, the TMS-neuroimaging methodology also has great value in neuroscience research. Some recent applications, such as TMS-EEG rhythmic approach, might provide precious insights into the brain-cognition-behaviour relationship.

Author details

Elias P. Casula, Vincenza Tarantino and Patrizia S. Bisiacchi*
Department of General Psychology, University of Padua, Italy

Demis Basso
Faculty of Education, Free University of Bozen-Bolzano, Bozen-Bolzano, Italy
CENCA – Centro di Neuroscienze Cognitive Applicate, Rome, Italy

---

[4] Theta-burst stimulation is a high-frequency TMS protocol in which 3 pulses at 50 Hz frequency are delivered 5 times in a second for 20 or 40 seconds (for details see [124])

* Corresponding Author

9. References

[1] Barker AT, Jalinous R, Freeston IL (1985) Non-invasive magnetic stimulation of human motor cortex. Lancet, 1:1106-1107

[2] Walsh V, Cowey A (2000) Transcranial magnetic stimulation and cognitive neuroscience. Nat. Neurosci., 1:73-79

[3] Shapiro KA, Pascual-Leone A, Mottaghy FM, Gangitano M, Caramazza A (2001) Grammatical distinctions in the left frontal cortex. J. Cognitive Neurosci., 13:713–720

[4] Cappa SF, Sandrini M, Rossini PM, Sosta K, Miniussi C (2002) The role of the left frontal lobe in action naming: rTMS evidence. Neurology, 59:720-723

[5] Pascual-Leone A, Tormos JM, Keenan J, Tarazona F, Cañete C, Català MD (1998) Study and modulation of human cortical excitability with transcranial magnetic stimulation. J. Clin. Neurophysiol., 15:333-343

[6] Bestmann S (2008) The physiological basis of transcranial magnetic stimulation. Trends Cogn. Sci., 12:81-83

[7] Miniussi C, Ruzzoli M, Walsh V (2010) The mechanism of transcranial magnetic stimulation in cognition. Cortex, 46:128-130

[8] Walsh V, Rushworth M (1998) A primer of magnetic stimulation as a tool for neuropsychology. Neuropsychologia, 37:125-135

[9] Ridding MC, Rothwell JC (2007) Is there a future for therapeutic use of transcranial magnetic stimulation? Nat. Neurosci., 8:559-567

[10] Miniussi C, Pellicciari MC, Rossini PM (2010) New prospects of transcranial electrical stimulation (tES) from bench to bed side. Neuropsychological Trends, 8:31-35

[11] Walsh V, Cowey A (1998) Magnetic stimulation studies of visual cognition. Trends Cogn. Sci., 2:103-110

[12] Amassian VE, Cracco RQ, Maccabee PJ, Cracco JB (1992) Cerebello-frontal cortical projections in humans studied with the magnetic coil. Electroencephalogr. Clin. Neurophysiol., 85:265-272

[13] Mottaghy FM, Hungs M, Brugmann M, Sparing R, Boroojerdi B, Foltys H et al. (1999) Facilitation of picture naming after repetitive transcranial magnetic stimulation. Neurology, 53:1806-1812

[14] Allen EA, Pasley BN, Duong T, Freeman RD (2007) Transcranial magnetic stimulation elicits coupled neural and hemodynamic consequences. Science, 317:1918-1921

[15] Wagner T, Rushmore J, Eden U, Valero-Cabre A (2009) Biophysical foundations underlying TMS: Setting the stage for an effective use of neurostimulation in the cognitive neurosciences. Cortex, 45:1025-1034

[16] Miniussi C, Ruzzoli M, Walsh V (2010) The mechanism of transcranial magnetic stimulation in cognition. Cortex, 46:128-130

[17] Ilmoniemi RJ, Virtanen J, Ruohonen J, Karhu J, Aronen HJ, Näätänen R et al. (1997) Neuronal responses to magnetic stimulation reveal cortical reactivity and connectivity. Neuroreport, 8:3537-3540

[18] Kähkönen S, Komssi S, Wilenius J, Ilmoniemi RJ (2005) Prefrontal TMS produces smaller EEG responses than motor-cortex TMS: implications for rTMS treatment in depression. Psychopharmacology, 181:16-20

[19] Poldrack RA (2005) Can cognitive processes be inferred from neuroimaging data? Trends Cogn. Sci., 10:59-63

[20] Aguirre GK (2003) Functional imaging in behavioral neurology and cognitive neuropsychology. In: Feinberg TE, Farah MJ Behavioral neurology and cognitive neuropsychology, 35–46, McGraw-Hill pp. 35-46.

[21] Raichle ME (1998) Behind the scenes of functional brain imaging: a historical and physiological perspective. Proc. Natl. Acad. Sci. USA, 95:765–772

[22] Sack AT, Linden EJD (2003) Combining transcranial magnetic stimulation and functional imaging in cognitive brain research: possibilities and limitations. Brain Res. Rev., 43:41-56

[23] Schiff S, Bardi L, Basso D, Mapelli D (2011) Timing spatial conflict within the parietal cortex: a TMS study. J. Cogn. Neurosci., 23:3998-4007

[24] Rothwell JC (2010) Using transcranial magnetic stimulation methods to probe connectivity between motor areas of the brain. Hum. Movement Sci., 30:906-915

[25] Chen R (2004) Interactions between inhibitory and excitatory circuits in the human motor cortex. Exp. Brain Res., 154:1-10

[26] Kujirai T, Caramia MD, Rothwell JC, Day BL, Thompson PD, Ferbert A et al. (1993) Corticocortical inhibition in human motor cortex. J. Physiol., 471:501-519

[27] Valls-Solé J, Pascual-Leone A, Wassermann EM, Hallett M (1992) Human motor evoked responses to paired transcranial magnetic stimuli. Electroencephalogr. Clin. Neurophysiol., 85:355-364

[28] Hanajima R, Ugawa Y, Machii K, Mochizuki H, Terao Y, Enomoto H et al. (2001) Interhemispheric facilitation of the hand motor area in humans. J. Physiol., 531:849-859

[29] Rossi S, Hallett M, Rossini PM, Pascual-Leone A, The safety of TMS Consensus Group (2009) Safety, ethical considerations, and application guidelines for the use of transcranial magnetic stimulation in clinical practice and research. Clin. Neurophysiol., 120:2008-2039

[30] Cohen LG, Celnik P, Pascual-Leone A, Corwell B, Falz L, Dambrosia J et al. (1997) Functional relevance of cross-modal plasticity in blind humans. Nature, 389:180-183

[31] George MS, Wassermann EM, Williams WA, Callahan A, Ketter TA, Basser P et al. (1995) Daily repetitive transcranial magnetic stimulation (rTMS) improves mood in depression. Neuroreport, 6:1853-1856

[32] Koch G, Brusa L, Caltagirone C, Peppe A, Oliveri M, Stanzione P et al. (2005) rTMS of supplementary motor area modulates therapy-induced dyskinesias in Parkinson disease. Neurology, 65:623-625

[33] Konishita M, Ikeda A, Begum T, Yamamoto J, Hitomi T, Shibasaki H (2005) Low-frequency repetitive transcranial magnetic stimulation for seizure suppression in patients with extratemporal lobe epilepsy – A pilot study. Seizure, 14:387-392

[34] Bohning DE, Pecheny AP, Epstein CM, Speer AM, Vincent DJ, Dannels W et al. (1997) Mapping transcranial magnetic stimulation (TMS) fields in vivo with MRI. Neuroreport, 8:2535-2538

[35] Rossini PM, Barker AT, Berardelli A, Caramia MD, Caruso G, Cracco RQ et al. (1994) Non-invasive electrical and magnetic stimulation of the brain, spinal cord and roots—basic principles and procedures for routine clinical application. Electroencephalogr. Clin. Neurophysiol., 91:79-92

[36] Fuhr P, Agostino R, Hallett M (1991) Spinal motor neuron excitability during the silent period after cortical stimulation. Electroencephalogr. Clin. Neurophysiol., 81:257-262
[37] Sadato N, Pascual-Leone A, Grafman J, Ibañez V, Deiber MP, Dold G et al. (1996) Activation of the primary visual cortex by Braille reading in blind subjects. Nature, 380:526-528
[38] Komssi S, Aronen HJ, Huttunen J, Kesäniemi M, Soinne L, Nikouline VV et al. (2002) Ipsi- and contralateral EEG reactions to transcranial magnetic stimulation. Clin. Neurophysiol., 113:175–184
[39] Siebner HR, Bergmann TO, Bestmann S, Massimini M, Johansen-Berg H, Mochizuki H et al. (2009) Consensus paper: Combining transcranial magnetic stimulation with neuroimaging. Brain Stimul., 2:58-80
[40] Lee L, Siebner HR, Rowe JB, Rizzo V, Rothwell JC, Frackowiak RSJ et al. (2003) Acute remapping within the motor system induced by low-frequency repetitive transcranial magnetic stimulation. J. Neurosci., 23:5308-5318
[41] Cracco RQ, Amassian VE, Maccabee PJ, Cracco JB (1989) Comparison of human transcallosal responses evoked by magnetic coil and electrical stimulation. Electroencephalogr. Clin. Neurophysiol., 74:417-424
[42] Virtanen J, Ruohonen J, Naatanen R, Ilmoniemi RJ (1999) Instrumentation for the measurement of electric brain responses to transcranial magnetic stimulation. Med. Biol. Eng. Comput., 37:322-326
[43] Miniussi C, Thut G (2010) Combining TMS and EEG Offers New Prospects in Cognitive Neuroscience. Brain Topogr., 22:249-256
[44] Thut G, Northoff G, Ives JR, Kamitani Y, Pfennig A, Kampmann F et al. (2003) Effects of single-pulse transcranial magnetic stimulation (TMS) on functional brain activity: a combined event-related TMS and evoked potential study. Clin. Neurophysiol., 114:2071-2080
[45] Lioumis P, Kičić D, Savolainen P, Mäkelä JP, Kähkönen S (2009) Reproducibility of TMS—Evoked EEG Responses. Hum. Brain Mapp., 30:1387-1396
[46] Komssi S, Kähkönen S, Ilmoniemi RJ (2004) The effect of stimulus intensity on brain responses evoked by transcranial magnetic stimulation. Hum. Brain Mapp., 21:154-164
[47] Hämäläinen MS and Ilmoniemi RJ (1994) Interpreting magnetic fields of the brain: minimum norm estimates. Med. Biol. Eng. Comput., 32:35-42
[48] Kähkönen S, Kesäniemi M, Nikouline VV, Karhu J, Ollikainen M, Holi M et al. (2001) Ethanol modulates cortical activity: direct evidence with combined TMS and EEG. Neuroimage, 14:322-328
[49] Massimini M, Ferrarelli F, Huber R, Esser SK, Singh H, Tononi G (2005) Breakdown of cortical effective connectivity during sleep. Science, 309:2228-2232
[50] Iramina K, Maeno T, Nohaka Y, Ueno S (2003) Measurement of evoked electroencephalography induced by transcranial magnetic stimulation. J. Appl. Phys., 93:6718-6720
[51] Bonato C, Miniussi C, Rossini PM (2006) Transcranial magnetic stimulation and cortical evoked potentials: a TMS/EEG coregistration study. Clin. Neurophysiol., 117:1699-1707
[52] Mills KR, Boniface SJ, Schubert M (1992) Magnetic brain stimulation with a double coil: the importance of coil orientation. Electroencephalogr. Clin. Neurophysiol., 85:17-21

[53] Brasil-Neto JP, Cohen LG, Panizza M, Nilsson J, Roth BJ, Hallett M (1992) Optimal focal transcranial magnetic activation of the human motor cortex: effects of coil orientation, shape of the induced current pulse, and stimulus intensity. J. Clin. Neurophysiol., 9:132-136

[54] Taylor PCJ, Nobre AC, Rushworth MFS (2006) FEF TMS Affects Visual Cortical Activity. Cereb. Cortex, 17:391-399

[55] Taylor PC, Nobre AC, Rushworth MF (2007) Subsecond changes in top down control exerted by human medial frontal cortex during conflict and action selection: a combined transcranial magnetic stimulation electroencephalography study. J. Neurosci., 27:11343-11353

[56] Eriksen BA, Eriksen CW (1974) Effects of noise letters upon the identification of a target letter in nonsearch task. Percept. Psychophys., 16:143-149

[57] Johnson SJ, Hamidi M, Postle BR (2010) Using EEG to Explore How rTMS Produces Its Effects on Behavior. Brain Topogr., 22:281-293

[58] Sauseng P, Klimesch W, Gerloff C, Hummel FC (2009) Spontaneous locally restricted EEG alpha activity determines cortical excitability in the motor cortex. Neuropsychologia, 47:284-288

[59] Brignani D, Manganotti P, Rossini PM, Miniussi C (2008) Modulation of Cortical Oscillatory Activity During Transcranial Magnetic Stimulation. Hum. Brain Mapp., 29:603-612

[60] Klimesch W, Sauseng P, Gerloff C (2003) Enhancing cognitive performance with repetitive transcranial magnetic stimulation at human individual alpha frequency. European J. Neurosci., 17:1129-1133

[61] Neubauer A, Freudenthaler HH, Pfurtscheller G (1995) Intelligence and spatiotemporal patterns of event-related desynchronization (ERD). Intelligence, 20:249-266

[62] Romei V, Brodbeck V, Michel C, Amedi A, Pascual-Leone A, Thut G (2008) Spontaneous fluctuations in posterior alpha-Band EEG activity reflect variability in excitability of human visual areas. Cereb. Cortex, 18:2010-2018

[63] Paus T, Castro-Alamancos MA, Petrides M (2001) Cortico-cortical connectivity of the human mid-dorsolateral frontal cortex and its modulation by repetitive transcranial magnetic stimulation. Eur. J. Neurosci., 14:1405-1411

[64] Bender S, Basseler K, Sebastian I, Resch F, Kammer T, Oelkers-Ax R et al. (2005) Transcranial Magnetic Stimulation Evokes Giant Inhibitory Potentials in Children. Ann. Neurol., 58:58-67

[65] Ferreri F, Pasqualetti P, Määttä S, Ponzo D, Ferrarelli F, Tononi G et al. (2010) Human brain connectivity during single and paired pulse transcranial magnetic stimulation. Neuroimage, 54:90-102

[66] Kiers L, Cros D, Chiappa KH, Fang J (1993) Variability of motor potentials evoked by transcranial magnetic stimulation. Electroencephalogr. Clin. Neurophysiol., 89:415-423

[67] Nikulin VV, Kičić D, Kähkönen S, Ilmoniemi RJ (2003) Modulation of electroencephalographic responses to transcranial magnetic stimulation: evidence for changes in cortical excitability related to movement. Eur. J. Neurosci., 18:1206-1212

[68] Litvak V, Komssi S, Scherg M, Hoechstetter K, Classen J, Zaaroor M, et al. (2007) Artifact correction and source analysis of early electroencephalographic responses

evoked by transcranial magnetic stimulation over primary motor cortex. Neuroimage, 37:56-70

[69] Veniero D, Bortoletto M, Miniussi C (2009) TMS-EEG co-registration: On TMS-induced artifact. Clin. Neurophysiol., 120:1392-1399

[70] Thut G, Ives JR, Kampmann F, Pastor MA, Pascual-Leone A (2005) A new device and protocol for combining TMS and online recordings of EEG and evoked potentials. J. Neurosci. Meth., 141:207-217

[71] Morbidi F, Garulli A, Prattichizzo D, Rizzo C, Manganotti P, Rossi S (2007) Off-line removal of TMS-induced artifacts on human electroencephalography by Kalman filter. J. Neurosci. Meth., 162:293-302

[72] Berg P, Scherg M (1994) A multiple source approach to the correction of eye artifacts. Electroencephalogr. Clin. Neurophysiol., 90:229-241

[73] Ilmoniemi RJ, Kičić D (2010) Methodology for Combined TMS and EEG. Brain Topogr., 22:233-248

[74] Roth BJ, Pascual-Leone A, Cohen LG, Hallett M (1992) The heating of metal electrodes during rapid-rate magnetic stimulation: a possible safety hazard. Electroencephalogr. Clin. Neurophysiol., 85:116-123

[75] Wassermann EM (1998) Risk and safety of repetitive transcranial magnetic stimulation: report and suggested guidelines from the International Workshop on the Safety of Repetitive Transcranial Magnetic Stimulation, June 5–7, 1996. Electroencephalogr. Clin. Neurophysiol., 108:1-16

[76] Tallgreen P, Vanhatalo S, Kaila K, Voipio J (2005) Evaluation of commercially available electrodes and gels for recording of slow EEG potentials. Clin. Neurophysiol., 116:799-806

[77] Ives JR, Rotenberg A, Poma R, Thut G, Pascual-Leone A (2006) Electroencephalographic recording during transcranial magnetic stimulation in humans and animals. Clin. Neurophysiol., 117:1870-1875

[78] Kammer T, Beck S, Thielscher A, Laubis-Hermann U, Topka H (2001) Motor thresholds in humans: a transcranial magnetic stimulation study comparing different pulse waveforms, current directions and stimulator types. Clin. Neurophysiol., 112:250-258

[79] Sommer M, Arànzazu A, Rummel M, Speck S, Lang N, Tings T et al. (2006) Half sine, monophasic and biphasic transcranial magnetic stimulation of the human motor cortex. Clin. Neurophysiol., 117:838-844

[80] Julkunen P, Pääkkönen A, Hukkanen T, Könönen M, Tiihonen P, Vanhatalo S et al. (2008) Efficient reduction of stimulus artifact in TMS–EEG by epithelial short- circuiting by mini-punctures. Clin. Neurophysiol., 119:475-481

[81] Sekiguchi H, Takeuchi S, Kadota H, Kohno Y, Nakajima Y (2011) TMS-induced artifacts on EEG can be reduced by rearrangement of the electrode's lead wire before recording. Clin. Neurophysiol., 122:984-990

[82] Starck J, Rimpiläinen I, Pyykkö I, Toppila E (1996) The noise level in magnetic stimulation. Scand. Audiol., 25:223-226

[83] Terao Y, Ugawa Y, Suzuki M, Sakai K, Hanajima R, Gemba-Shimuzu K et al. (1997) Shortening of simple reaction time by peripheral electrical and submotor-threshold magnetic cortical stimulation. Exp. Brain Res., 115:541-545

[84] Nikouline V, Ruohonen J, Ilmoniemi RJ (1999) The role of the coil click in TMS assessed with simultaneous EEG. Clin. Neurophysiol., 110:1325-1328

[85] Tiitinen H, Virtanen J, Ilmoniemi RJ, Kamppuri J, Ollikainen M, Ruohonen J et al. (1999) Separation of contamination caused by coil clicks from responses elicited by transcranial magnetic stimulation. Clin. Neurophysiol., 110:982-985

[86] Fuggetta G, Pavone EF, Walsh V, Kiss M, Eimer M (2006) Cortico-Cortical Interactions in Spatial Attention: A Combined ERP/TMS Study. J. Neurophysiol., 95:3277-3280

[87] Di Lazzaro V, Oliviero A, Profice P, Dileone M, Pilato F, Insola A et al. (2009). Reduced Cerebral Cortex Inhibition in Dystonia: Direct Evidence in Humans. Clin. Neurophysiol., 120:834-839

[88] Levy R, Lozano AM, Lang AE, Dostrovsky JO (2010) Event-Related Desynchronization of Motor Cortical Oscillations in Patients with Multiple System Atrophy. Exp. Brain Res., 206:1-13

[89] Casarotto S, Määttä S, Herukka SK, Pigorini A, Napolitani M, Gosseries O et al. (2011) Transcranial Magnetic Stimulation-Evoked EEG/Cortical Potentials in Physiological and Pathological Aging. Neuroreport, 22:592-597

[90] Schutter DJ, Hortensius R (2011) Brain Oscillations and Frequency-Dependent Modulation of Cortical Excitability. Brain Stimul., 4:97-103

[91] Basar-Eroglu C, Brand A, Hildebrandt H, Karolina Kedzior K, Mathes B, Schmiedt C (2007) Working Memory Related Gamma Oscillations in Schizophrenia Patients. Int. J. Psychophysiol., 64:39-45

[92] Cho RY, Konecky RO, Carter CS (2006) Impairments in Frontal Cortical Gamma Synchrony and Cognitive Control in Schizophrenia. PNAS USA, 103:19878-19883

[93] Manganotti P, Fuggetta G, Fiaschi A (2004) Changes of motor cortical excitability in human subjects from wakefulness to early stages of sleep: a combined transcranial magnetic stimulation and electroencephalographic study. Neurosci. Lett., 362:31-34

[94] Ferrarelli F, Massimini M, Sarasso S, Casali A, Riedner BA, Angelini G et al. (2010) Breakdown in Cortical Effective Connectivity During Midazolam-Induced Loss of Consciousness. PNAS, 107:2681-2686

[95] Manganotti P, Bongiovanni LG, Fuggetta G, Zanette G, Fiaschi A (2006) Effects of Sleep Deprivation on Cortical Excitability in Patients Affected by Juvenile Myoclonic Epilepsy: A Combined Transcranial Magnetic Stimulation and EEG Study. J. Neurol. Neurosurg. Psychiatry, 77:56-60

[96] Del Felice A, Fiaschi A, Bongiovanni GL, Savazzi S, Manganotti P (2011) The Sleep-Deprived Brain in Normals and Patients with Juvenile Myoclonic Epilepsy: A Perturbational Approach to Measuring Cortical Reactivity. Epilepsy Res., 96:123-131

[97] Valentin A, Arunachalam R, Mesquita-Rodrigues A, Garcia Seoane JJ, Richardson MP, Mills KR et al. (2008) Late EEG responses triggered by transcranial magnetic stimulation (TMS) in the evaluation of focal epilepsy. Epilepsia, 49:470-480

[98] Bohotin V, Fumal A, Vandenheede M, Gérard P, Bohotin C, Maertens de Noordhout A et al. (2002) Effects of Repetitive Transcranial Magnetic Stimulation on Visual Evoked Potentials in Migraine. Brain, 125:912-922

[99] Boorman ED, O'Shea J, Sebastian C, Rushworth MF, Johansen-Berg H (2007) Individual differences in white-matter microstructure reflect variation in functional connectivity during choice. Curr. Biol., 17:1426-1431

[100] Sach M, Winkler G, Glauche V, Liepert J, Heimbach B, Koch MA et al. (2003) Diffusion tensor MRI of early upper motor neuron involvement in amyotrophic lateral sclerosis. Brain, 127:340-350

[101] Sparing R, Hesse MD, Fink GR (2010) Neuronavigation for transcranial magnetic stimulation (TMS): Where we are and where we are going. Cortex, 46:118-120

[102] Bungert A, Chambers CD, Phillips M, Evans CJ (2012) Reducing image artefacts in concurrent TMS/fMRI by passive shimming. Neuroimage, 59:2167-2174

[103] Weiskopf N, Josephs O, Ruff CC, Blankenburg F, Featherstone E, Thomas A et al. (2009) Image artifacts in concurrent transcranial magnetic stimulation (TMS) and fMRI caused by leakage currents: Modeling and compensation. J. Magn. Reson. Imaging, 29:1211-1217

[104] Bestmann S, Baudewig J, Frahm J (2003) On the synchronization of trans- cranial magnetic stimulation and functional echo-planar imaging. J. Magn. Reson. Imaging, 17:309-316

[105] Bohning DE, Shastri A, Nahas Z, Lorberbaum JP, Andersen SW, Dannels WR et al. (1998) Echoplanar BOLD fMRI of brain activation induced by concurrent transcranial magnetic stimulation. Invest. Radiol., 33:336-340

[106] Bestmann S, Baudewig J, Siebner HR, Rothwell JC, Frahm J (2004) Functional MRI of the immediate impact of transcranial magnetic stimulation on cortical and subcortical motor circuits. Eur. J. Neurosci., 19:1950-1962

[107] Sack AT, Kohler A, Bestmann S, Linden DEJ, Dechent P, Goebel R et al. (2007) Imaging the brain activity changes underlying impaired visuospatial judgments: simultaneous fMRI, TMS, and behavioural studies. Cereb. Cortex, 17:2841-2852

[108] Tegenthoff M, Ragert P, Pleger B, Schwenkreis P, Förster AF, Nicolas V et al. (2005) Improvement of tactile discrimination performance and enlargement of cortical somatosensory maps after 5 Hz rTMS. PLoS Biol., 3:e362

[109] Li X, Nahas Z, Kozel FA, Anderson B, Bohning DE, George MS (2004) Acute Left Prefrontal Transcranial Magnetic Stimulation in Depressed Patients is Associated with Immediately Increased Activity in Prefrontal Cortical as well as Subcortical Regions. Biol. Psychiatry, 55:882-890

[110] Li X, Large CH, Ricci R, Taylor JJ, Nahas Z, Bohning DE et al. (2011) Using Interleaved Transcranial Magnetic Stimulation/Functional Magnetic Resonance Imaging (fMRI) and Dynamic Causal Modeling to Understand the Discrete Circuit Specific Changes of Medications: Lamotrigine and Valproic Acid Changes in Motor or Prefrontal Effective Connectivity. Psychiatry Res., 194:141-148

[111] Hamzei F, Liepert J, Dettmers C, Weiller C, Rijntjes M (2006) Two Different Reorganization Patterns After Rehabilitative Therapy: An Exploratory Study with fMRI and TMS. Neuroimage 31:710-720

[112] Paus T, Jech R, Thompson CJ, Comeau R, Peters T, Evans AC (1997) Transcranial magnetic stimulation during positron emission tomography: a new method for studying connectivity of the human cerebral cortex. J. Neurosci., 17:3178-3184

[113] Schall JD, Morel A, King DJ, Bullier J (1995) Topography of visual cortex connections with frontal eye field in macaque: convergence and segregation of processing streams. J. Neurosci., 15:4464-4487

[114] Mottaghy FM, Krause BJ, Kemna LJ, Töpper R, Tellmann L, Beu M et al. (2000) Modulation of the neuronal circuitry subserving working memory in healthy human subjects by repetitive transcranial magnetic stimulation. Neurosci. Lett., 280:167-170

[115] Speer AM, Kimbrell TA, Wassermann EM, D Repella J, Willis MW, Herscovitch P et al. (2000) Opposite Effects of High and Low Frequency rTMS on Regional Brain Activity in Depressed Patients. Biol. Psychiatry, 48:1133-1141

[116] Speer AM, Benson BE, Kimbrell TK, Wassermann EM, Willis MW, Herscovitch P et al. (2009) Opposite Effects of High and Low Frequency rTMS on Mood in Depressed Patients: Relationship to Baseline Cerebral Activity on PET. J. Affect. Disord., 115:386-394

[117] Nadeau SE, McCoy KJ, Crucian GP, Greer RA, Rossi F, Bowers D et al. (2002) Cerebral Blood Flow Changes in Depressed Patients after Treatment with Repetitive Transcranial Magnetic Stimulation: Evidence of Individual Variability. Neuropsychiatry Neuropsychol. Behav. Neurol., 15:159-175

[118] Strafella AP, Ko JH, Grant J, Fraraccio M, Monchi O (2005) Corticostriatal Functional Interactions in Parkinson's Disease: A rTMS/[11C]raclopride PET Study. Eur. J. Neurosci., 22:2946-2952

[119] Oliviero A, Di Lazzaro V, Piazza O, Profice P, Pennisi MA, Della Corte F et al. (1999) Cerebral blood flow and metabolic changes produced by repetitive magnetic brain stimulation. J. Neurol., 246:1164-1168

[120] Noguchi Y, Watanabe E, Sakai KL (2003) An event-related optical topography study of cortical activation induced by single-pulse transcranial magnetic stimulation. Neuroimage, 19:156-162

[121] Mochizuki H, Ugawa Y, Terao Y, Sakai KL (2006) Cortical hemoglobin concentration changes under the coil induced by single-pulse TMS in humans: a simultaneous recording with near-infrared spectroscopy. Exp. Brain Res., 169:302-310

[122] Chiang TC, Vaithianathan T, Leung T, Lavidor M, Walsh V, Delpy DT (2007) Elevated haemoglobin levels in the motor cortex following 1 Hz transcranial magnetic stimulation: a preliminary study. Exp. Brain Res., 181:555-560

[123] Mochizuki H, Furubayashi T, Hanajima R, Terao Y, Mizuno Y, Okabe S et al. (2007) Hemoglobin concentration changes in the contralateral hemisphere during and after theta burst stimulation of the human sensorimotor cortices. Exp. Brain Res., 180:667-675

[124] Huang YZ, Edwards MJ, Rounis E, Bhatia KP, Rothwell JC (2005) Theta Burst Stimulation of the Human Motor Cortex. Neuron, 45:201-206

Section 3

Legal Implementations of Modern Neuroimaging

Chapter 9

Intraoperative Imaging for Verification of the Correct Level During Spinal Surgery

Claudio Irace

Additional information is available at the end of the chapter

http://dx.doi.org/10.5772/52055

1. Introduction

One of main problems in current medical practice is the rocketing conflict patient *vs* physician, generally popularized with the term malpractice; this is particularly true in the field of surgical activity. When dealing with errors occurring in different specialties one of the first and embarrassing event is to deliver surgery at the incorrect (not affected!?) side or level; as the wrong-side in most cases may be prevented by means of strict application of a protocol consisting of vocal identification, cross-check with clinical chart and unequivocal skin marking before incision, avoiding the wrong-level in spinal surgery requires some additional in-depth measures.

When performing a lumbar microdiscectomy or a one-level decompression (even endoscopically assisted), the exploration of a wrong disc space may be not considered a relevant error; nevertheless it can become a true ordeal for the patient in terms of acute or late-occurring complications [1]. Medico-legal implications are easily understood, although such a matter is ill-defined. Some authors have identified the wrong-level as the second most common reason for reoperation for lumbar disc herniation [2]; and this grim event has been recognized as one of the starting-points of the cascade of symptoms leading to the well-known failed back surgery syndrome (FBSS); nevertheless many surgeons deem wrong-disc surgery as inconsequential [3] and not necessarily involving a worsening of patient's symptoms.

Concerning the anterior approach to the cervical spine it's mandatory to have an intraoperative x-ray confirmation of the disc space before performing discectomy; indeed no anatomical bony points may lead the surgeon to the correct disc space undoubtedly. When operating upon the thoracic spine via a posterior approach the problem of level identification is more complex and several x-ray images could be required; in these cases surgical incisions and approaches are longer and it's rare to mistake the spinal level. The posterior approach to the lumbar spine involves the highest risk of level-error if the surgeon does not perform routinely an intraoperative x-ray. As you can see, at any spinal level plain x-ray study or standard fluoroscopy done intraoperatively are the pivotal step to avoid a wrong-level operation.

2. Verification of the correct level

2.1. Surgical localization in the cervical spine

If one considers medico-legal reports about malpractice for wrong level in spinal surgery, two main groups may be recognized: cervical and lumbar. Concerning anterior cervical spine surgery, cases referred for malpractice due to level error are few; this is quite easy to explain, because standard surgical strategy includes mandatorily a x-ray control before violating the disc space. The following is what we perform in this kind of surgery.

A preliminary x-ray image is obtained after having applied a metallic tool on the lateral area of the neck; this mark will serve as a better indication of the skin fold in which the horizontal skin incision will be done [Figure 1]. After having performed surgical dissection along the carotido-oesophageal plane a fluoroscopic control will be delivered before making disc incision [Figure 2]. These two steps allow the surgeon to explore the correct disc space in almost every case.

The only true problem may arise when operating at a lower cervical level in a patient with a short neck and/or prominent shoulders. In such cases, before skin incision, it's helpful to pull patient's shoulders down to try obtaining a better visualization of the lower cervical spine on lateral x-ray view. It must be remembered that prolonged and excessive cranio-caudal pulling of the shoulders may cause injury of the spinal accessory nerve entering the trapetius muscle fibers; so, it is safe to remove shoulder traction as soon as having obtained x-ray confirmation of the disc space to be explored, without waiting the surgical procedure be completed. If even such a measure does not allow to visualize the disc space to be explored – which is usually is the C6-C7 or C7-Th1 one – nothing remains that to identify the lowest disc space, by placing a wire in the disc space and obtaining a fluoroscopic check; then, the surgeon will perform the planned discectomy at the one or two more caudal segment. It goes without saying that a postoperative computed tomography (CT) scan must be obtained as soon as possible at the end of surgery, to confirm the correctness of the disc space operated just before.

Although rare another cause of wrong-level in anterior cervical spine surgery may be related to error in compilation or interpretation of patient's clinical charts. When compiling the medical chart the physician may not clearly identify the pathological level to be operated, and this is due to hasty transcription and observation (if done!) of magnetic resonance (MR) and/or CT scans. Or it frequently occurs that neuroimaging studies report cervical disc herniations or foraminal stenosis at two or more levels, and these findings are then reported in clinical charts without specifying the level to be operated; in the operating room the surgeon starting the planned cervical discectomy will approach that level which is not the one correlated to patient's symptoms and signs. Therefore we recommend that before skin incision patient's neuroimaging reports and medical charts be matched one another as first, and then compared with neurodiagnostic images, so to have an unequivocal confirmation of the disc space to be explored.

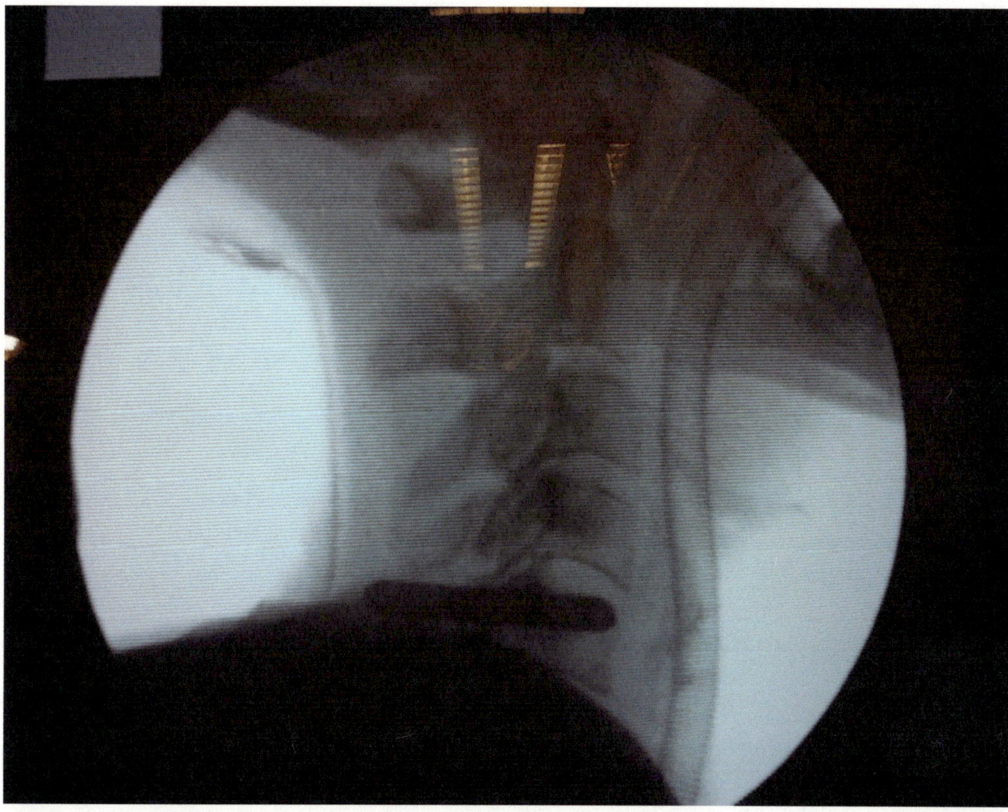

Figure 1. Intraoperative lateral cervical fluoroscopy. A metallic tool applied over the skin points the C4-C5 disc space. As you can see patient's prominent shoulders do not allow an optimal visualization of the lower cervical spine.

2.2. Global introduction to lumbar spine microsurgery

The scenario becomes dangerously grey when the wrong-level occurs at lumbar spine surgery: the rate of this kind of error sadly increases and medical and medico-legal consequences become potentially dramatic. Well keeping in mind this complication when performing microsurgery at the lumbar spine, one of the most important principles in microsurgery must be here remembered: the surgical scar formation, which is considered the main cause of the FBSS, is less extended when a more reduced approach is used. Following this principle, the skin incision for a one-level lumbar spine microsurgical procedure is 2.5 to 4.0 cm: **no external landmarks may convoy the surgeon to the correct level through such a narrow corridor**. Nevertheless some surgeons perform operations at the L5-S1 level making no intraoperative x-ray control [4], only by recognizing anatomical features of sacrum; and in the same way they operate upon upper lumbar levels simply 'counting' from L5-S1. Such an attitude has to be rejected. First, one cannot approach a lumbar upper level (for example, L3-L4) simply 'counting' from L5-S1, without making a long skin incision and extended skeletonization of paravertebral muscles. Second, anatomical variations (*e.g.*, a transitional vertebra) may contribute to miss the interspace to be explored. As a final point, even an L5-S1 disc space in a hyperlordotic spine may be missed if the superficial dissection and the operative microscopy are not oriented in an oblique enough direction [1].

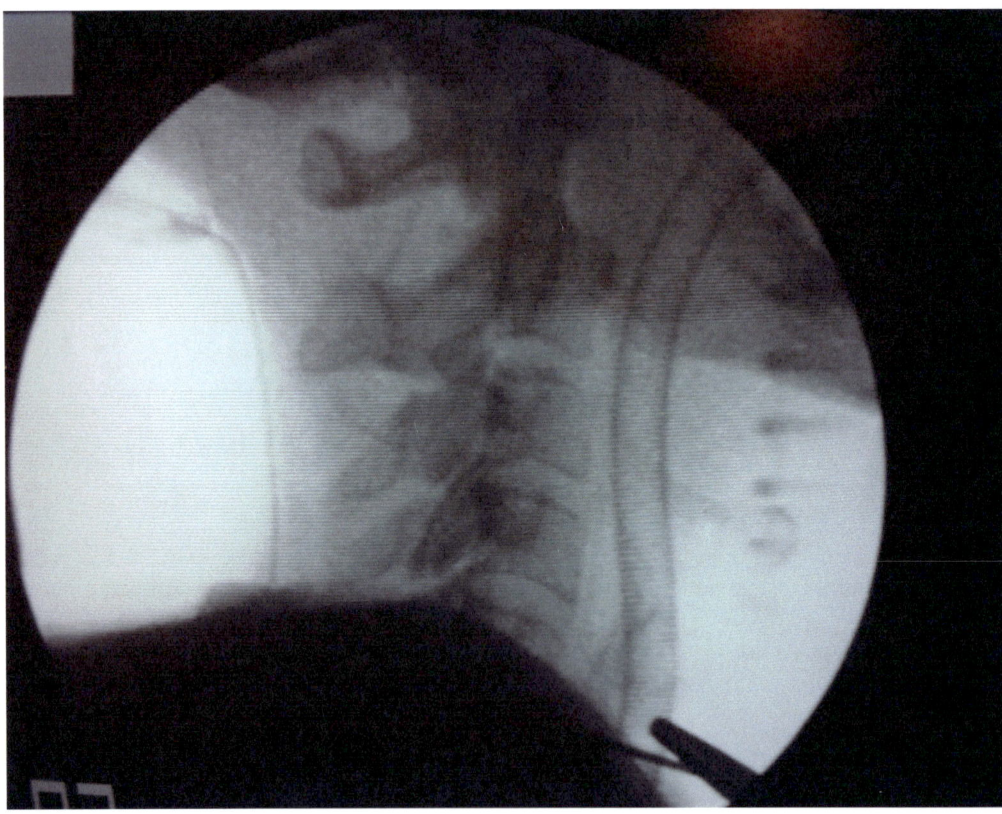

Figure 2. Intraoperative lateral cervical fluoroscopy. Before disc incision a wire is inserted in the correct disc space C5-C6, which may be seen even if partially obscured by superimposing shoulders.

Therefore the basic rule to perform a microsurgical one-level operation at the correct lumbar interspace is to obtain a good-quality x-ray intraoperative confirmation; a lateral view provided by a C-arm fluoroscopic machine, well placed over the patient lying prone and with a metallic tool applied to a bony marker (*e.g.*, the spinous process), allows the surgeon to direct the dissection toward the correct space to be explored, even if working in a tubular-like surgical corridor.

2.3. Surgical localization in the lumbar spine

The strategy of utilizing a lumbar radiopaque tool on a bony landmark to indicate the level to be explored, checked by fluoroscopy before and, if required, after skin incision has been adopting by our School for about forty years. Moreover we have identified three further 'crucial aspects': global strategy, attention, precision in level identification; and the corresponding starring are: the surgeon, the circulating nurse, the (neuro)radiologist.

Basing upon this background we have designed a 3-step method to avoid the level (but the wrong-side too!) error in lumbar spine surgery; this method was called IRACE, meaning Intraoperative Radiograph And Confirming Exclamation [1]. (**Step 1**) In the operating room, with the patient in the prone position, a wire is applied to the cranial spinous process of the level to be explored and a fluoroscopic control is delivered [Figure 3a]; if the level is confirmed by the radiologist, the superficial part of the wire is cut away. (**Step 2**) Before skin incision the surgeon asks out loud for level confirmation; the circulating nurse reads aloud the level and side reported on the patient's medical chart [Figure 3b]. (**Step 3**) Additional fluoroscopy is utilized when anatomical landmarks appear confounding or when subtotal arthrectomy (for foraminal or extraforaminal disc herniations) is planned, and the articular process to be drilled is marked for further confirmation. Before skin closure the scrub nurse reminds the surgeon to remove the wire if not already done; he pulls it out saying 'Tip!', meaning that the wire has been removed as a whole.

The ISO system defines the rules ensuring the delivery of a elevated standard of care; our Department received an official certificate attesting our accomplishment of the requirements of the ISO 9001:2000 standards [Figure 4]. This ISO system requires several procedures describing core activities of each function; about lumbar disc surgery a specific procedure was designed to avoid level error and this procedure is the pivot of the 3-step IRACE method we have just described.

2.4. Field of application of the IRACE method

The IRACE method may be mainly used in four kinds of operation at the lumbar spine. Of course the first and most frequent and important procedure is microdiscectomy; in this procedure we think that the wire placed in the spinous process of the cranial vertebra, previously confirmed fluoroscopically, is a valuable guide to perform all subsequent surgical steps in a tubular-like corridor. Another surgical intervention in which our method can help the surgeon is the one-level uni- or bilateral foraminotomy or decompression for spinal stenosis; in these cases bone spurs, osteophytes and thickening of ligamentum flavum make the skeletonization and bone decompression at the correct level difficult; if a scoliosis or a degree of obesity coexist, hence an intraoperative radiograph interpreted by a neuroradiologist becomes fundamental. A third context in which we suggest using this method is the endoscopic foraminotomy; in this procedure the correct localization is a critical point and posteroanterior and lateral fluoroscopies are performed before, during and after surgery [5]. At last a fourth procedure is the interspinous stabilization; even in this case a level error may occur [Figure 5] and therefore our method is advisable too.

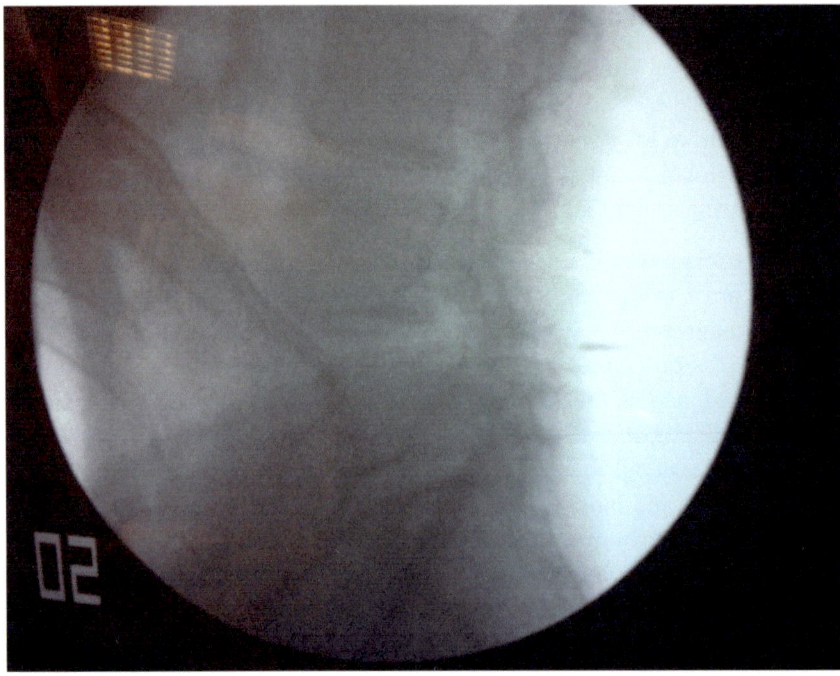

a

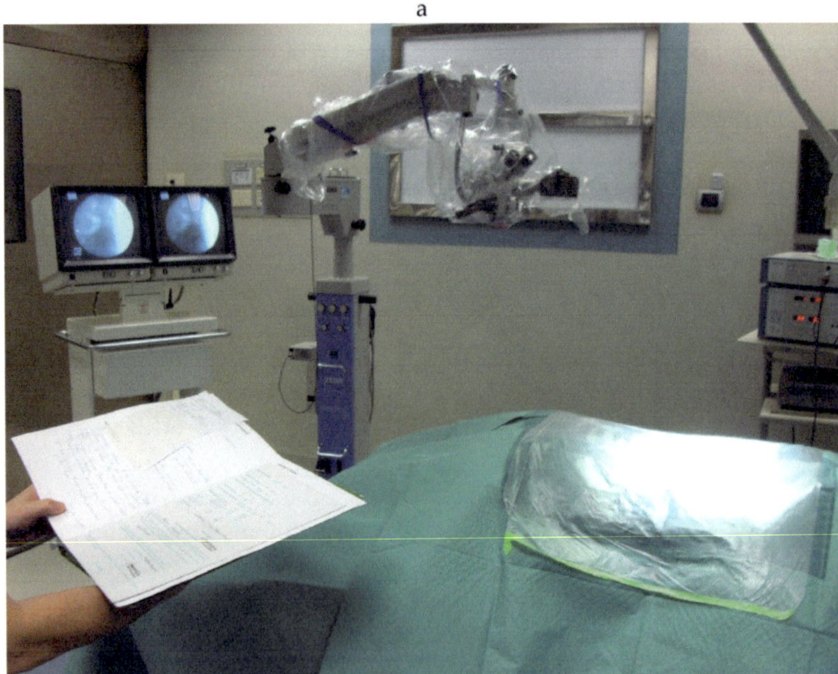

b

Figure 3. (a) Intraoperative lateral fluoroscopy obtained before skin incision; the wire placed in the spinous process of L-4 is demonstrated. (b) Before skin incision the circulating nurse reads patient's medical chart aloud to remember level and side of lumbar disc to be explored.

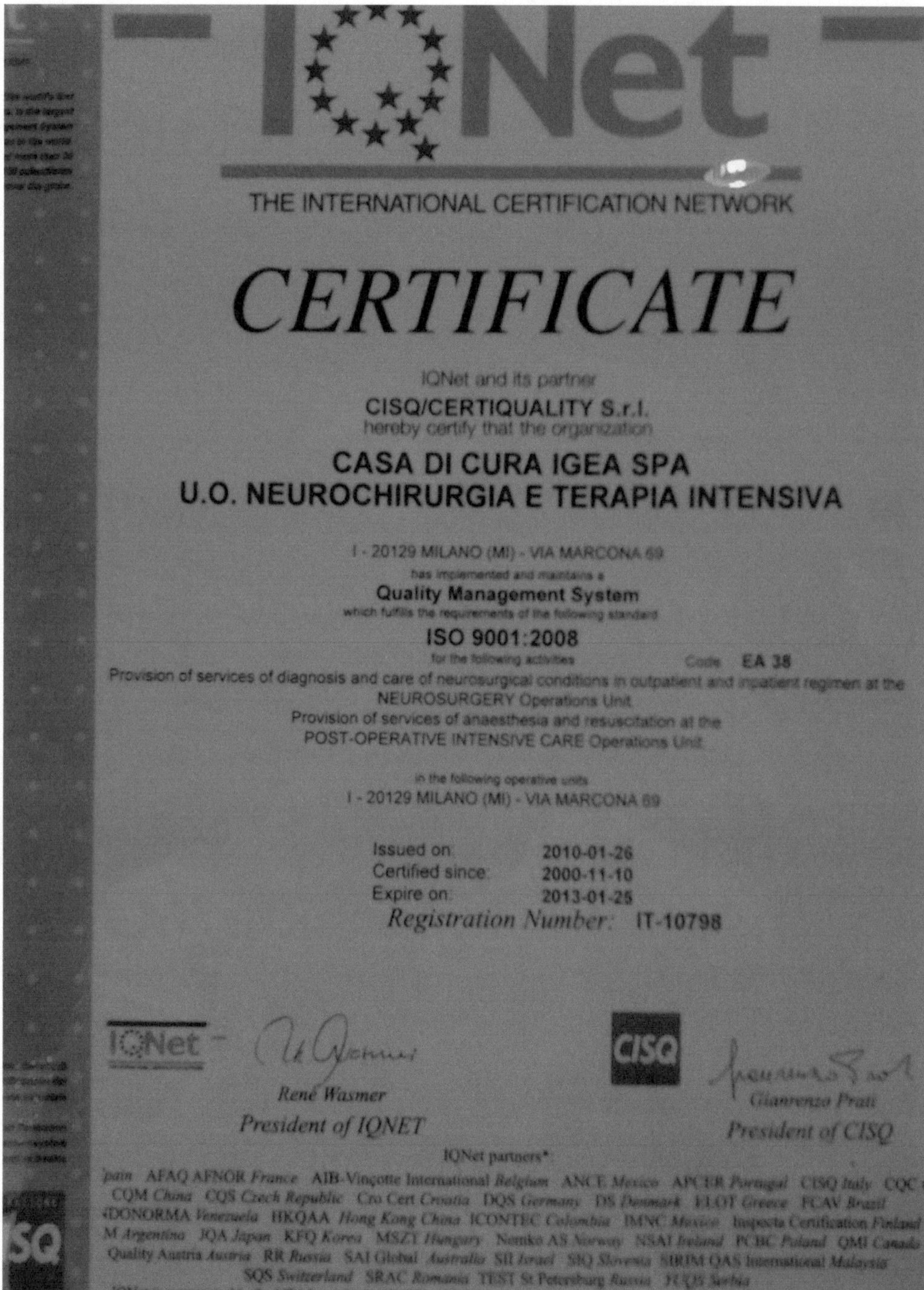

IQNet

THE INTERNATIONAL CERTIFICATION NETWORK

CERTIFICATE

IQNet and its partner

CISQ/CERTIQUALITY S.r.l.

hereby certify that the organization

CASA DI CURA IGEA SPA

U.O. NEUROCHIRURGIA E TERAPIA INTENSIVA

I - 20129 MILANO (MI) - VIA MARCONA 69

has implemented and maintains a

Quality Management System

which fulfills the requirements of the following standard

ISO 9001:2008

for the following activities Code EA 38

Provision of services of diagnosis and care of neurosurgical conditions in outpatient and inpatient regimen at the NEUROSURGERY Operations Unit

Provision of services of anaesthesia and resuscitation at the POST-OPERATIVE INTENSIVE CARE Operations Unit

in the following operative units

I - 20129 MILANO (MI) - VIA MARCONA 69

Issued on:	2010-01-26
Certified since:	2000-11-10
Expire on:	2013-01-25

Registration Number: IT-10798

René Wasmer
President of IQNET

CISQ

Gianrenzo Prati
President of CISQ

IQNet partners*:

Figure 4. Reproduction of the renewal of certification ISO 9001:2000, issued to the Unit of Neurosurgery, Casa di Cura Igea, Milan, Italy

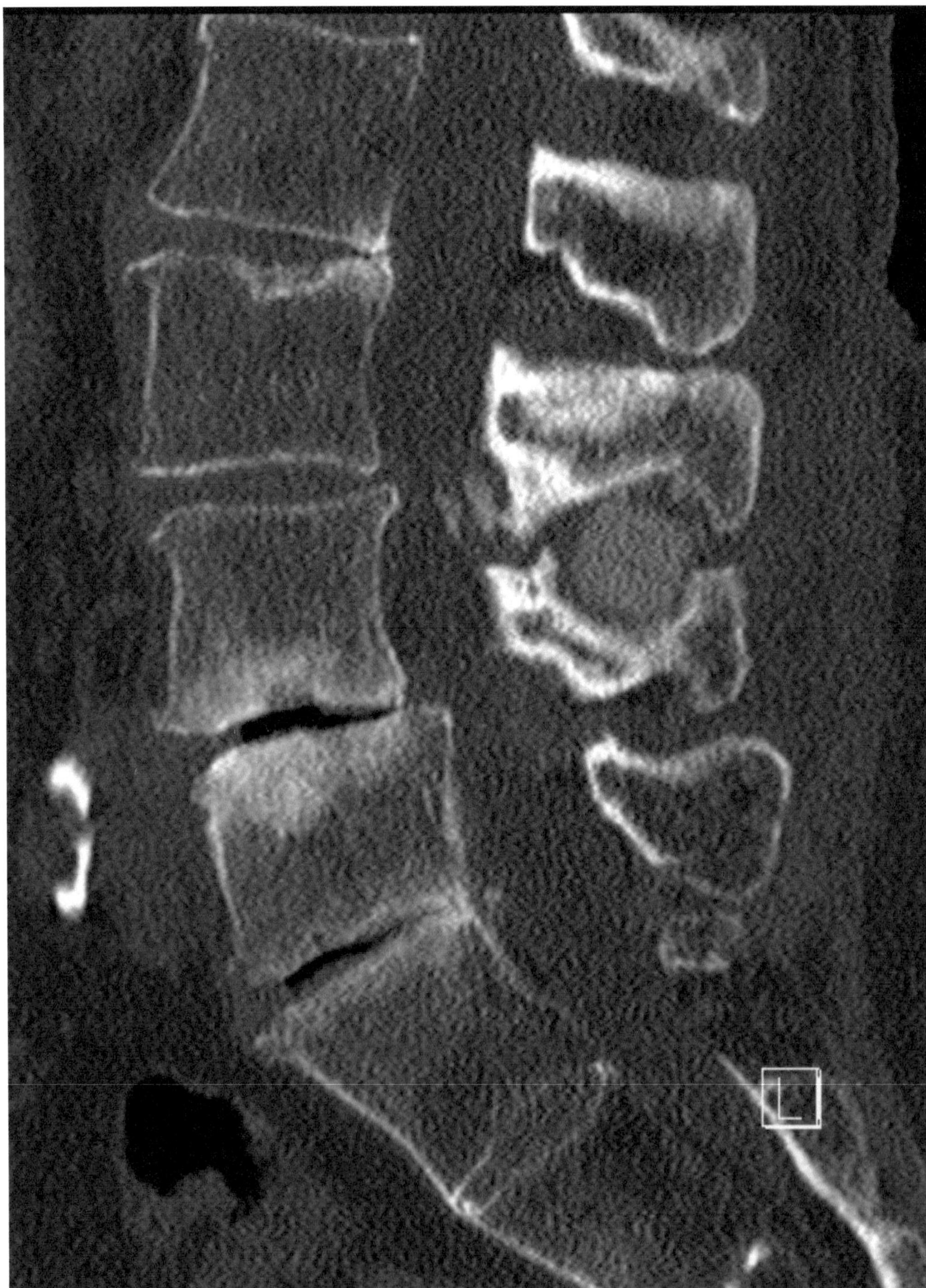

a

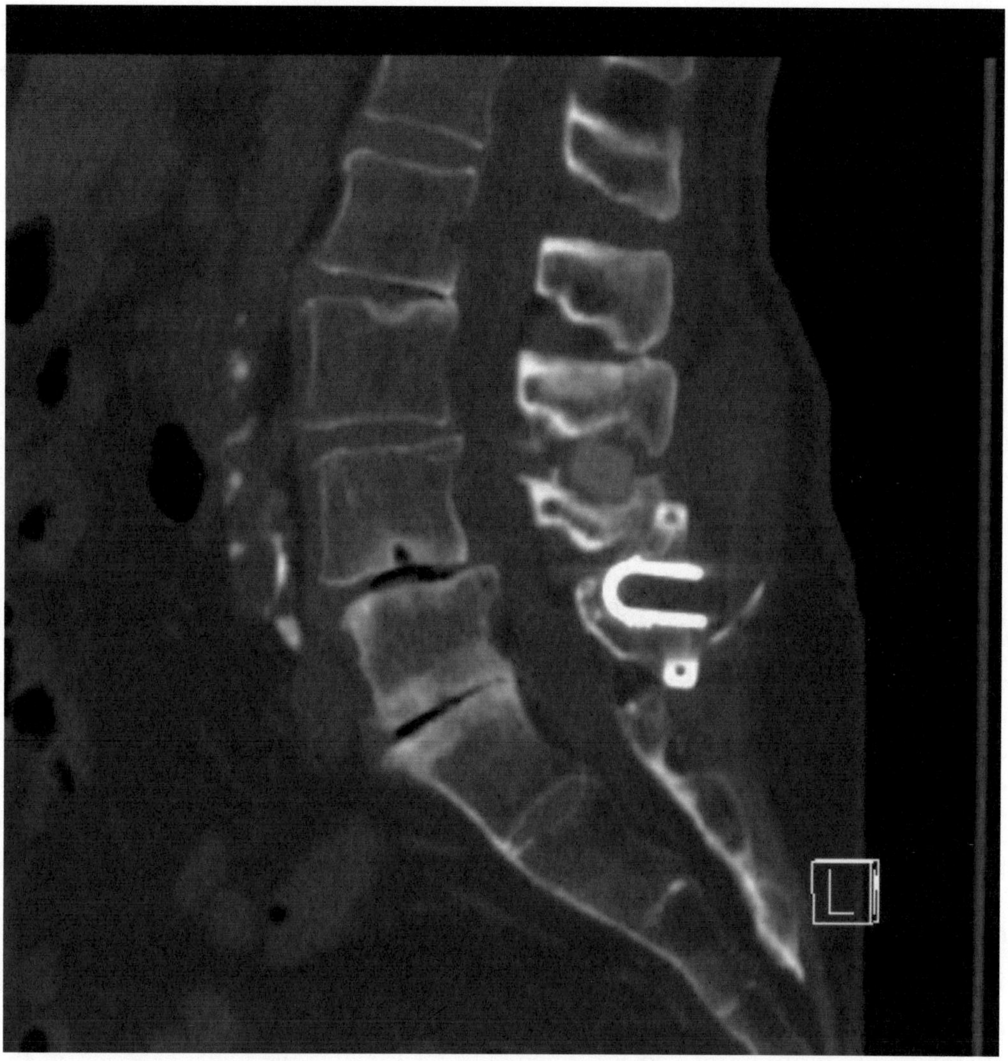

b

Figure 5. (a) Preoperative sagittal reconstruction CT scan. This patient came to our attention after having performed a "interspinous stabilization L4-L5" elsewhere, as reported in medical discharging chart; soon after this surgery her bilateral claudicatio radicolaris started to worsen; the CT scan clearly shows the DIAM interspinous device applied at the L3-L4 interspinous space (wrong). (b) Postoperative CT scan. The COFLEX device correctly inserted at L4-L5 is well visualized; the DIAM at L3-L4 was intentionally left in place to avoid late compromise of segmental stability.

2.5. Other strategies to avoid the wrong-level operation

Different methods and protocols have been suggested to avoid wrong-level or wrong-side errors, aiming to identify and correct the potential causes of this problem. Three main methods adopted to avoid the error of level are currently used. 1) The **'Sign, Mark and Xray (or SMaX) Program'**. It has designed by the North American Spine Society and it is included in a wider checklist addressing the problem of performing the right operation in the right patient at the right site. This program consists of signing the level and side before surgery, marking the level in the operating room using a metallic instrument on a bony landmark, performing a lumbar radiograph with the marker in place [6]. 2) The Joint Commission on the Accreditation oh Healthcare Organizations **'JCAHO Protocol'**. It articulates a 3-step process: preoperative verification involving the patient, marking the operative site, a time-out before starting surgery [7]. 3) The **'ABCD pause'**. It's basically a preincision step during with the surgical team re-analyzes the operative schedule and diagnostic imaging [8].

If we compare the above strategies with the IRACE method, we can observe that concerning the SMaX Program, our method seems more detailed and integrated because of the subsequent oral confirmation. The JCAHO Protocol appears effective when applied to other fields of surgery, but it is less specific than the IRACE method when utilized in lumbar spine surgery. The ABCD pause does not identify the single person dedicated to the oral check; moreover the time-out *per se* does not address the problem of level error which may derive from incorrect direction of dissection during microsurgery [1].

3. What we feel about the matter of wrong level

Going back to the 'crucial aspects' involved in level error lumbar spine surgery, the first to be matched is surgical strategy. An elective microsurgical procedure in lumbar spine region starts well before disc space exploration and refers to what we have called as the "atmosphere" of the operation. This means that the surgeon starting a lumbar microdiscectomy (or another one-level procedure) must participate in the positioning of the patient and personally choose the diagnostic neuroimages deemed necessary for a correct surgery; we strongly feel that the habit of the surgeon of coming into the surgical suite once the patient has already been positioned and draped must be abandoned [1].

The second point is attention. Loss of concentration, fatigue, sense of inferiority, or a mix of these aspects, can lower the degree of attention, particularly in those steps of the operative procedure which are considered less important, for example the initial exposure of the interlaminar space and the lamino-arthrotomy. In the operative theatre we have identified the circulating (or assistant) nurse as the one who is able to better remember to the surgeon the level to be explored just before skin incision. Indeed the assistant nurse is not directly engaged in the procedure (as the scrub nurse really is), moves freely all around so having easy access to neurodiagnostic images and medical charts.

The third and perhaps central point is the precision in lumbar spine identification and, hence, the importance of the (neuro)radiologist. All spine surgeons well know how regional anatomy sometimes may be difficult to interpret, due to congenital anomalies or local abnormalities induced by previous surgeries. Surgeon's skill is a *conditio sine qua non*, but the correct lane to engage may be correctly indicated only by a lateral x-ray image obtained intraoperatively. The (neuro)radiologist will also be able to provide a correct interpretation of a poor quality x-ray image, for example due to obesity of the patient; last he will provide a decisive correlation between the intraoperative fluoroscopy and the preoperative neurodiagnostic images; the typical example is the presence of a transitional vertebra, which may be called in MR or CT report differently from what reported on medical charts.

4. 360°-considerations

We feel the problem of wrong level or side still exists and it is far to be eliminated; it's hard to admit but many spine surgeons are reluctant to face this issue and such an attitude does not contribute to its solution. It's difficult to quantify the true dimension of the wrong-level, but it may be assumed that this error rate ranges from 0.14 to 5.3 percent [1]. Several studies demonstrated that most of wrong-level spinal operations occur at the lumbar level.

A lot of conditions has been identified as potentially leading to a wrong-level operation; when dealing with spinal surgery it must be remembered that these condition have been amplified by the fast increasing number of "spinal" procedures. Currently we think that the use of an intraoperative neuroimaging study should be mandatory. We have to remember here once again that this matter mainly addresses one-level microsurgical procedures (indeed the most frequent one) and endoscopic operations, which involve short skin incisions and tubular-like surgical corridors, directed only to the disc space or the neural foramen to be explored.

Fatigue, often coupled with external forces which press all the surgical team to complete a crowded operative session quickly, represent an explosive cocktail. In current spinal surgical activity it is not difficult to encounter repeat lumbar discectomies, scheduled on the same day; cases involving same-level, different-side disc herniations or vice versa strongly ressemble an assembly line, which involves an increased potential gross error [9]; the surgeon is in a hurry and the first step he disregards to spare time is fluoroscopic control for level identification.

From philosophical and practical points of view the microsurgical approach constitutes another potential cause of error. It has been demonstrated that the wider the surgical approach the more extended the scar formation [10]; basing upon the finding that scar formation is perhaps the main cause of the FBSS, hence it appears clear that the microsurgical approach is to be preferred strongly to standard 'opener sky' surgery (further multiple advantages of lumbar spine microsurgery go beyond the scope of this chapter). But, this having said, it must be stressed that the attitude to work in a finger-like often deep surgical field, which is indeed the microsurgical field, constitutes a peculiar ability, that needs a long-lasting learning curve. In lumbar spine microsurgery, even if performed by experienced 'good hands', the error of level is always behind the corner, mainly because the fatigued surgeon trusts of his 'dissecting' finger too much; and once the self-retractor is being in place, subsequent surgical steps progress forcedly toward a single disc space, which may be correct or not. How to avoid such a highly undesired event?

5. The neuroradiologist

Our experience using the IRACE method in over 1000 lumbar spine microsurgical procedures has showed that the better way to start a lumbar spine one-level microsurgical operation is performing an intraoperative radiography with a wire placed in the cranial spinous process of the level to be explored. This lateral x-ray image will be easily read by the surgeon himself, but in most of cases the presence or the remote interpretation by the neuroradiologist is fundamental.

First, the reading of a radiograph is really his own job, and, at least in the Italian code, a radiological report can be signed exclusively by a medical doctor who obtained the specialization in Radiology (and medico-legal consequences are obviously understood).

Second, local conditions such as scoliosis, obesity, coexistence of internal metallic instrumentation easily obscure the radiographic appearance; the neuroradiologist is the one who can correctly extricate among all different 'greys', appearing close to the wire applied to the spinous process.

Third, the neuroradiologist is free from surgery's stressing pulse, as on the contrary is the surgeon; therefore he can provide a correct, shining and ultimate interpretation of the intraoperative radiographic image (or ask for repeating it, if required) stressless.

6. Lessons learned

As a final consideration we can state that the attention we paid to the matter of wrong-level is so strong, that our strategy starting with a fluoroscopy performed after having placed a wire in the spinous process has become the starting point of any one-level lumbar spine surgical procedure.

Keeping in mind the somewhat abandoned "ancient doctor-patient relationship" [11], we wish to point out the current surgical activity of academic institutions and large hospitals, in which many patients are globally managed by multiple treating physicians and nurses; it means that, in the global process of assistance to the patient, cardinal steps of indication for surgery, compilation of medical charts and elucidation of the informed consent, and the operation itself are performed by different physicians [12]. If all this is true, hence **strict cooperation between neuroradiologist and spine surgeon, to have a useful x-ray study performed and interpreted intraoperatively in a short time, is one of the clues for a successful spinal operation.**

7. The future

If we assume that in lumbar spine microsurgery a localizing intraoperative image before skin incision is essential, two ways may be anticipated at the moment. On one side we can expect a technological advancement of radiological equipment, in order to deliver better spine images utilizing very low radiations. On the other side, different neurodiagnostic techniques are to be adopted and in this light intraoperative CT scan seems to be the most promising. It is currently used in stabilization surgical procedures and since its introduction a substantial decrease of the rate of pedicle screw malpositioning has been reported. The next obvious step could be its implementation in the routine daily spine surgical activity, although high costs and additional radiation exposure to the patient markedly limit its diffusion.

Author details

Claudio Irace *

Department of Neurosurgery, Hospital "IGEA", Milan, Italy

Acknowledgement

Our huge thanks run to Dr Claudio Corona, our current Head Department: under his illuminating, open-minded daily guide, deriving from a near-40year neurosurgical career mainly devoted to spinal surgery, we had and have the chance to go on clinical research in the management of patients affected by spine diseases.

8. References

[1] Irace C, Corona C (2010) How to avoid wrong-level and wrong-side errors in lumbar microdiscectomy. J Neurosurg Spine 12: 660-665.

[2] WN Harsha (1990) Medical malpractice: handling orthopaedic cases. Colorado Springs, CO, USA: Shepard's/McGraw-Hill.

[3] Rampersaud YR, Moro ERP, Neary MA, White K, Lewis SJ, Massicotte EM, et al (2006) Intraoperative adverse events and related postoperative complications in spine surgery: implications for enhancing patient safety founded on evidence-based protocols. Spine 31: 1503-1510.

[4] Maroon JC, Abla AA (1986) Microlumbar discectomy. Clin Neurosurg 33: 407-417.

[5] Pao J-L, Chen W-C, Chen P-Q (2009) Clinical outcomes of microendoscopic de compressive laminotomy for degenerative lumbar spinal stenosis. Eur Spine J 18: 672-678

[6] Wong DA, Watters WC III (2007) To err is human: quality and safety issues in spine care. Spine 32 (11 Suppl): S2-S8.

[7] Joint Commission on the Accreditation of Healthcare Organizations (USA) 2004 Universal Protocol. Available: http://www.jointcommissionorg/PatientSafety/National PatientSafety-Goals/04_npsgs.htm Accessed 2010 February 2.

[8] Jhawar BS, Mitsis D, Duggal N (2007) Wrong-sided and wrong-level neurosurgery: a national survey. J Neurosurg Spine 7: 467-472.

* Corresponding Author

[9] Irace C, Giannachi L, Usai S, Corona C (2008) Wrong-sided surgery. J Neurosurg Spine 9: 107-108 (letter).
[10] Krämer J (1995) Micro- or macrodiscectomy for open lumbar disc surgery? Eur Spine J 4: 69-70.
[11] van den Brink W (2011) Wrong level. J Neurosurg Spine 15(6): 689 (letter) (published online August 12, 2011; DOI: 10.3171/2011.3.SPINE10886).
[12] Irace C (2011) Wrong level. J Neurosurg Spine 15(6): 689-690 (reply to letter) (published online August 12, 2011; DOI: 10.3171/2011.3.SPINE10886).

Chapter 10

Neuroimaging in Narcolepsy

A. Bican, İ. Bora, O. Algın, B. Hakyemez, V. Özkol and E. Alper

Additional information is available at the end of the chapter

http://dx.doi.org/10.5772/25077

1. Introduction

Narcolepsy is a chronic neurological disorder, has no specific cause, and is characterized by excessive daytime sleepiness and uncontrollable sleep attacks. In case of strong emotions such as laughter, anger or joy, a cataplexy (sudden loss of muscle tone, lasting for a short period of time) may occur (1, 2). Other symptoms of narcolepsy include sleep paralysis and hypnagogic hallucinations (3, 4). Narcolepsy can occur in both men and women at any age. The prevalence of narcolepsy shows similar values in North America and Western Europe, varying from 0.02% to 0.05% (5, 6). HLA DQB1-0602 ratio 85% and HLA DQA-102 95% ratios of people with narcolepsy were found (7, 8). In spite of the fact that 99% of the cases develops sporadically, the risk is 30 to 40 times higher in the first-degree relatives than in the normal population (6).

Hypocretin-1 is reduced in cerebrospinal fluid (CSF) in most people with narcolepsy. Neurons, which contain hypocretins, are widely found in pons, thalamus and cerebral cortex (9). Recent findings indicate a reduction or full-loss of hypocretin cell development in the lateral thalamus of people with narcolepsy (10). Cases are mostly idiopathic (11). Rarely, symptomatic episodes may develop accompanied by brainstem or diencephalon lesions.

There is no gold standard test for the diagnosis of narcolepsy (12). The disorder is often diagnosed on clinical basis (13). A Polysomnogram is appropriate for assessing night-time sleep, while the Multiple Sleep Latency Test (MLST) is employed to evaluate daytime sleep attacks lasting for a short period of time (14).

There is currently a paucity of research evidence relating to magnetic resonance spectroscopy (MRS) and single-photon emission tomography (SPECT) findings in narcolepsy (9, 11, 15-17). The routine magnetic resonance imaging (MRI) performed on the patients with narcolepsy showed particular differences in various parts of the brain and in pons, while MR indicated variations in T2 weighted images, signal intensity (17, 18). Furthermore, according to cerebral perfusion studies, perfusion variations were detected in hippocampus, frontal-premotor cortex, pons and thalamus (15). Our purpose in this study is to find out the role of MRI, MRS and SPECT examinations in determining the structural changes in cerebrum and brainstem of people with narcolepsy. In addition, our purpose is also to explore the relationship of clinical and laboratory tests with the results of imaging tests.

2. Materials and method

2.1. Study population

10 patients with diagnosed narcolepsy (6 males, 4 females) as well as 11 control cases (8 males, 3 females) of similar age group were subjected to MRI, MRS and cerebral SPECT examinations. Average age of people with diagnosed narcolepsy and control group was respectively 37.1 years (range: 23-50 years) and 46 years (range: 34-55 years). Estimated starting age of the patients with disorder was 13.7 years in average (range: 5-25 years). Study protocol was examined and approved by the Ethics Committee of Uludag University. Demographical, clinical and laboratory values of patients with Narcolepsy are given in Table 1.

Patients	Sexuality	Age	Symptomatology	Cataplexy	Sleep Paralysis	Family history	HLA DQ B1O602
1	F	49	25 year	absent	existing	existing	positive
2	M	37	20 year	existing	existing	absent	positive
3	M	32	16 year	existing	existing	absent	negative
4	F	31	10 year	absent	existing	absent	negative
5	M	32	10 year	absent	existing	absent	negative
6	M	42	15 year	existing	existing	existing	negative
7	F	50	10 year	absent	existing	absent	negative
8	M	29	5 year	existing	absent	existing	negative
9	M	23	6 year	absent	existing	absent	negative
10	F	46	20 year	absent	absent	existing	positive

Table 1. Demographical, clinical and laboratory values of patients with Narcolepsy.

2.2. Polysomnogram

After being assessed in the sleep clinic, the patients were scheduled for nocturnal polysomnograms with subsequent MSLTs. In the meantime, they were advised to avoid having caffeinated foods or drinking alcohol. All nocturnal polysomnograms and next-day sleepiness tests were conducted by means of Grass Telefactor (AS 40 Amplifier system). In the standard polysomnogram, four-channel EEG (C3/A2; C4/A1; O1/A2; O2/A1), two-channel electrooculogram (EOG), submental and anterior tibial muscle electromyogram (EMG), and electrocardiogram (EKG) electrodes were used. Thermistor (oronasal airflow), pulsoxymetry, abdominal and thoracic body sensors were also available.

The images of the patients were observed through an infrared video camera by a sleep technician, and the records kept. The patients were put to bed at 11:00 pm and waken up at 07:00 am. Sleep stages were scored for each 30-second epoch according to Rechtshaffen and Kales criteria. In MSLT, again four-channel EEG, two-channel EOG, and single-channel EMG records were kept by Grass Telefactor device, accompanied by imaging process by a sleep technician. MSLT was started at 09:00 am in the morning of long nocturnal process, with repetition for 5 times with a 20-minute sleep followed by 20-minute wakefulness. During MSLT, every 30-second sleep epochs were scored considering Sleep-Onset REM, in supervision of a doctor. The patients were diagnosed with narcolepsy according to the International Classification of Sleep Disorders. All of the patients diagnosed with narcolepsy, who had been involved in the study, had short daytime sleep attacks and had not undergone a specific sleep treatment.

2.3. Cerebral SPECT examinations

Brain Perfusion SPECT imaging was performed from 02:00 pm to 06:00 pm. All patients were asked to urinate, followed by a 10-minute relaxation period in supine position in an unlit and silent imaging room, and 15 mCi (555 MBq) ^{99m}Tc-HMPAO injected intravenously. Imaging process was initiated 10 minutes later than injection. In this study, the low-energy, high-resolution, parallel-hole collimator, double detector gamma camera (Millenium VG, GE Medical Systems) was used. Data was gathered with the settings 1.2 zoom, 128x128-matrix and centre at 140 keV, 20% window interval, at every 5° rotation angle in step mode for 25 seconds, in total at 360° rotation in 2x36 projection; and imaging process lasted 30 minutes. No attenuation or scattering correction is applied. Raw data so gathered was transferred to data-processing and evaluation unit (Entegra Workstation, GE Medical Systems), processed through Butterworth filter (cut-off frequency 0,55 rev./cm; order, 8) and reconstructed in cross-sections with thickness of 3.68 mm, which were parallel to the orbitomeatal line. SPECT cross-sections were evaluated visually at first in orbitomeatal, coronal and sagittal cross-sections. In case of presence of the increased or decreased ^{99m}Tc-HMPAO retention compared to symmetric areas, the symmetric identical cross-sectional and volumetric areas of interest were determined, semi-quantitative evaluation done, and a standard deviation of 2 or over accepted significant.

2.4. MR imaging and MR spectroscopy

All the examinations were performed using 1.5 Tesla MR equipment (Siemens, Magnetom Vision Plus, Erlangen, Germany) with standard head coils, and the study protocol consisted of the following sequences, respectively. Axial-coronal T2-weighted (W) fast spin-echo (FSE) (TR/TE 5400/99), sagittal fluid attenuated inversion recovery (FLAIR) (TR/TE/TI 8400/114/2150), axial-sagittal T1W spin-echo (SE) sequences (TR/TE 550/18), were applied. Field of view (FOV) 24 cm, 256×256 matrix, 5mm slice thickness and 1mm inter slice gap were obtained. Subsequent to these sequences, a 8 cm^3 VOI (volume of interest) was put in frontal cortex, hippocampus, thalamus and pons, and MRS obtained with PRESS sequence

(TE: 135 ms, TR: 2000 ms, number of acquisitions: 136). Total duration of MR examinations was approximately 20 minutes.

Once imaging process was completed, the routine MR and MRS data available in the MR equipment workstation was analysed by a radiologist (O.A.), who had been unaware of clinical and laboratory findings. The peak values of N-acetyl aspartate (NAA), choline (Cho) and creatine (Cr) as well as their respective ratios were obtained. Total duration of MR examinations was about 10 minutes. All MRI and MRS examinations were evaluated by 2 radiologists (O.A., B.H.), on a randomized basis.

2.5. Statistical analysis

The routine MRI, MRS and cerebral SPECT data obtained from the whole cases was compared with clinical and laboratory findings, while the contribution of such examinations to diagnosis evaluated statistically. All statistical analysis was done with statistical programme of SPSS 13.0 software (SPSS Inc., Chicago, IL, USA). The concordance of the data to the normal variation was evaluated with Shapiro-Wilk test. Concordance of normal distribution of all continuous variables was calculated through Shapiro-Wilk test. The relationship between two groups was evaluated with Mann-Whitney U test. The level of statistical significance was set at $P < 0.05$.

3. Results

The presence of cataplexy was 40% (4/10), sleep paralysis 80% (8/10), and family history 40% (4/10). Two of the patients were brothers. HLA DQ B10602 was positive at a ratio of 30% (3/10). Average total sleep time of the patients was 397 min. (range: 370-438 min.), average sleep latency 6.5 min. (range: 3-8 min.). Average Epwort sleepiness test was concluded as 10.

The routine cranial MRIs for all cases involved in the study showed no pathological signal variation (Picture 1). In the MRS examinations from frontal cortex and thalamus, no significant statistical difference between NAA/Cr, NAA/Cho, Cho/Cr values of people with narcolepsy and of control group was found ($p>0.05$) (Picture 2). Measurements from pons and hippocampus indicated NAA/Cho ratios for narcolepsy group (1.17±0.2 and 0.78±0.26, respectively) and for control group (2.1±0.76 and 1.12±0.15, respectively) were significantly lower ($p<0.05$). Cho/Cr ratios in the level of pons for people with narcolepsy pons (1.89±0.52) were higher than that for control cases (1.2±0.3) significantly ($p<0.05$). In terms of pontine NAA/Cr values, no significant difference was detected between narcolepsy group (2.21±0.68) and control group (2.46±0.78) ($p>0.05$) (Picture 3). Measurement from hippocampus showed no significant variation in NAA/Cr and Cho/Cr values between narcolepsy group and control group ($p>0.05$). MRS values for all cases involved in the study are given in Table 2.

In SPECT examinations, the parietal lobe showed hypoperfusion for one case (Picture 4). SPECT examinations for other cases with diagnosed narcolepsy and for control group were evaluated normal. SPECT data for narcolepsy group is given in Table 3.

MRS localization	Groups	NAA/Cho	NAA/Cr	Cho/Cr
Pons	Patient with narcolepsy	1.17±0.2	2.21±0.68	1.89±0.52
	Controls	2.1±0.76	2.46±0.78	1.2±0.31
	Statistical significance	P<0.05	P>0.05	P<0.05
Hippocampus	Patient with narcolepsy	0.78±0.26	0.95±0.43	1.19±0.21
	Controls	1.12±0.15	1.33±0.21	1.19±0.15
	Statistical significance	P<0.05	P>0.05	P>0.05
Frontal lobe	Patient with narcolepsy	2.05±0.52	2.5±0.74	1.23±0.2
	Controls	1.76±0.42	2.26±1.02	1.09±0.35
	Statistical significance	P>0.05	P>0.05	P>0.05
Thalamus	Patient with narcolepsy	1.74±0.18	1.93±0.28	1.12±0.2
	Controls	1.95±0.48	1.9±0.18	0.97±0.19
	Statistical significance	P>0.05	P>0.05	P>0.05

Table 2. All cases result of MRS

Patients	Serebral SPECT (Tc 99m-HMPAO)
1	Normal
2	Parietal lobe showed hypoperfusion
3	Normal
4	Normal
5	Normal
6	Normal
7	Normal
8	Normal
9	Normal
10	Normal

Table 3. SPECT result of patients with Narcolepsy.

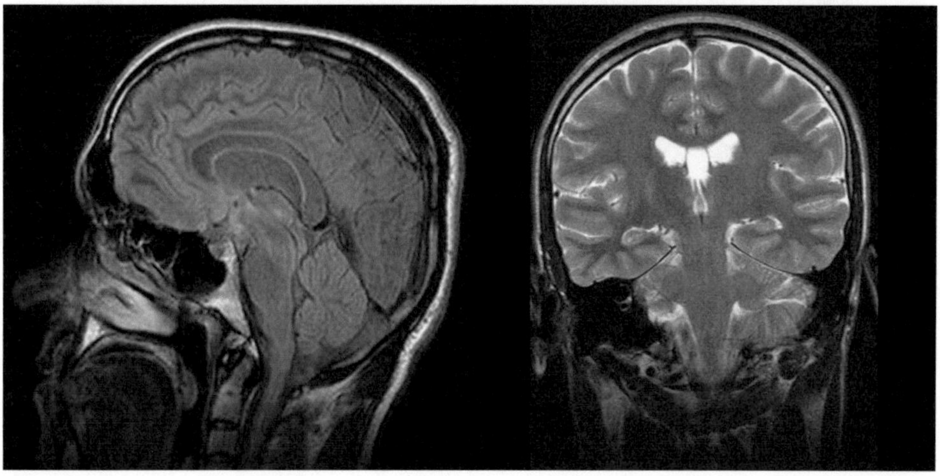

Picture 1. Normal cranial MRI images (sagittal FLAIR and coronal T2W images, respectively) in patient with narcolepsy.

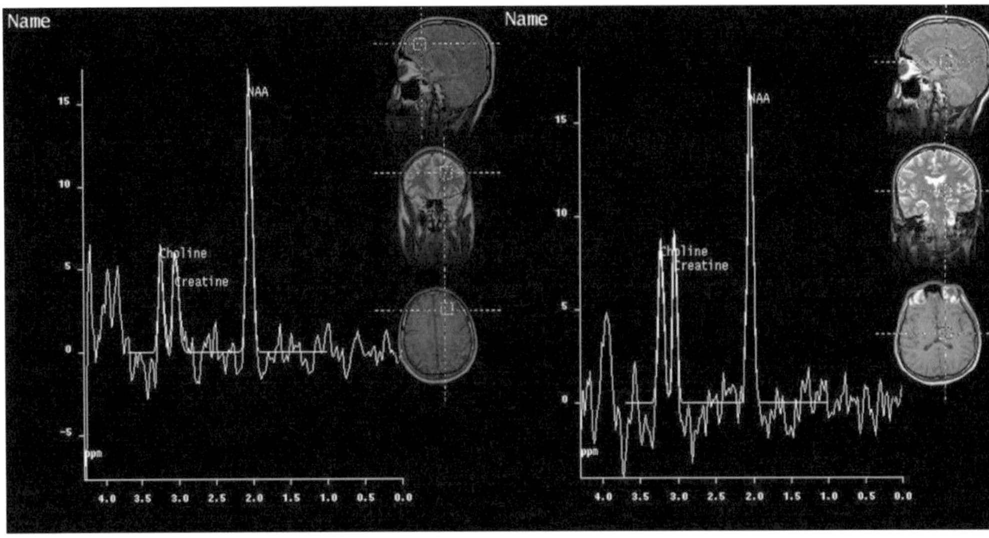

Picture 2. Normal MRS examinations from frontal cortex and thalamus.

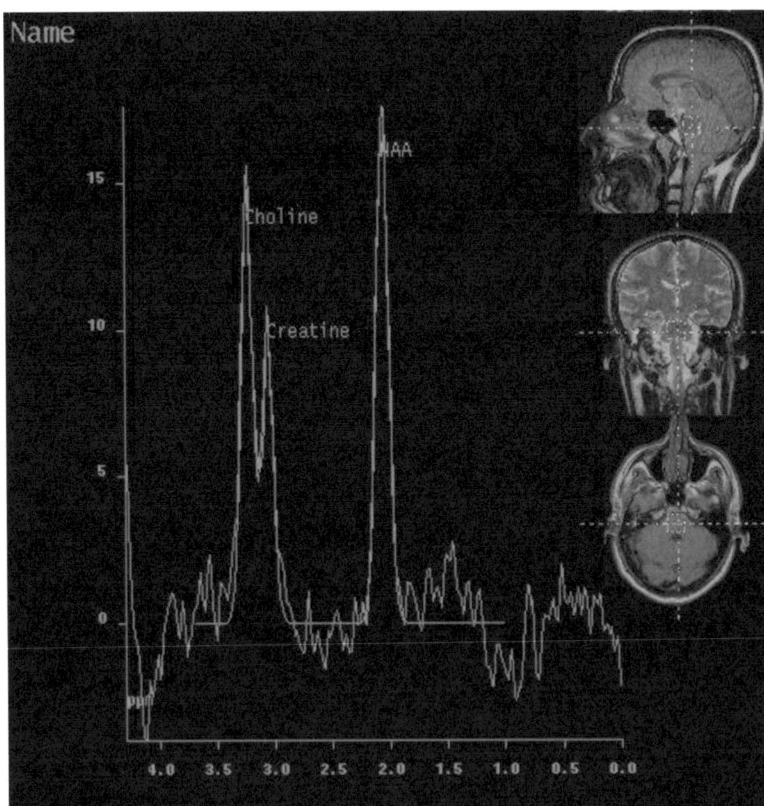

Picture 3. Proton MR spectra in the patient with narcolepsy. N-acetylaspartate (NAA), choline, and creatine peaks are observed. NAA/Cho ratio in this patient was decreased comparing to controls. Also, Cho/Cr ratio was increased comparing to controls.

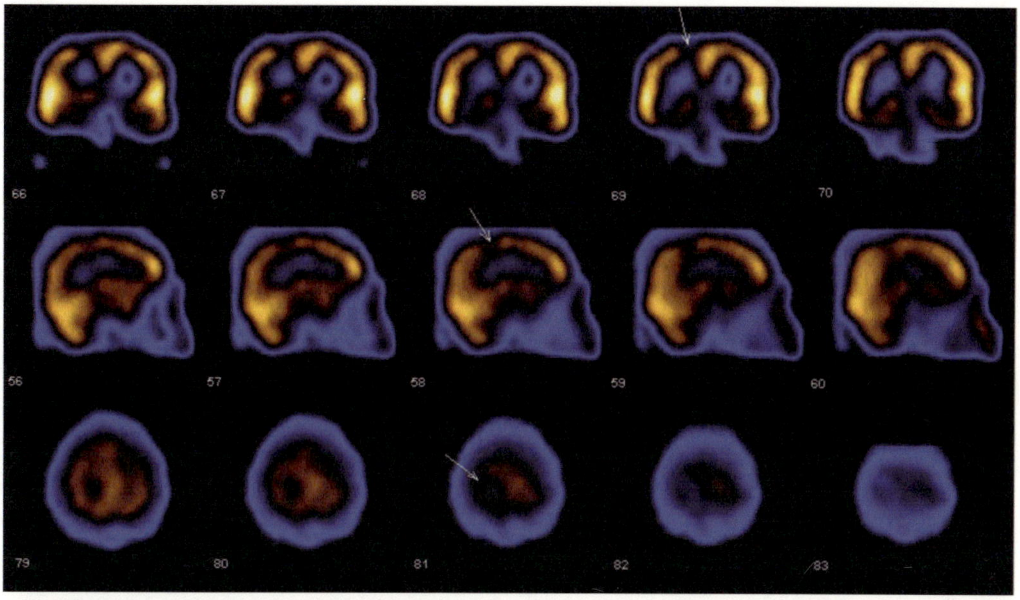

Picture 4. Parietal lobe showed hypoperfusion (2. Patient)

4. Discussion

Narcolepsy is mostly an idiopathic disease, and clinical findings are used in diagnosing narcolepsy. There is no gold standard test for the diagnosis of narcolepsy (9, 12). Diagnosis criteria include clinical, polysomnogram, multiple sleep latency test (MSLT), and measurement of hypocretin level in cerebrospinal liquid (CSF), which is an invasive method (15). There are a limited number of literatures regarding the use of MRS and SPECT on people with narcolepsy (11, 15, 17). In most of these literatures the results are controversial (15, 16). This may be attributed to the inadequacy of both number and homogeneity of the cases. Our purpose in this study narcolepsy is to find out the role of MRI, MRS and SPECT examinations in determining the structural changes in cerebrum and brainstem in the patients with narcolepsy.

Brain SPECT imaging is a nuclear medicine procedure that allows the clinicians to evaluate the brain function (15, 16). Brain perfusion SPECT gives information regarding blood build-up of various anatomic regions in the brain (12, 15, 16). Reduced activity in hypothalamus, thalamus, prefrontal cortex, parahipocampal gyrus and hippocampus localizations was found during SPECT examinations performed to investigate brain perfusion changes for patients with narcolepsy (15). Specific changes in cerebral blood flow cannot be shown regularly, since the sleep stages in narcolepsy are not fully stabilized (19). In the cataplexic status, high activity was observed in singular gyrus, orbitofrontal and putaminal regions; while, unlike other studies, no activation was shown in pons, amygdala and occipital cortex (20). According to our study, in 9 of 10 cases with diagnosed narcolepsy no perfusion change was detected during SPECT examination. 1 patient showed hypoperfusion in in the right cerebral hemisphere parietal lobe. Based on these findings, it may be suggested that

SPECT examination has limited contribution to the evaluation of the cases with diagnosed narcolepsy.

One of the most interesting practices of MR procedure is the proton MRS. Based on this technique, information regarding microscopic environments in which protons are available is obtained through chemical shift effect. Protons in the water indicate different release frequencies than those in lactate, adipose tissue or other important biological structures (21, 22). Thus, by the aid of MRS, we are able to determine, on a non-invasive basis, the concentrations of metabolites in brain as well as the metabolite variations occurring for various reasons (21). Today, MRS is used in diagnosing many diseases. MRS plays an important role in the differential diagnosis of infectious, metabolic, ischemic and tumoral diseases (22). Furthermore, by the help of MRS, neuronal damages and metabolite variations, which cannot be shown in brain through the routine MRI, may be also indicated. NAA is a metabolite especially found in neurons and is generally accepted as neuronal marker (23). Reduction in NAA reveals neuronal damage and loss, since the regeneration capacity of neurons is extremely limited (22, 23).

In consideration of the fact that narcolepsy may be attributed to neuronal loss or damage in hypothalamus, MRS examinations were performed in relation to hippocampuses for people with narcolepsy. In these studies involving limited number of cases, hypothalamic NAA/Cr was found lower in patients with narcolepsy, compared to control group. Based on this finding, it was emphasized that the central pathology in narcolepsy might be the neuronal loss in hippocampus (16, 17). In another study performed through MRS, ventral pontine regions of patients with diagnosed idiopathic narcolepsy were investigated and no variation observed from those of control group (11, 16). Certain studies conducted by means of MRI showed variations in several regions of brain and in pons, while those performed through MRI revealed changes in T2-weighted images and in signal intensity (16-18). In the cerebral SPECT study over 25 patients with narcolepsy, Joo, et. al. suggested that hypoperfusion had been found in parahipocampal gyrus, hippocampus, frontal cortex, pons and thalamus. These regions probably reflect cerebral hypocretin system (15, 16). For such reasons, MRS measurements from pons, frontal lobe, thalamus and hippocampus were used in our study.

Pontine tegmentum regulates the transition among sleep stages (16). Pons contains reticular formation regulating REM sleep (18). Neuronal damage in this stage is expressed as the main reason of narcolepsy (16). Plazzi, et. al. (18) suggested that pontine T2 hyperintensities detected through MRI are significant in terms of narcolepsy. There are also counter-literatures suggesting that such signal variations are age-dependent non-specific ischemic-degenerative changes (1, 16). In the cranial MRI examinations on patients with diagnosed narcolepsy, we detected no significant variation in signal intensity in the pons stage or a pathological finding. Our findings make us think that the routine MRI has no considerable contribution to the diagnosis of narcolepsy. MRI may contribute to the exclusion of other organic lesions, restricting the list of dissepimental diagnoses. In MRS examinations performed with respect to pons, we determined a reduction in NAA/Cho ratios and an increase in Cho/Ch rations for patients with narcolepsy, compared to those for control group. These findings reveal the neuronal damage in the pons stage. In a MRS study conducted by Ellis, et. al., no significant variation was found between control group and narcolepsy group in terms of metabolite values (11). That study is inconsistent with our findings; however, another MRS study carried out from the pons stage is found to be consonant to our data.

In our study, NAA/Cho ratios in hippocampus were found significantly lower than those of control group. This result makes think that there is a neuronal loss in hippocampuses of patients with narcolepsy for several reasons. Neuronal damage in hippocampus, which is a part of the limbic system, may reveal the emotional instability in patients with narcolepsy. SPECT examinations on people with narcolepsy showed hypoperfusion in the structures forming the limbic system (15, 16). Hypoperfusion of the limbic system may become the reason of neuronal damage detected in our study.

The main limitation of our study is the relative adequacy of the number of cases. Furthermore, failure to perform MRS examinations from other regions excluding frontal lobe and from hypothalamus may also feature another limitation of us. We failed to carry out multivoxel MRS due to technical deficiencies in our MR equipment. New wide-series studies in which brain is evaluated globally, also containing multivoxel MRS examinations, and where cases are followed for a long period of time, are required.

As a result, MRI and SPECT examinations have limited contribution to the diagnosis of narcolepsy. MRS appears to be beneficial in diagnosing narcolepsy, indicating those structural changes that cannot be detected through the routine cranial MRI.

Author details

A. Bican
Uludag University School of Medicine, Departments of Neurology, Görükle, Bursa, Türkiye
Uludag Universitesi Tip Fakultesi, Nöroloji ABD, Görükle, Bursa, Türkiye

İ. Bora
Uludag University School of Medicine, Departments of Neurology, Görükle, Bursa, Türkiye

O. Algın and B. Hakyemez
Uludag University School of Medicine, Departments of Radiology, Görükle, Bursa, Türkiye

V. Özkol and E. Alper
Uludag University School of Medicine, Departments of Nuclear Medicine, Görükle, Bursa, Türkiye

5. References

[1] Bassetti C, Aldich MS, Quint DJ. MRI findings in narcolepsy. Sleep 1997; 20:630-631
[2] Aldrich MS. The neurobiology of narcolepsy-cataplexy. Prog Neurobiol 1993;41:533-541
[3] Honda Y. Clinical features of narcolepsy. In: Honda Y, Juji T, ed. HLA in narcolepsy. Berlin: Springer-Verlag, 1988:24-57
[4] Diagnostic Classification Steering Committee. Thorpy MJ CASDA. ICSD-International classification of sleep disorders. Diagnostic coding manual. Rochester, MN: American Sleep Disorders Association; 1990

[5] National Institutes of Health. National Heart L, and Blood Institute. Narcolepsy. Bethesda: National Institutes of Health, National Heart, Lung and Blood Institute; NIH Publication No. 96-3649,1996
[6] Mignot E. Genetic and familial aspects of narcolepsy. Neurology 1998;50:16-22
[7] Kadatoni H, Faraco J, Mignot E. Genetic studies in the sleep disorder narcolepsy. Genome Res 1998;8:427-434
[8] Mignot E, Hayduk R, Black J, et al. HLA DQB1-602 is associated with cataplexy in 509 narcoleptic patients. Sleep 1997;20:1012-1020
[9] C. Brenneis, E. Brandauer, B. Frauscher, M. Schocke, T.Trieb, W. Poewe, B.Högl Voxel-based morphometry in narcolepsy. Sleep Medicine 2005; 531–536
[10] Nishino S, Ripley B, Overeem S, et al. Hypocretin (orexin) deficiency in human narcolepy. Lancet 2000; 355:39-40
[11] Ellis CM, Simmons A, Lemmens G, Williams SC, Parkes JD. Proton spectroscopy in the narcoleptic syndrome. Is there evidence of a brainstem lesion? Neurology. 1998;50:23-6.
[12] Sturzenegger C, Bassetti CL. The clinical spectrum of narcolepsy with cataplexy: a reappraisal . J. Sleep Res. 2004;13,395–406
[13] Khatami R, Bassetti CL. Narcolepsy. Schweiz Arch Neurol Psychiatr 2003;154:339-348.
[14] Aldrich, M. S, Chervin, R. D and Malow, B. A. Value of the multiple sleep latency test (MSLT) for the diagnosis of narcolepsy. Sleep 1997, 20: 620–629.
[15] Hong SB, Tae WS, Joo EY. Cerebral perfusion changes during cataplexy in narcolepsy patients. Neurology 2006 13;66:1747-9
[16] Dang-Vu TT, Desseilles M, Petit D, Mazza S, Montplaisir J, Maquet P. Neuroimaging in sleep medicine. Sleep Medicine 2007;8:349–372
[17] Lodi R, Tonon C, Vignatelli L, Iotti S, Montagna P, Barbiroli B, Plazzi G.M In vivo evidence of neuronal loss in the hypothalamus of narcoleptic patients. Neurology 2004 26;63:1513-5
[18] Plazzi G, Montagna P, Provini F, Bizzi A, Cohen M, Lugaresi E. Pontine lesions in idiopathic narcolepsy. Neurology 1996;46:1250-4
[19] Asenbaum S, Zeithofer J, Saletu B, Frey R, Brücke T, Podreka I, Deecke L. Technetium-99m-HMPAO SPECT imaging of cerebral blood flow during REM sleep in narcoleptics. J Nucl Med. 1995;36:1150-5
[20] Chabas D, Habert MO, Maksud P, Tourbah A, Minz M, Willer JC, Arnulf I. Functional imaging of cataplexy during status cataplecticus. Sleep. 2007;30:153-6
[21] Bonavita S, Di Salle F, Tedeschi G. Proton MRS in neurological disorders. Eur J Radiol 1999; 30:125-131
[22] Yerli H, Ağıldere AM, Özen O, Geyik E, Atalay B, Elhan AH. Evaluation of cerebral glioma grade by using normal side creatine as an internal reference in multi-voxel 1H-MR spectroscopy. Diagn Interv Radiol 2007;13:3-9
[23] Kubas B, Kulak W, Sobaniec W, Walecki J, Lewko J. Proton magnetic rasonance spectroscopy in patients with normal pressure hydrocephalus. The Neuroradiology Journal 2006;19:597-602

Chapter 11

Forensic Issues in the Structural or Functional Neuroimaging of Traumatic Brain Injury

Robert P. Granacher, Jr.

Additional information is available at the end of the chapter

http://dx.doi.org/10.5772/51978

1. Introduction

1.1. Application area

1.1.1. Forensic differences between examinations by a treating physician and examinations for the purpose of legal testimony

It is not possible to provide a comprehensive forensic neuropsychiatric assessment of a person following traumatic brain injury (TBI) without also including within the examination, at a minimum, structural brain imaging (e.g., magnetic resonance imaging (MRI), or computed tomography (CT)). Functional brain imaging such as positron emission tomography (PET) or single photon emission computed tomography (SPECT) may be useful in very particular or special circumstances, but they should never be the modality of first choice following TBI. [1-2] Table 1 is a listing of the common structural and functional procedures available to the forensic examiner for a TBI assessment. The need for neuroimaging within a forensic assessment of TBI is based on two principles: (1) The first principle is the pathogenesis of TBI generally results in at least some organic changes to the brain, and (2): in the second principle, the forensic physician has an ethical obligation to provide the soundest opinions possible to the trier-of-fact, judge or jury. In light of the possible organic pathology associated with a TBI, the examination of a head trauma patient is incomplete without examination of the integrity of the brain if the data is to be presented in a court of law. Another very important forensic principle in a legal case of alleged TBI is that a very high percentage of those claiming mild traumatic brain injury (MTBI), may in fact be malingering or symptom magnifying. [4] If malingering of a TBI or symptom magnification of complaints to the physicians is probable, obviously the forensic examiner's opinion will be buttressed by the absence of lesions consistent with TBI on neuroimaging.

Structural Imaging:	• Computed Tomography (CT) • Magnetic Resonance Imaging (MRI)
Functional Imaging :	• Single Photon Emission Computed Tomography (SPECT) • Positron Emission Tomography (PET) • Functional Magnetic Resonance Imaging (fMRI) • Magnetic Resonance Spectroscopy (MRS)

Table 1. Methods for Imaging Traumatic Brain Injury

Physicians of all specialties carry an ethical obligation to assist in the application of the judicial process and to assist the courts in carrying out matters brought to them. Physicians also have an ethical obligation to testify on behalf of their patients if asked to do so, but when testifying as a treating physician, the physician is a fact witness, not an opinion witness. In particular, for forensic neuroimaging of TBI, this means that the physician will testify about the facts of the neuroimaging and how it relates to the physician's patient including the clinical findings, treatment plan, and outcomes. As a general rule, a physician examining a TBI patient where it is known that the patient is in a legal context, should avoid issues of malingering, ratable disability impairment, whether or not the patient is telling the truth, and other factors that will have special importance in a legal forum. If the treating physician ventures into these areas, it puts at risk the doctor-patient relationship, and this should never be allowed to happen.

On the other hand, the physician who has been asked to examine a patient claiming to have been injured by TBI should never imply to the examinee that a doctor-patient relationship exists. Most persons who have suffered a TBI, and then are forensically examined by neuroimaging, are generally not familiar with the exceptions to the doctor-patient relationship, which exists before the law in most modern countries. Thus, the examinee is placed in a very disadvantageous position. The examinee may incorrectly assume that the neuroimaging is being obtained to provide assistance in the diagnosis or treatment for the brain injury. This is absolutely not the case in a forensic examination; the physician is acting as an agent for the entity or person who hired him/her to perform the neuroimaging. The physician examiner in a forensic case should treat the examinee with compassion and appropriate respect, but there should be no doubt left in the examinee's mind for whom the physician is employed. In this case, it is obviously not the patient. The examinee should always be advised of this difference within the context of the examination at the outset, and it is suggested that this be done in writing as well as verbally. [5]

1.2. Rules of scientific evidence in the court room

As a general rule following TBI, if the person who sustained the injury is being assessed to determine the level of cognitive impairment or rehabilitation outcome, the most likely individuals who will order neuroimaging well after the acute TBI will include: neurologists, rehabilitation medicine specialists, neuropsychiatrists, general psychiatrists, internists, pediatricians, and possibly other medical specialties as well. Physicians possessing these specialties or subspecialties are not expected to master neuroimaging techniques at the level of radiologists or nuclear medicine physicians. However, a general principle of medical practice is that a physician who orders a laboratory test will have the requisite experience and knowledge to use that laboratory test as part of the assessment of an examinee. In other words, use of neuroimaging within a forensic assessment requires that the physician should have a fundamental understanding of the principles of neuroimaging specific to the particular case, when and when not to order neuroimaging, familiarity with the radiologic anatomy of the brain, and that physician should possess an ability to use neuroimaging data in the overall analysis of an examinee following alleged TBI. Thus, it is recommended that a physician ordering neuroimaging following TBI should have a professional relationship with radiologists and/or nuclear medicine physicians who will be providing interpretive reports to the examining physician.

In general, when a non-radiologic physician is asked to examine persons within a court setting to determine if they have damage from an alleged TBI, it is recommended that the examining physician collect reports of the original injury and/or digital discs of previous neuroimaging, and that these be sent to the radiologist or nuclear medicine physician prior to the neuroimaging ordered by the examining physician. This will be very useful to the radiological physician at the time the examinee undergoes neuroimaging, and it will enable a clinical correlation to be determined between the chronic neuroimaging and the acute neuroimaging at the time of injury. Obviously, the examining physician should ask that a computer disc (CD) of the images of the examinee be prepared and sent to this physician with the report. The forensic physician should review the CD of the images, over-read them, and ensure that the forensic physician agrees with the interpretation of the radiologist. This is very important in a court case, because occasionally typographic errors are made in a radiological report. For instance, it is possible that a lesion in the right temporal lobe could be mistakenly reported as being present in the left temporal lobe. The forensic physician should then provide clinical correlation between the neuroimaging he/she orders of the examinee and relate this to the further analysis of medical records, mental examinations, neurological examinations, and neuropsychological test findings to determine the level of functional brain injury.

It is rare that a forensic physician is asked to evaluate a TBI victim during the acute phases following TBI. Almost all forensic medical assessments are made either in the subacute or chronic phase of the TBI. The forensic physician will generally focus upon neurologic, cognitive and behavioral changes following TBI, and any obvious negative neurological or orthopedic outcomes represented peripherally in the cranial nerves, arms or legs. Therefore, in order for the examining physician to provide testimony within reasonable medical probability, it is generally wise not to make outcome diagnoses and predictions about an examinee until at least six months, and up to 1-½ years following the TBI. Precise predictions are difficult with a TBI, but some generalizations can be made: [6]

1. The more severe the injury, the longer the recovery period, and the more impairment a survivor will have once recovery has plateaued.
2. Recovery from diffuse axonal injury takes longer than recovery from focal contusions.

3. Recovery from TBI with associated hypoxic injury is less complete than absent significant hypoxic injury.
4. The need for intracranial surgery does not necessarily indicate a worse outcome. For example, a patient requiring the removal of a subdural hematoma may recover cognition as completely as one who never needed surgery.

The length of time an examinee spends in coma correlates to both posttraumatic amnesia (PTA) and recovery times: [6]

1. A coma lasting seconds to minutes results in PTA that lasts hours to days; the recovery plateau occurs over days to weeks.
2. A coma that lasts hours to days results in PTA lasting days to weeks; the recovery plateau occurs over months.
3. A coma lasting weeks results in PTA that lasts for months; the recovery plateau occurs over months to years.

The aforementioned points about recovery periods and posttraumatic amnesia are extremely important when testifying in court about functional outcome of the TBI. Clearly, these periods of recovery and posttraumatic amnesia allow the forensic physician to testify to the trier-of-fact reasonable predictions about recovery time and outcomes. The litigation of a traumatic brain injury case for worker's compensation benefits or compensation for damages, often requires the forensic physician to provide the court with statements as to how long the individual will need medical assistance, how long the victim of the TBI will require rehabilitation, and to what level the TBI victim can be expected to return to his/her prior baseline.

2. Pathophysiology of traumatic brain injury

The forensic physician is often required to provide the court with a description of how a blunt force, a penetrating force, or an explosion can render the victim with a TBI. Much is known about the organic pathogenesis of TBI. The biomechanical forces commonly involved in TBI are usually of three main types: (1) blunt force trauma to the head and/or (2) penetrating injuries to the head and/or (3) blast overpressure brain injury from improvised explosive devices (IEDs), bombs, industrial explosions, and other sources of blast overpressure. The kinetic injury from blunt force trauma or blast overpressure translates into passive parenchymal damage and secondary brain insults. Brain tissue is injured by compressive, tensile and shearing strains, which in turn produce contusions, lacerations, or diffuse axonal injury. [6] The passive damage to brain tissue is generally instantaneous, but secondary brain insults are associated with post-trauma factors including ischemic blood flow, hypoxic injury, and metabolic changes at the cellular level. This cascade of events can occur over hours to several days after TBI and may significantly alter the level of damage and thus the prognosis. [7]

At the moment of blunt force trauma or blast overpressure injury, and less so with penetrating injuries, microporation of the lipid bilayer cell membrane occurs, leading to cell rupture. This activates voltage- and ligand-gated channels, which in turn produces ischemia. This enables the entry of calcium ions and sodium ions into neurons with egress of potassium ions. The resulting ionic shift produces an altered state of consciousness. [8] Even with a concussion that does not produce evidence of structural brain injury, the concentration of extracellular potassium can be increased for a short period, up to 50 times baseline. For the more severely injured person, excess potassium in the extracellular fluid is sequestered, and there is a direct relationship between extracellular potassium and mortality. [9] As potassium is sequestered, this may produce ischemia secondary to cerebral edema. Another important development of tissue damage is associated with disturbances of calcium homeostasis. The cellular movement of calcium ions into the cell results in metabolic cascades. As the level of intracellular calcium dramatically increases, this in turn, causes the outer membrane of the mitochondria to develop permeability pores, which allows the calcium to interfere with electron transport in the cell. This may result in cell necrosis. [10] The neurochemical cascade that activates certain intracellular enzymes can cause the mitochondria to release proteins that result in programmed cell death (apoptosis). [11] The long-term effect of this confluence of compromise in ionic and molecular transport along the axonal sheath, is cytoskeletal damage. This, in turn, produces axotomy (disruption of the axon) and Wallerian degeneration. [11]

3. Structural neuroimaging of traumatic brain injury

From a forensic standpoint, almost all cases of evaluation of traumatic brain injury will be completed well after the original injury. These evaluations are generally completed by a psychiatrist, neurologist, or physiatrist. Therefore, Variant 5: subacute or chronic closed head injury, the American College of Radiology (ACR) Appropriateness Criteria, enable the physician to determine a rating of appropriateness for examination of an injury by neuroimaging within the period after acute injury. [3] Variant 5 is for persons who demonstrate cognitive and/or neurological deficits at the time of the examination. Table 2 lists the ACR Appropriateness Criteria for Variant 5: closed head injury, subacute or chronic. It is important to note that at this time, the ACR Appropriateness Criteria for acute injuries following closed head injury invariably list CT of the head as the most appropriate neuroimaging modality. On the other hand, the reader should note in Table 2 that for the subacute and chronic head injury with cognitive and/or neurological deficits, MRI now becomes a preferred neuroimaging modality.

3.1. Computed Tomography (CT)

Neuroradiologists and neurosurgeons generally agree that CT is the most common means used for intracranial evaluation in the emergency department or acute care setting. While this opinion is changing with the evolving nature of high-speed MRI, it continues presently to be the accepted way to manage acute head injuries from a neuroradiological perspective. [12]

Radiologic Procedure	Rating	Comments	RRL*
MRI head without contrast	8		0
CT head without contrast	6		3
Tc-99m HMPAO SPECT head	4	For selected cases.	4
FG-PET head	4	For selected cases	4
MRA head and neck without contrast	4	For selected cases	0
MRA head and neck without and with contrast	4	For selected cases	0
CTA head and neck	4	For selected cases	3
MRI head without and with contrast	3		0
CT head without and with contrast	2		3
X-ray and/or CT cervical spine without contrast	2	Assuming there are no spinal neurologic deficits.	2
X-ray head	2		1
Functional (MRI) head	2		0
US transcranial with Doppler	1		0
Arteriography cervicocerebral	1		3
Rating Scale: 1,2,3 = Usually not appropriate; 4,5,6 = May be appropriate; 7,8,9 = Usually appropriate			* Relative Radiation Level
MRI = Magnetic Resonance Imaging CT = Computed Tomography SPECT = Single photon emission computed tomography FDG-PET = Fluorodeoxyglucose positron emission tomography MRA = Magnetic resonance angiography CTA = Computed tomographic angiography US = Ultrasound			

Table 2. American College of Radiology (ACR) Appropriateness Criteria: Variant 5. Subacute or Chronic Closed Head Injury with Cognitive and/or Neurological Deficit(s) [3]

It will be rare that the post-acute injury examination will require CT evaluation unless the examinee has a contraindicated metallic implant or other medical device such as prosthetic cardiac valves, cardiac pacemaker, etc. It is recommended that the examining physician, where possible, get a copy of the original CD of the CT head imaging from the acute care setting so that one can compare the possible pathology at the time the individual was evaluated on an emergency basis with the imaging of a current evaluation. This is because in order to provide the soundest of opinions to the trier-of-fact, upon the assessment of TBI, it is best wherever possible for the examining physician to clinically correlate the neuroimaging findings with that originally obtained at the time of the injury. For example, Figure 1 shows an initial CT following head trauma revealing a contusion of diffuse axonal injury in the left inferior temporal lobe, contusion in the right temporal tip, and an accompanying subarachnoid hemorrhage in the posterior fossa. It can be noted on a CT made approximately six weeks later (Figure 2), that there is now evidence of encephalomalacia in the left temporal lobe and right temporal lobe, indicated by reduced attenuation of the brain parenchyma, and the subarachnoid blood is absent. As noted in the magnetic resonance imaging section below, it is important to determine later if indicia of injury still remain when the person is examined within the subacute or chronic phase.

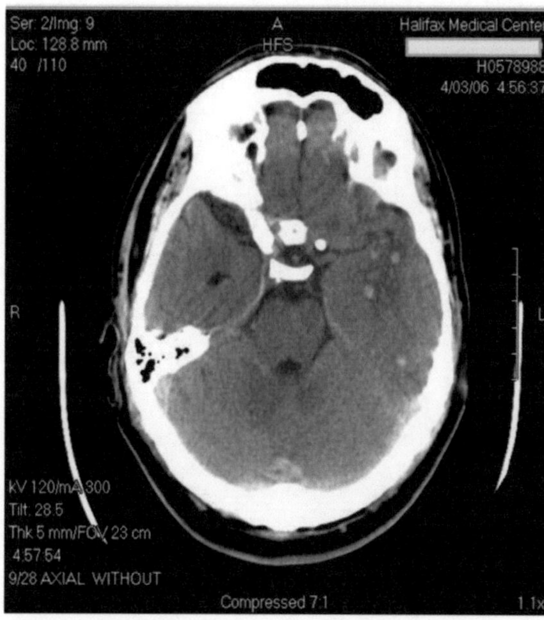

Figure 1.

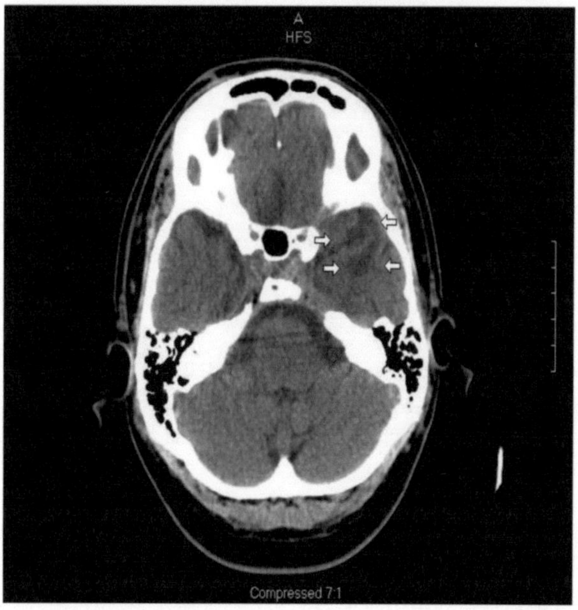

Figure 2.

Figure 3 shows CT evidence of a shear injury in the left frontal lobe of an adolescent following a fall from a moving vehicle onto the ground. When an MRI was obtained three years after injury, it is noteworthy that on the axial T2 gradient echo imaging, evidence of hemosiderin remains in the same anatomic area as a marker of the original shear injury, and the resultant bleeding has left hemosiderin behind (Figure 4). Figures 3 and 4 clearly demonstrate the usefulness of having initial CT imaging for comparison with postinjury MRI.

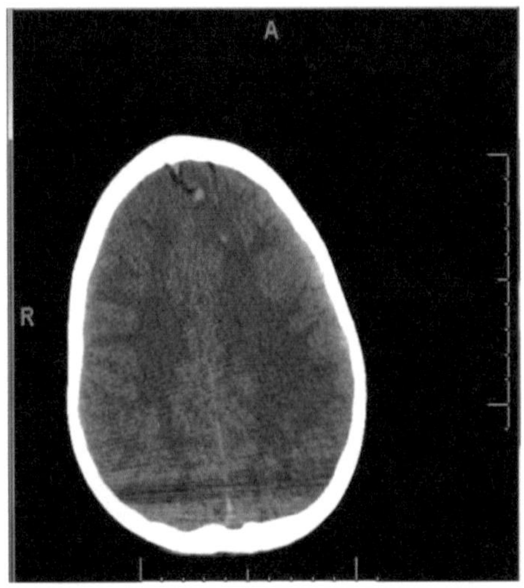

Figure 3.

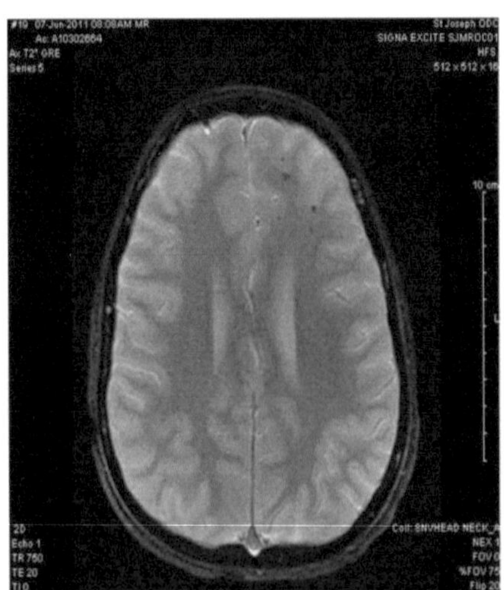

Figure 4.

3.2. Magnetic Resonance Imaging (MRI)

MRI has become a powerful tool in the assessment of the aftereffects of traumatic brain injury. From a medico-legal perspective, it is the complex behavioral and cognitive changes that occur following TBI that will be of most interest. It is hoped that the forensic evaluation of traumatic brain injury will enable a positive medical correlation to be made between the evidence of injury on the MRI and the major changes in cognition that can be detected by neuropsychological assessment. [1] For instance, Figure 5 is an example of the appearance of encephalomalacia on a T2 MRI obtained in a young man who was brutally harmed in a backyard beating. The coronal image (Figure 6) delineates the extensive depth of this lesion on the lateral surface of the anterior left frontal lobe. It correlated very highly with mood changes that are often associated with left anterior frontal injuries as well as alterations of complex executive function confirmed on neuropsychological assessment.

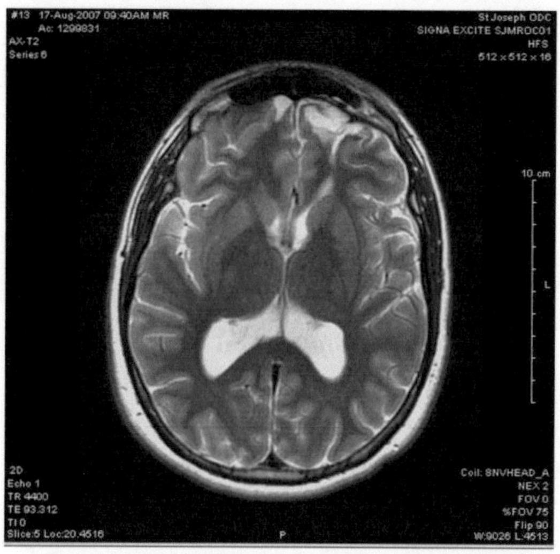

Figure 5.

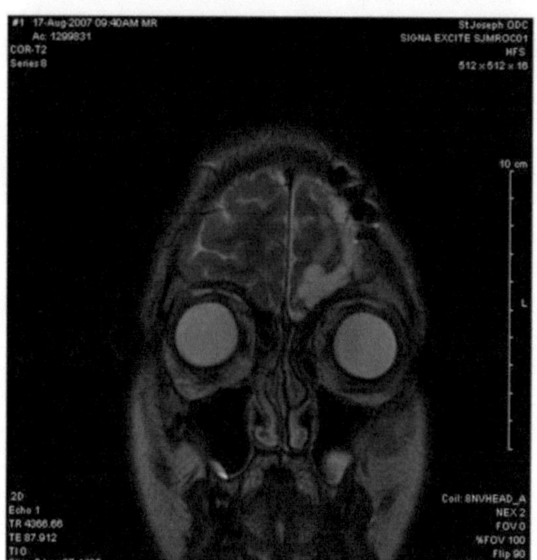

Figure 6.

Another example of the severe trauma that can occur following inflicted head injury is seen in Figures 7 and 8. Severe traumatic brain injury often causes substantial shrinkage of hippocampal structures. This shrinkage will often correlate with a substantial drop in memory skill. Figure 7, a coronal T-2 MRI image, shows significant encephalomalacia overlying the right cerebral hemisphere, which correlates very highly with a substantial enlargement of the hippocampal cistern on the right, following a reduction in hippocampal volume of almost two-thirds. This, in turn, correlates with volume loss in the brain, as demonstrated by the enlarged lateral ventricles. The level of encephalomalacia was quite massive, particularly in the right cerebral hemisphere, which is well demonstrated on the axial FLAIR MRI image in Figure 8.

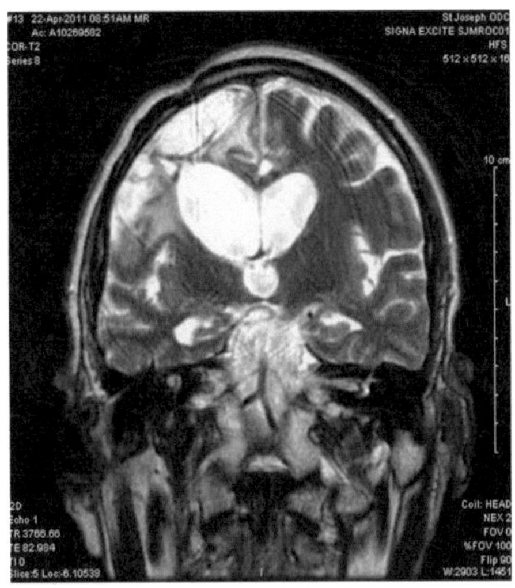

Figure 7.

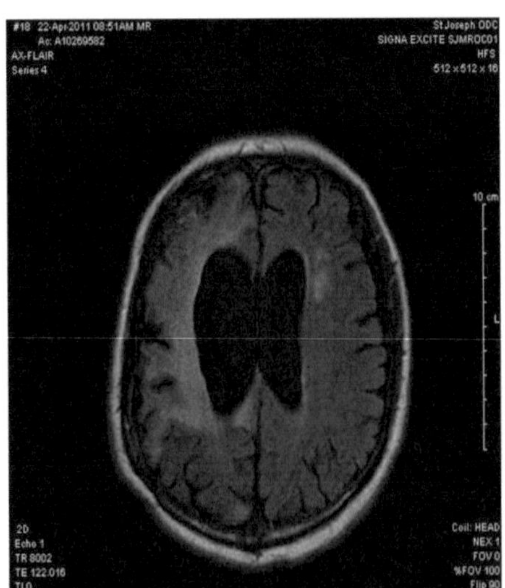

Figure 8.

A perplexing problem often seen in medico-legal evaluations of traumatic brain injury is that of an individual who had a preexisting brain insult and then sustained a second brain trauma. Distinguishing these from each other can be quite complex after the fact. Figure 9 represents a woman who had lung cancer metastatic to the brain 17 years prior to the image in Figure 9. The metastatic lesion was treated with whole-brain radiation, and the resulting white matter gliosis following radiation is demonstrated in Figure 9. The radiation was administered following the surgical excision of the left cerebral hemisphere metastatic lesion from the primary cancer in the lung. This is noted in Figure 10. Lastly, Figure 9 reveals in the right frontal brain, two areas of abnormal signal on axial FLAIR, which probably represents prior small nodes of tumor that were killed by whole-brain radiation, and then ex vacuo lesions developed when the metastatic tumors dissolved. Seventeen years following successful treatment of lung cancer metastatic to brain, her vehicle was struck by a very large tractor-trailer truck. She was seriously injured and required extraction from her automobile and transport to a Level I trauma center by helicopter. When received at the university hospital, her *Glasgow Coma Scale* = 10. She was making incomprehensible sounds and would localize to pain, but otherwise she was not speaking or answering questions. Her chronic phase examination at the time the MRI exemplars in Figures 9 and 10 were obtained, revealed her to be demented. Interviews with her family indicated that following successful treatment for lung cancer, she worked as a clerk for the Internal Revenue Service in the United States. She was able to continue that employment following brain surgery and brain irradiation. As often occurs with individuals who have significant preexisting cerebral disease, a substantial subsequent traumatic brain injury can markedly aggravate or exacerbate the underlying organic brain condition and produce a dementia that was not present prior to trauma. That appears to have occurred in this case.

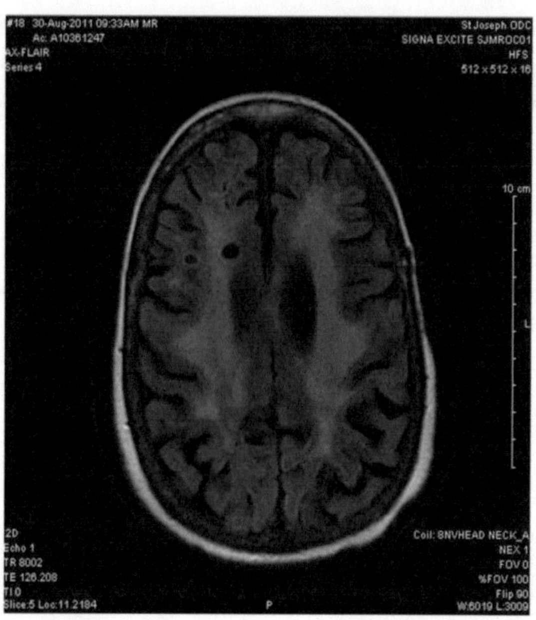

Figure 9.

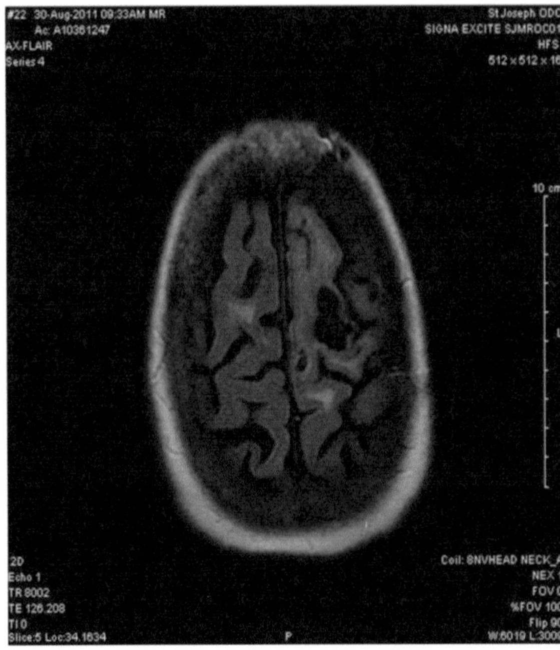

Figure 10.

As stated earlier, while CT of the head has been the imaging modality of choice for the acute care of TBI, MRI is now being used in the acute phase more frequently due to the availability of the newer sequences. Figure 11 reveals a CT image of a man who fell 40 feet down a flight of stairs. His initial *Glasgow Coma Scale* = 7. He was found unconscious, lying facedown when Emergency Medical Services arrived. The initial CT depicted in Figure 11 indicates a focal hyperdensity in the left parietal lobe. Blood was accumulating in the left occipital horn, consistent with intraventricular hemorrhage. It is well known that intraventricular hemorrhage is a primary marker for diffuse axonal injury [1]. A few hours later, a diffusion-weighted image was made by MRI of the same patient. Figure 12 reveals evidence of ischemia near the left corpus callosum.

Returning to the issue of separate TBIs in the same individual with a significant time interval between, Figure 13 gives a graphic example of two independent brain injuries separated by a three-year interval. The first injury occurred in a motor vehicle accident in 2006. The injury can be seen in the lateral margin of the right inferior temporal lobe. Three years later, in 2009, she sustained a slip-and-fall at work and received injury to the inferior pole of the left temporal lobe found by CT. The 2006 injury caused significant orthopedic fractures. No follow-up imaging was ever obtained after injury. It is obvious that the 2006 injury played a substantial role in causing the right inferior temporal encephalomalacia, and this became a significant issue in the apportionment of damages to the 2009 injury.

Not only is it critical to obtain neuroimaging through prior medical evaluations at the time of the forensic examination of traumatic brain injury, but also it is also important to gather any significant preinjury medical information that may be present. A case in point is made by reviewing Figures 14 and 15. In this case, a 30-year-old man was injured during a fall of more than 15 feet in a grain silo at a river offloading facility. The *Glasgow Coma Scale* = 5T when he arrived at a university hospital trauma center. The initial CT in Figure 14 reveals evidence of a right frontal contusion, a right lenticular contusion, and bilateral intraventricular bleeding, with bilateral effacement. Figure 15 reveals evidence of a midbrain hematoma. Following his injury, he had substantial cognitive complaints, which were corroborated by neuropsychological testing. However, the importance of securing other medical information became clear when it was learned that he was severely beaten at age 7 by his mother's boyfriend; he was found to be learning disabled; during his primary and secondary education, he had difficulty sitting still in school; he could not keep his mind on tasks as a child; he consumed 24 bottles of beer daily over more than a three-year period as a young adult; he had been convicted of two driving-under-the-influence charges; and he had been arrested three times for alcohol intoxication. Moreover, he had spent at least 180 days incarcerated on various occasions for alcohol-related offenses; he used cocaine more than 50 times in his life; he used lysergic acid eight to ten times in his life; and he admitted to using methamphetamine more than 200 times in his life. Had the images in Figures 14 and 15 been the sole information in the case, it is obvious that erroneous or incomplete conclusions could have been presented to a trier-of-fact.

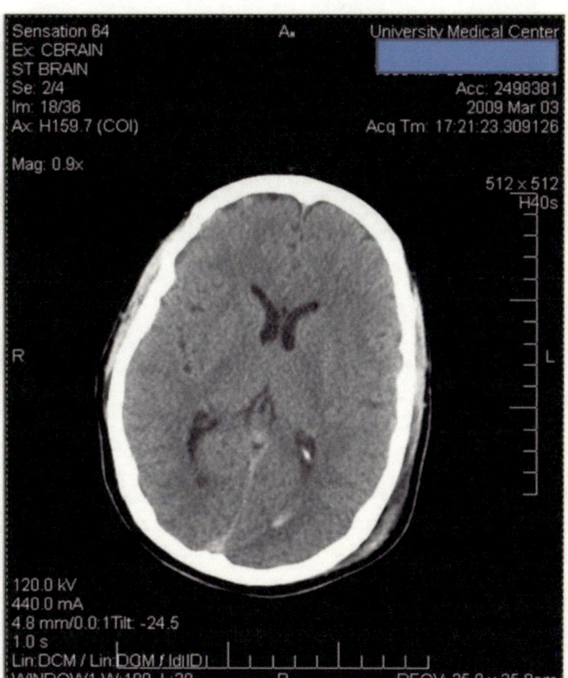

Figure 11.

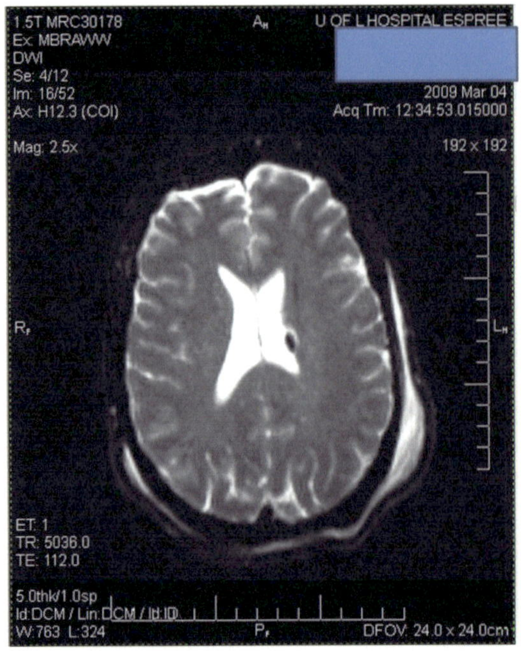

Figure 12.

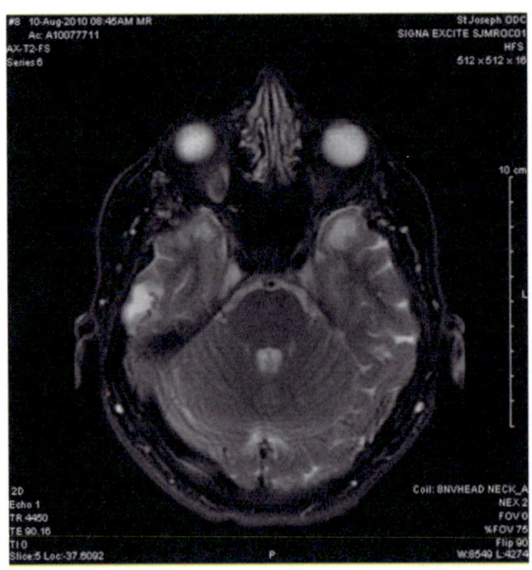

Figure 13.

As was noted above, there are three major causes of traumatic brain injury. Blunt force trauma has been discussed, and the second cause is penetrating injury. The issues with penetrating injury are different than those associated with blunt force trauma. The extent of injury from impalement of the head is extremely variable and depends on (1) the size, shape and number of impaling projectiles; (2) the velocities of the projectiles when they enter the skull; and (3) the entry/exit sites and the course of the projectile through the brain. [13] The most prominent cause of penetrating brain trauma in the United States is gunshot wounds to the head. Individuals who receive injuries from large caliber, high velocity weapons, rarely survive. The neuroimaging in those who survive rarely, if ever, correlates in an anatomical fashion to the neuropsychological testing used to measure residual brain function.

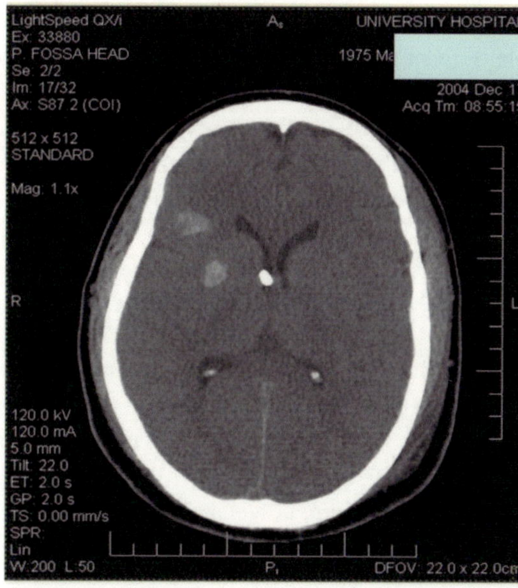

Figure 14.

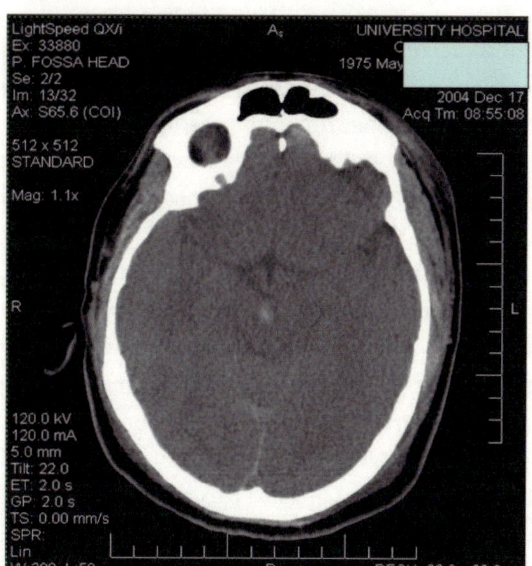

Figure 15.

The third major cause of TBI is blast overpressure brain injury. This is a worldwide phenomenon that has been dramatically changed in terms of outcome to survivors as a result of improvised explosive devices and other high-velocity explosive materials that are now in common usage by terrorists throughout the world. The evaluation of blast overpressure brain injury within a forensic medical setting generally reveals little on neuroimaging unless there has been an association between the type of explosive charge and whether or not it contained projectiles, which could be sent by high velocity as the blast force moves in a radius beyond the explosion site. Little is found on neuroimaging if no penetration of the skull occurs. Table 3 gives a description of the phenomenology of blast overpressure trauma. The forensic physician should be aware of these facts in any person who has sustained a significant blast injury with associated multiple body trauma. As Table 3 demonstrates, head injuries rarely occur in isolation in these kinds of injuries, and it is expected that injuries to the lung, brain, auditory system, bowel and testicle may all occur in single or multiple combinations. A lung or bowel rupture is seen with powerful blast injuries, as gas-filled organs are particularly susceptible to injury by a blast. The cognitive and emotional changes can be quite extensive following blast overpressure head injury and often quite dramatic. [14]

- Intense overpressurization impulse (at the speed of sound > 700 mph) causes primary, secondary, tertiary, and quaternary injuries.
- High-order explosives: TNT, C-4, Semtex, nitroglycerin, dynamite and ammonium nitrate/fuel oil.
- Injuries to lung, brain, auditory system, bowel, and testicles.
- Cognitive and emotional changes common.

Table 3. Blast or Explosion Overpressure Trauma [1]

Of the many sequences available in MRI, diffusion tensor imaging (DTI) is becoming one of the more prominent new techniques, particularly for evaluating brain white matter. However, there is a word of caution about the forensic uses of this new tool. The legal profession is being transformed by neuroimaging as applied to civil litigation, particularly in traumatic brain injury cases. A whole new area has developed called Neurolaw. [15] The reader is referred to a recent analysis of diffusion tensor imaging applied in mild traumatic brain injury litigation. [16]. DTI is an MRI-based data-analysis technique, which fundamentally relies on the clinically well established technique of diffusion-weighted imaging (DWI), a common sequence used in MRI to detect strokes and ischemia. DTI is a more refined adaptation of DWI that allows for the determination of the directionality as well as the magnitude of water diffusion in the brain, and more specifically within and between different brain tissue types. [17] A scaled value between 0 and 1 describes the degree of a diffusion process. A value of 0 means that the diffusion is unrestricted in all directions. Tractography is a method using DTI to assess the structural integrity of white matter tracts within the brain. [18-19]

Since 2007, in the United States, DTI has been allowed in court proceedings were TBI is litigated by state court judges on a reasonably regular basis with inability by most defense lawyers to challenge this concept based on *Daubert* criteria. Wortzel, et al. have concluded that careful analysis of DTI in mild traumatic brain injury literature, guided by *Daubert* criteria, suggests that presently the admission of DTI evidence in mild TBI litigation is seldom medically appropriate.[16] Under the best of circumstances, with DTI data generated by highly experienced laboratories and from patients with clinically unambiguous mild traumatic brain injury, the imaging data may add a quantifiable measure of white matter integrity to the body of evidence describing such patients. However, in these cases, DTI would serve as superfluous evidence. More alarming, though, is the potential use of DTI to prove mild traumatic brain injury in cases where other forms of more reliable and accepted clinical evidence fail to uphold, or directly refute such conclusions, such as the standard MRI sequences, T1, T2 and FLAIR. The compelling visual images of DTI do not add any useful data to whether or not the alleged TBI victim can think, reason, calculate, analyze, or even speak or read. This data cannot be determined from DTI images and requires careful face-to-face neuropsychiatric examination as well as corroborating neuropsychological test data. If misused and left unchallenged, DTI imaging findings in mild TBI may be misleading. An expert witness is required ethically to acknowledge this fact, and particularly for the diagnosis of mild traumatic brain injury. At the single patient level, data are not available in peer reviewed scientific journals and at a generally accepted standard within the medical field.[16] In fact, there is currently no evidence in the medical literature that enables a correlation to be drawn from DTI findings in order to relate this to neuropsychological data, and provide an anatomical relationship between the DTI data and the neuropsychological data. Figure 16 demonstrates the beauty of the images obtained by DTI. However, as noted, it is not possible at this time to draw a fundamental positive correlation between elements of the DTI image and the functional capacity of a person's brain after TBI. In other words, DTI images cannot tell a jury if a person can think, reason, calculate, remember, or speak.

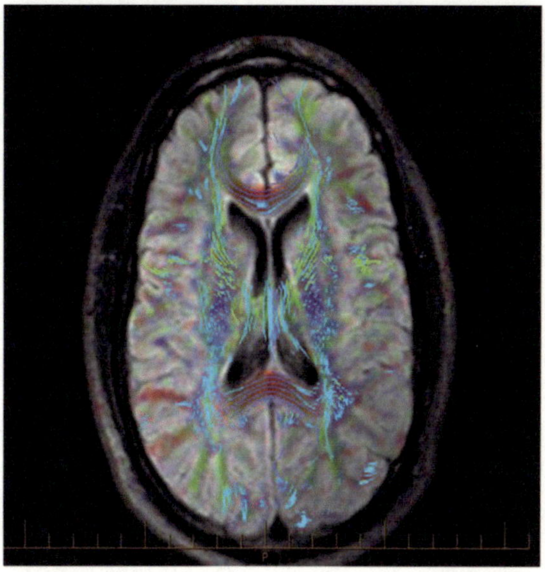

Figure 16.

Susceptibility-weighted imaging (SWI) is a high-resolution 3D echo MR imaging technique with phase post-processing that accentuates the paramagnetic properties of blood products such as deoxyhemoglobin, intracellular methemoglobin, and hemosiderin. It is particularly useful for detecting intravascular venous deoxygenated blood as well as extravascular blood products. It is also quite sensitive to the presence of other substances such as iron, some forms of calcification, and air. In traumatic brain injury, its greatest use is for the detection of posttraumatic blood products. It may be useful for detecting some of the secondary manifestations of traumatic brain injury such as hypoxic/anoxic injury. Figure 17 depicts significant evidence of multiple microhemorrhages in the left frontal cerebral hemisphere with a few hemorrhages in the posterior right cerebral hemisphere. These images were obtained following a high-speed, single vehicle collision into a tree by a teenager operating his automobile at high speed. These images were made many months after the original impact, indicating the ability of SWI to detect hemosiderin deposits well after the trauma. [20]

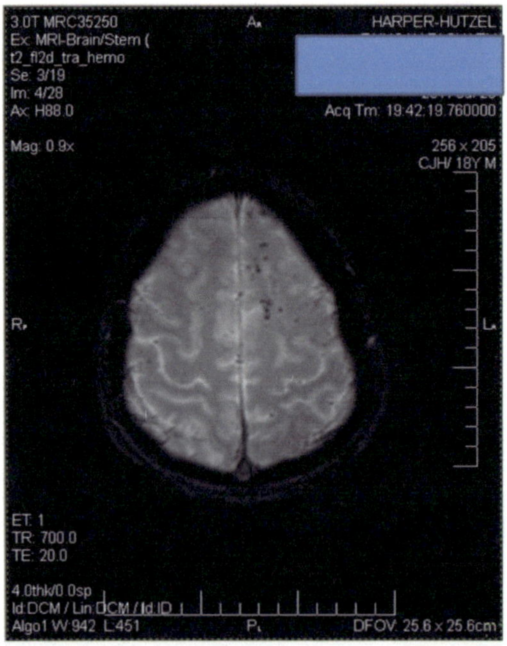

Figure 17.

4. Functional neuroimaging

Functional neuroimaging as applied to TBI, is of two general types: (1) tomographic images based on nuclear scanning using radioactive isotopes, and (2) imaging using functional aspects of magnetic resonance. Nuclear imaging consists primarily of single photon emission computed tomography (SPECT) and positron emission tomography (PET). The functional imaging using magnetic resonance is functional MRI (fMRI) and magnetic resonance spectroscopy (MRS).

4.1. Single Photon Emission Computed Tomography (SPECT)

SPECT is based upon an indirect determination of blood flow in the brain using the distribution of a radiopharmaceutical agent within the brain to approximate almost on a 1:1 basis, regional cerebral blood flow. The commonest tracer used today is Technetium-99 m-hexamethylpropyleneamine oxime (Tc-99 mHMPAO). Other tracers are available for use in SPECT as well, and all are known nuclear medicine pharmaceuticals. To obtain a SPECT brain image, the radioactive tracers are injected into the venous blood of the person to be imaged. After appropriate distribution, the tracer decays, emitting a photon that is detected and recorded by a gamma camera. The data from the gamma camera are then reconstructed by computer, and tomographic sectioning is undertaken.

SPECT has numerous sources of potential measurement error, which are important in a legal case. SPECT imaging requires that regional radiation counts be normalized to a brain area that is theoretically free from injury. This sets a standard of relative flow values (RFV) in SPECT. Nuclear medicine physicians commonly base these relative values upon an anatomical region such as the thalamus or cerebellum, which is assumed theoretically to be uninjured in TBI. (It is not uncommon for either of these structures to be injured in TBI.) The reader is advised to again review Table 2, the American College of Radiology Appropriateness Criteria for subacute or chronic closed head injury. [3] This table demonstrates that for the subacute or chronic closed head injury, SPECT is considered appropriate 4/9 on a 1-9 rating scale. Recently, the appropriateness of SPECT imaging has been reviewed in the forensic psychiatric literature when used with testimony in TBI cases. These reviews have concluded that SPECT uses a sole diagnostic imaging modality, lacks scientific merit, and may actually breach the ethics of expert testimony when SPECT is presented to a trier-of-fact as a sole neuroimaging instrument to demonstrate that a TBI has occurred. [21, 22] Currently, the state of the art for SPECT neuroimaging in TBI, particularly in mild traumatic brain injury, is that there is no SPECT profile that is pathognomonic for any level of TBI. [23] Moreover, SPECT imaging is routinely positive in a variety of medical and neurological disorders. Thus, false positives are very high including such common issues as substance abuse, depression, and attention deficit disorder.

4.2. Positron Emission Tomography (PET)

Current PET studies of brain tissue generally utilize intravenous tracers such as 18F-fluorodeoxyglucose (FDG) for quantification of regional brain metabolism. This is based on giving the brain a sugar analog. The brain then attempts to metabolize in the same fashion as it would for glucose. The decay particles from the 18F-FDG are detected and then converted to digital images, which are further converted to colors corresponding to regional differences in 18F-FDG metabolism. Thus, similar to SPECT, PET is a radioisotope-based imaging technology. Its most common current application is for the detection of metastatic cancer or recurrence of cancer.

Using PET for the evaluation of chronic cognitive symptoms potentially related to TBI seems an intuitive choice for the physician. PET has been used for the evaluation of TBI since 1970, but to this date, more than 40 years later, few studies can be found that directly relate functional imaging findings between PET and cognition following TBI.[1] Moreover, the majority of studies found within the neuropsychological literature and other psychological assessments where PET has been used, have been obtained at time points that were quite disparate from the time at which the imaging occurred. It is rare to find studies where the neuropsychological testing was done at time points that correspond to when the PET images were obtained. [24] Additionally, when one reviews the ACR Appropriateness Guidelines for using PET following TBI (Table 2) to evaluate chronic head trauma with cognitive and neurological deficits, PET is rated 4/9 for that use. [3]

There are a few carefully designed studies, which do find localized abnormal cerebral metabolism rates in the frontal and temporal regions that correlate with subjective complaints and neuropsychological test results obtained during the chronic phase of recovery. [25] However, there are almost no contemporary studies and no significant studies in the last 15 years that find strong correlations between PET neuroimaging of TBI and concurrent correlation with neuropsychological cognitive data. For the forensic examiner, though, there is one situation where PET may be the imaging modality of choice when evaluating a TBI. This would be a patient who may have Alzheimer's disease present before or closely associated with a concurrent TBI. In those cases, PET might be quite useful to differentiate the lesions of Alzheimer's disease from the lesions of TBI, as the current neuroimaging data of Alzheimer's disease using PET is quite specific for the regions that generally are metabolically abnormal. These regions of abnormality in Alzheimer's disease are not regions generally damaged in patients who have sustained cortical injury from traumatic brain injury. It is not recommended that PET be used as a sole neuroimaging modality in assessing a TBI case, especially mild TBI. [22]

4.3. Functional Magnetic Resonance Imaging (fMRI)

Functional magnetic resonance imaging is used routinely to study cognition, and it has become the neuroimaging modality of choice for such studies. Moreover, there is a significant body of medical literature that demonstrates strong correlations between fMRI findings and neuroanatomical areas specific for various domains of cognition. [26] However, while fMRI represents a very advanced approach to brain neuroimaging, this advanced approach does not meet the criteria of real-world data usage to evaluate TBI in a single case. Functional magnetic resonance imaging has not reached an efficient threshold of scientific evidence for routine use for testimony at any level of injury severity after head trauma. Reviewing Table 2, it can be seen that the American College of Radiology rates this technique 2/9 for appropriateness in evaluating subacute or chronic closed head injury. [3]

Functional MRI (fMRI) is a variant of structural MRI. The primary differences between the two are that the dependent variable of interest in fMRI is the change in magnetic susceptibility related to increases in blood flow. These changes occur due to a presumed alteration in neural activity. The focus of fMRI is on regional changes in brain activity rather than anatomic structure, such as noted using classical MRI techniques. The excess blood flow to the region of interest results in a localized surplus of oxyhemoglobin relative to deoxyhemoglobin in the central venous and capillary beds. Oxyhemoglobin is naturally diamagnetic, while deoxyhemoglobin is paramagnetic. There is a net decrease in the paramagnetic material resulting in an increased signal intensity that can be detected externally (BOLD: blood oxygen level dependent). It is not recommended that fMRI be used for the routine evaluation of traumatic brain injury.[3]

4.4. Magnetic Resonance Spectroscopy (MRS)

MRS offers an examination of the cellular and metabolic status after TBI, toxic insults to the brain, infections, or other conditions wherein the monitoring of chemical changes detectable by MRS can be used. The capability of MRS to quantify neuronal and glial metabolites makes it useful for repeated studies in survivors of injury. However, there are a very small number of studies in TBI that enable one to translate MRS findings to clinical practice and rehabilitation. The current spectroscopic data available by MRS can provide information about the cellular injury that is often seen neuropathologically, but is rarely observed by conventional radiologic assessment. MRS has been used for three categories of assessment following TBI: (1) acute post-injury phase observation of elevated lactate (la) suggesting hypoxic injury; (2) evidence of decreased N-acetyl aspartate (NAA) suggesting neuronal loss or dysfunction; elevated choline (Cho) and myo-inositol (mI) suggesting inflammation; and altered glutamate (Glu) and glutamine (Glm) suggesting excitotoxicity, which is related to severity of injury; and (3) prediction of behavioral outcome. [27] Figure 18 shows a voxel of interest over the left temporal area for an MRS analysis. Note the coronal MRI with the spectroscopic pattern displayed across the coronal view.

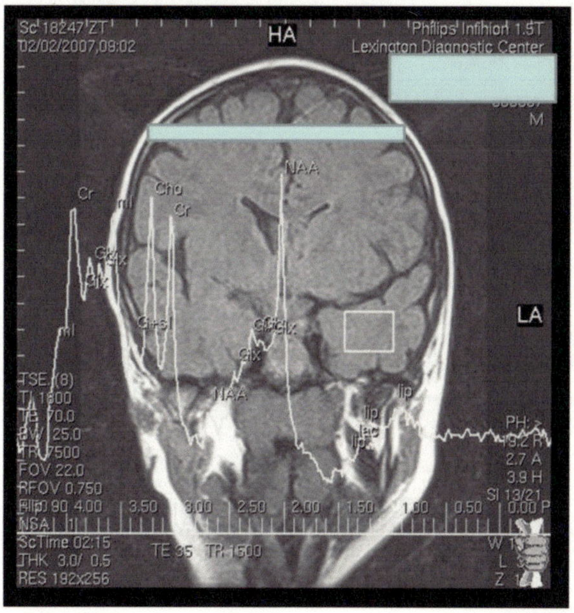

Figure 18.

Figure 19 shows a more readable spectroscopic graph of the chemicals of interest. Other data are collected numerically and displayed in this case in Figure 20. It is the evidence of decreased N-acetyl aspartate (NAA) that may be the most promising for evaluating neuronal loss and dysfunction in forensic TBI assessment. MRS can be obtained in a standard MRI system by obtaining appropriate software for the analysis. In diffuse axonal injury (DAI), the main abnormalities found using MRS to evaluate TBI are reductions in NAA levels and a reduction in the NAA/creatine ratio. DAI is also associated with an increase in Cho levels and an increase in the Cho/creatine ratio. Choline is associated with myelin and membrane breakdown. Neuronal damage is usually characterized by a reduction in the NAA/creatine ratio in parietal white matter near the corpus callosum. It can be detected by MRS in the more acute phase from the second day forward, and in the chronic phase up to three years post-trauma. [28] Proton MRS is the most widely applicable form of MRS. MRS has been approved by the United States Food and Drug Administration as a noninvasive method providing metabolic information about the brain in general. [29]

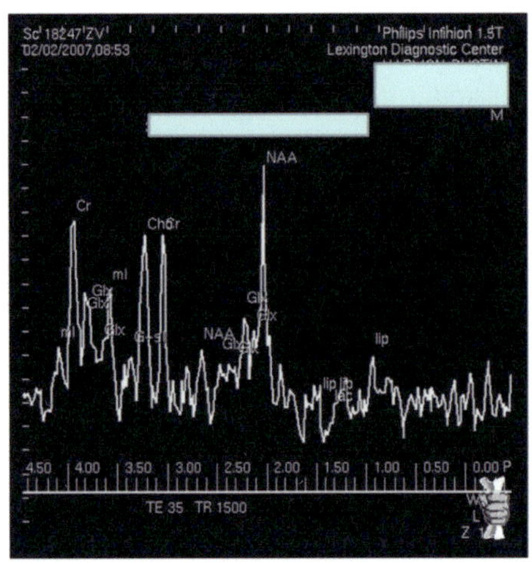

Figure 19.

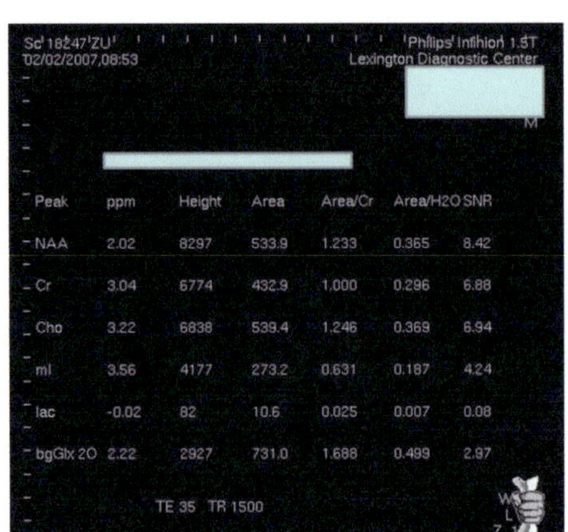

Figure 20.

Author details

Robert P. Granacher, Jr.
Department of Psychiatry, University of Kentucky College of Medicine,
Lexington Forensic Neuropsychiatry, Lexington, KY, USA

5. References

[1] Granacher RP. The Use of Structural and Functional Imaging in the Neuropsychiatric Assessment of Traumatic Brain Injury. In: Granacher, RP. *Traumatic Brain Injury: Methods for Clinical and Forensic Neuropsychiatric Assessment.* 2nd ed. Boca Raton: CRC Press; 2008. p. 207-246.

[2] Granacher RP. Neuroimaging in Traumatic Brain Injury. In: Simpson J, editor. *Neuroimaging in Forensic Psychiatry.* Cambridge: Cambridge University Press; 2012. p. 41-61.

[3] American College of Radiology [home page on the Internet]. Reston, Virginia: ACR Appropriateness Criteria [updated 2008; cited 2012 March 17]. Available from: http://www.ACR.org/

[4] Mittenberg W, Patton C, Craynock E, et al., Base Rates of Malingering and Symptom Exaggeration. *J Clin Exp Neuropsychol.* 2002; 24: 1094-1102.

[5] Granacher RP. Forensic Issues and TBI. In: *Clinical Manual of Adults with Traumatic Brain Injury.* Washington D.C.: American Psychiatric Press; 2012. [In press]

[6] Blumbergs P, Reilly P, Vink R. Trauma. In: Love S, Lewis D, Ellison D, editors. *Greenfield's Neuropathology.* 8th ed. London: Hodder Arnold; 2008. p. 733-812.

[7] Aarabi B, Eisenberg H, Murphy K, et al. Traumatic Brain Injury: Management and Complications. In: Layon A, Gabrielli A, Friedman W, editors. *Textbook of Neurointensive Care.* Philadelphia: Saunders; 2004. p. 771-794.

[8] Bullock R, Zauner A, Woodward J, et al. Early Insults to the Injured Brain. *J Neurosurg* 1998; 89: 507-518.

[9] Marshall L. Head Injury: Recent Past, Present, and Future. *Neurosurg.* 2000; 47: 546-561.

[10] Maxwell W, Povlishock J, Graham D. A Mechanistic Analysis of Nondisruptive Axonal Injury: A Review. *J Neurotrauma.* 1997; 14: 419-440.

[11] Buki A, Okonkwo D, Povlishock, J. Postinjury Cyclosporine-A Administration Limits Axonal Damage and Disconnection in Traumatic Brain Injury. *J Neurotrauma.* 1999; 16: 511-521.

[12] Quisling R, Sohn-Williams L. Neuroradiologic Imaging. In: Layon A, Gabrielli A, Friedman W, editors. *Textbook of Neurointensive Care.* Philadelphia: Saunders; 2004. p. 41-101.

[13] Osborne A, Salzman K, Barkovich A, editors. *Diagnostic Imaging: Brain.* 2nd ed. Salt Lake City: Amirsys; 2010. p. I2.2 – I2.75.

[14] Taber K, Warden D, Hurley R. Blast Related Traumatic Brain Injury: What is Known? *J Neuropsychiatry Clin Neurosci.* 2006; 18: 141-145.

[15] Rozen J. The Brain on the Stand: How Neuroimaging is Transforming the Legal System. *The New York Times Magazine*. 2007; March 11. p. 48.

[16] Wortzel H, Kraus M, Christopher M, et al. Diffusion Tensor Imaging in Mild Traumatic Brain Injury Litigation. *J Am Acad Psychiatry Law*, 2011; 511-523.

[17] Kraus MF, Susmaras T, Caughlin BP, et al. White Matter Integrity and Cognition in Chronic Traumatic Brain Injury: A Diffusion Tensor Imaging Study. *Brain.* 2007; 130: 2508-2519.

[18] Sidaros A, Engberg A, Sidaros K, et al. Diffusion Tensor Imaging During Recovery from Severe Traumatic Brain Injury and Relation to Clinical Outcome: A Longitudinal Study. *Brain*. 2008; 131: 559-572.

[19] Rutgers D, Toulgoat F, Kazejust J., et al. White Matter Abnormalities in Mild Traumatic Brain Injury: A Diffusion Tensor Imaging Study. *AJNR Am J Neuroradiol*. 2008; 29: 514-519.

[20] Tonga K, Ashwalb S, Obenause A, et al. Susceptibility-weighted MR Imaging: A Review of Clinical Applications in Children. Annual Meeting of the American Society of Neuroradiology, Toronto, Ontario, Canada; April – May 2005.

[21] Wortzel H, Filley C, Anderson C, et al. Forensic Applications of Cerebral Single Photon Emission Computed Tomography in Mild Traumatic Brain Injury. *J Am Acad Psychiatry Law*. 2008; 36: 310-322.

[22] Granacher R. Commentary: Applications of Functional Neuroimaging to Civil Litigation of Mild Traumatic Brain Injury. *J Am Acad Psychiatry Law*. 2008; 36: 323-328.

[23] Ricker J. Functional Neuroimaging in Medical Rehabilitation Populations. In: Delisa, J, Gans B, editors. *Rehabilitation Medicine*, 4th ed. Baltimore: Williams and Wilkins; 2005. p. 229-242.

[24] Ruff R, Crouch J, Troester A, et al. Selective Cases of Poor Outcome Following Minor Brain Trauma: Comparing Neuropsychological and PET Assessment. *Brain Inj*. 1994; 8: 297-308.

[25] Gross H, Kling A, Henry G, et al. Local Cerebral Glucose Metabolism in Patients with Long-term Behavioral and Cognitive Deficits Following Mild Head Injury. *J Neuropsychiatr Clin Neurosci*. 1996; 8: 324-334.

[26] Mayberg HS. Towards the Use of Neuroimaging in the Management of Major Depression. The American Neuropsychiatric Association 23rd annual meeting; 2012 Mar 21-24; New Orleans, USA.

[27] Brooks W, Holshouser B. Magnetic Resonance Spectroscopy in Traumatic Brain Injury. In: *Clinical MR Neuroimaging: Physiological and Functional Techniques*, 2nd ed. Cambridge: Cambridge University Press; 2010. p. 656-662.

[28] Sinson G, Bagley L, Cecil K., et al. Magnetization Transfer Imaging in Proton MR Spectroscopy in the Evaluation of Axonal Injury: Correlation with Clinical Outcome After Traumatic Brain Injury. *AJNR Am J Neuroradiol*. 2001; 22: 143-151.

[29] Bandao L, Domingues R. *MR spectroscopy of the brain*. Philadelphia: Lipincott, Williams and Wilkins; 2004.